..., in writing or by telephone

last date shown below

Date due

DEC

THE MECHANICAL BASIS OF RESPIRATION
An Approach to Respiratory Pathophysiology

THE MECHANICAL

BASIS OF RESPIRATION
n Approach to Respiratory Pathophysiology

Richard M. Peters, M.D.

Professor of Surgery and Bioengineering,
and Head, Division of Cardiovascular
and Thoracic Surgery, University of
California, San Diego, School of Medicine

J. & A. Churchill Ltd., London

Library of Congress catalog card No. 76-82929

First Edition

Published in Great Britain by J. & A. Churchill Ltd., London
British Standard Book Number 7000 0158 1

Printed in the United States of America

To Ann, Joan, Deborah, Barbara, and Rick

PREFACE

THIS BOOK, with the exception of the chapter on transplantation, is my own creation. It is not an exhaustive compendium of respiratory pathophysiology. Rather, it is meant as a discussion of respiratory function and malfunction from the viewpoint of the medical mechanical engineer, the surgeon. Most American males love machines and at some time in their lives have tinkered with them. If the respiratory system is looked at from this familiar viewpoint, new understanding may be possible.

The Mechanical Basis of Respiration concentrates on the way the system runs, an approach that requires a more detailed discussion of the mechanical properties of the lungs and chest bellows than is common. The pulmonary circulation likewise is given greater emphasis because of my great interest in it and also because of my conviction that the function of the heart, lungs, and circulation must be considered and treated as an integrated system. Since elimination of CO_2 by pulmonary gas exchange and its transport by hemoglobin are major elements in the control of acid-base balance, a general but brief review of acid-base balance is included. The last five chapters, which deal with clinical aspects of pulmonary disease, are focused primarily on acute disease that can respond to mechanical manipulation by the surgeon or internist.

No exhaustive list of references or sources is included. Rather, selected supplemental reading is given by chapter at the end of the book. Basic resources are the sections Respiration and Circulation of the *Handbook of Physiology,* published by the American Physiological Society.

The chapter on transplantation was written by Dr. Peter Hutchin, a colleague, who is trained in both cardiothoracic surgery and immunology. He also was kind enough to read all the other chapters and to make helpful suggestions, as was Dr. Mark Hilberman.

The illustrations for the book were prepared by Miss Gwynne Moore who, with creativity and high standards, interpreted my rough sketches and produced meaningful drawings. Those used in the final text are only a portion of the many she made. These drawings also reflect my family's contribution to this book. My daughter Barbara and son Richard spent many hours running the machine that printed the labels for the figures.

Perhaps the most crucial force in completing this manuscript was Mrs. Dorothy Dysard, my capable and tolerant secretary. The early drafts of this book were collections of ideas until Mrs. Dysard used her editorial skill and tact not only to correct syntactical errors, but to raise questions of presentation and conception. In the final proofreading and assembly she was indispensable.

Mr. Fred Belliveau of Little, Brown gave me much encouragement, and all his editorial staff were very helpful.

I cannot close without mentioning the students and houseofficers who were subjected to trial runs of this material, and my colleagues who bore extra work to enable me to complete this task.

During the years this book was in the writing, my wife and children were patient and encouraging and were practically helpful in numerous ways.

R. M. P.

CONTENTS

Preface   vii

1. **FUNCTIONAL ANATOMY**   1
   THE RESPIRATORY APPARATUS   1
   THE CHEST BELLOWS   2
   THE MUSCULATURE   3
   THE PLEURAL CAVITIES   5
   THE UPPER AIRWAYS   5
   THE TRACHEA, BRONCHI, AND LUNGS   6

2. **BLOOD GASES AND ACID-BASE BALANCE**   9
   HEMOGLOBIN AND OXYGEN   10
   CARBON DIOXIDE AND CARBONIC ACID   16
   DISTURBANCES IN ACID-BASE BALANCE   26
   LABORATORY ASSESSMENT OF ACID-BASE BALANCE   30
   ANALYSIS OF ABNORMALITIES IN BLOOD GASES   33

3. **VENTILATION**   41
   THE UPPER AIRWAYS   41
   COMPOSITION OF GASES IN THE RESPIRATORY TRACT AND BLOOD   42
   DEFINITION OF LUNG VOLUMES   45
   MINUTE VENTILATION AND ALVEOLAR VENTILATION   45
   THE EFFECT OF RESIDUAL VOLUME ON COMPOSITION OF
       ALVEOLAR AIR AND BLOOD GASES   48
   THE ASSESSMENT OF ADEQUACY OF VENTILATION   51

4. **MECHANICAL PROPERTIES OF THE RESPIRATORY SYSTEM**   55
   THE PULMONARY MACHINE   56
   THE ELASTIC COMPONENTS OF THE PUMP   63
   DYNAMIC PROPERTIES OF THE LUNG   88

ix

5. PULMONARY CIRCULATION   103
FUNCTIONAL ANATOMY   103
RELATIONSHIP OF FLOW AND PRESSURE   107
PULMONARY CAPILLARY CIRCULATION   116
ABNORMAL PULMONARY CIRCULATORY DYNAMICS   122
NEWER CONCEPTS IN THE STUDY OF BLOOD FLOW AND
    PRESSURE RELATIONSHIPS   140

6. DIFFUSION   145
DIFFUSION OF GASES   145
THE ANATOMY AND PHYSIOLOGY OF DIFFUSION   148
PULMONARY DIFFUSING CAPACITY   150
FACTORS ALTERING DIFFUSING CAPACITY   152

7. COORDINATION OF VENTILATION AND PERFUSION   157
MIXING OF GAS AND BLOOD   157
FACTORS LEADING TO NONUNIFORM VENTILATION AND
    PERFUSION   158
VENTILATION-PERFUSION RATIOS   164
MEASUREMENT OF REGIONAL VENTILATION-PERFUSION RATIO
    DIFFERENCES   174
DISEASE AND THE VENTILATION-PERFUSION RATIO   175

8. CHEMICAL AND REFLEX REGULATION OF RESPIRATION   179
THE PERIPHERAL CHEMORECEPTORS   180
THE CENTRAL CHEMORECEPTORS   181
THE CHEMICAL REGULATION OF RESPIRATION   183
REFLEX REGULATION OF RESPIRATION   187
VENTILATORY RESPONSE TO EXERCISE, COLD, AND PAIN   189
SLEEP, ANESTHESIA, AND DRUGS   189
WORK OF BREATHING AND VENTILATORY RESPONSE   191

9. THE ENERGY COST (WORK) OF BREATHING   195
OXYGEN COST OF BREATHING   196
MECHANICAL WORK   197
A DIRECT METHOD OF CALCULATING MECHANICAL WORK   206
ENERGY COST OF BREATHING AND METABOLIC RATE   209

10. THE EFFECTS OF ENVIRONMENT AND THE LEVEL OF ACTIVITY   213
THE ENVIRONMENT   213
ACTIVITY LEVELS AND ENERGY REQUIREMENTS   222

11. AGE, HABITUS, AND DEGENERATIVE DISEASE   231
THE EFFECTS OF AGING   231
THE CONDITION OF THE CHEST WALL AND ABDOMEN   232
DEGENERATIVE LUNG DISEASE   237
CARDIAC DISEASE AND LUNG FUNCTION   241
PULMONARY EMBOLI   242

12. **THE EFFECT OF INJURY ON PULMONARY FUNCTION** 247
 EFFECTS OF TRAUMA ON PULMONARY FUNCTION 247
 INTRATHORACIC COMPLICATIONS OF INJURIES AND INFECTION 258
 PULMONARY RESECTION 267
 THE SHOCK LUNG SYNDROME 271

13. **RESPIRATORS** 281
 INDICATIONS FOR VENTILATORY SUPPORT 282
 RESPIRATORS 288
 SPECIAL CONSIDERATIONS FOR INFANTS AND CHILDREN 296
 LIMITATIONS OF AVAILABLE RESPIRATORS 297
 COMPLICATIONS OF ARTIFICIAL VENTILATION 298
 RESPIRATORS AND DERANGED RESPIRATORY MECHANICS 301

14. **PULMONARY TRANSPLANTATION**
 Peter Hutchin, M.D. 305
 TECHNICAL CONSIDERATIONS 305
 PULMONARY FUNCTION OF THE REIMPLANTED LUNG 307
 EXPERIMENTAL LUNG ALLOGRAFTS 310
 CLINICAL LUNG TRANSPLANTATION 312
 PROCUREMENT AND PRESERVATION 313

APPENDIX: THE PHYSICAL BASIS OF RESPIRATION 317
 DEFINITIONS OF SYMBOLS USED 317
 GAS LAWS AND KINETIC THEORY 318
 FLUID MECHANICS 324
 MECHANICS OF PULSATILE FLOW 338

References 357

Index 373

THE MECHANICAL BASIS OF RESPIRATION
An Approach to Respiratory Pathophysiology

1. FUNCTIONAL ANATOMY

GAS can be exchanged between gas and fluid media only by diffusion. Krogh has calculated that an organism with a radius of 0.5 mm. is the largest animal that can live if its respiration is dependent on diffusion alone. If the size of the animal increased to 1 cm. in diameter, the partial pressure of oxygen would have to be increased to 19,000 mm. Hg, or twenty-five atmospheres, and this would not provide a means for eliminating carbon dioxide. A gas exchange system avoids the limitations of respiration by diffusion by utilizing a circulatory system, to transport gases and food to and wastes from the tissues, and a gas exchange membrane with a large air-liquid surface area, for the diffusion of gases from the gas phase into the liquid blood and from blood into the gas phase.

While the circulation in various species of animals is quite similar, the gas exchange apparatus varies from gills in fish to lungs in mammals. Anatomical description of the gas exchange apparatus must relate gross and miscroscopic structure to function to assure complete appreciation of the importance of the various structural elements. The classic descriptions of the anatomy of the human respiratory system describe it as a dead structure. In this chapter no attempt is made to review the detailed gross and histological anatomy of the lungs, chest wall, and airways; rather, the relation of anatomical structure to the dynamic state of the system is presented.

THE RESPIRATORY APPARATUS

A functional respiratory apparatus must have two pumps: one, the heart, to move blood through the apparatus; and another, the chest bellows, to move air in and out of it. These pumps must have sets of pipes through which air and blood can be brought in contact across a large

1

surface area. The precapillary pulmonary circulatory system has some unique differences from the systemic circulation. These differences are described in the chapter on pulmonary circulation. The functional anatomy of chest bellows, upper airways, bronchi, alveoli, and alveolar capillaries will be considered in this chapter.

THE CHEST BELLOWS

The chest bellows must have a rigid structure, to prevent collapse when pressures in the chest cavities change, and a set of muscles to drive the bellows pump. The bony framework of the chest provides rigidity, which protects the viscera from injury and permits the thorax to withstand alterations in pressure within it without undue distortion of its shape. The framework is so arranged that the structural elements—twelve pairs of ribs, twelve vertebrae, the spine, and the sternum—can move to allow a change in volume. The twelve ribs articulate with the vertebrae posteriorly. Anteriorly the first seven ribs are connected to the sternum by the costal cartilages to provide a complete bony enclosure to the upper two-thirds of the chest. The eighth through tenth ribs do not extend anteriorly as far toward the midline as the first through seventh ribs. They connect to a cartilage plate which is in turn connected to the sternum. The eleventh and twelfth ribs are short, and the anterior ends have no bony or cartilaginous connections.

This bony framework has the shape of a truncated cone. At birth, the chest's bony framework is quite flexible; the chest is nearly circular in shape, and the plane of the ribs is nearly horizontal. As the child develops an erect posture, the shape of the chest changes so that the lateral dimension of the chest cavity exceeds the anteroposterior dimension and the ribs become structurally stronger.

In the adult (Fig. 1-1) the kidney-shaped superior orifice of the chest is about four inches in its lateral dimension and two inches in its anteroposterior dimension. This opening is not horizontal; the anterior extremity of the opening, the suprasternal notch, is at the second thoracic vertebra. The downward slope of the lower ribs is greater than that of the first rib, so that the anterior end of the seventh rib may be at the level of the tenth thoracic vertebra. The ribs articulate posteriorly with the dorsal vertebrae. At the point of articulation the ribs run dorsally; they then take a sharp lateral turn at the neck to run laterally for a short distance and then develop a gentle curve to reach their anterior articulations. The volume of the chest cavity is increased when the ribs are raised, which adds to both the anteroposterior and lateral dimensions of the chest. To rise, the ribs must rotate about the axis of the neck of

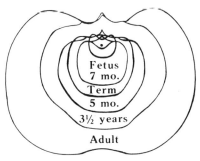

Fig. 1-1. Change in shape of thorax with growth. Concentric outlines are super-imposed. At birth the chest is nearly circular in shape; with growth the lateral diameter increases faster than the anteroposterior diameter. (From Vernon E. Krahl, "Anatomy of the Mammalian Lung." In Wallace O. Fenn and Hermann Rahn [Eds.], *Handbook of Physiology, Section 3: Respiration.* Vol. I. Baltimore: Williams & Wilkins, 1964. P. 229, Fig. 10.)

the rib; hence the principal motion at the costovertebral articulations is rotation. At their posterior articulation the ribs are so shaped that the greatest movement in the upper ribs is in the vertical direction and in the lower ribs in the lateral direction.

THE MUSCULATURE

The force to move the chest is supplied by the respiratory muscles—the external and internal intercostals and the diaphragm—and by the accessory muscles—the muscles of the shoulder girdle, neck, and abdomen. In quiet breathing only the diaphragmatic and intercostal muscles are used; as effort increases, the accessory muscles are called into play. How much of the motion of the ribs is achieved by contraction of the intercostals alone and how much is done by the accessory muscles is a matter of controversy. It is agreed, however, that the ribs are raised by contraction of the external intercostals and lowered by contraction of the internal intercostals and that contraction of both sets of these muscles provides rigidity to the intercostal spaces.

The muscles of the back brace the dorsal and cervical spine so that during inspiration the other cervical muscles, such as the sternocleidomastoids, can raise and fix the upper thorax. The action of the muscles of the shoulder girdle is less well understood, but interaction of these muscles can aid both inspiration and expiration. When the diaphragmatic muscle is relaxed, the position of the diaphragms is determined by the force across the diaphragms, which is the difference between the intra-abdominal and intrapleural pressures (see p. 76). Contraction of the diaphragms causes them to descend in the chest, increasing the volume of the chest cavity. To raise the diaphragms above the relaxation level requires contraction of the accessory muscles, principally the abdominal muscles, which raises the intraabdominal pressure above the intrathoracic pressure and passively pushes the diaphragms up.

In extreme expiration the diaphragms can be pushed up to the fourth rib posteriorly, and in extreme inhalation the dome can come down to the tenth or eleventh rib. As the diaphragms rise in the chest and the chest cage moves in, the lung is displaced out of the lower chest and the diaphragms lie closer to the lateral chest wall, so that the area of contact between visceral and parietal pleura is decreased. The volume of the chest cavity can be varied by 4,000 to 6,000 cc., and this is achieved by raising and lowering the ribs and diaphragms. (See Figure 1-2.)

In quiet breathing the muscles that act to decrease chest volume are not used. At the start of a quiet inspiration, inspiratory muscle activity begins and increases progressively during inspiration. During expiration the activity of the inspiratory muscles continues at a decreasing rate until it ceases at the midpoint of expiration; then, to limit collapse, the inspiratory muscles start to contract again just before the end of expiration. Thus, in quiet breathing the inspiratory muscles control the rate of expansion and contraction of the chest by counteracting the elastic recoil of the system. As the level of hyperventilation increases, the inspiratory muscles act for shorter and shorter periods during expiration. Eventually

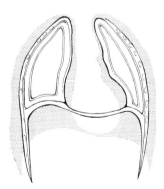

Fig. 1-2. The change in shape of the pleural cavities on expiration and inspiration. At inspiration (*stippled area*) there is a great increase in the total area of contact between visceral and parietal pleura as the lung moves down into the costophrenic angle. The mediastinum narrows, but the total mediastinal pleural surface changes very little. (From H. Braus, *Anatomie des Menschen,* 3rd Ed. Berlin: Springer-Verlag, 1956. Vol. 2.)

the inspiratory muscles cease acting at all during expiration, and the muscles of expiration are called upon to actively contract to expel air. The change in volume induced by the muscles alters the shape of and pressures within the pleural cavities.

THE PLEURAL CAVITIES

The two pleural cavities are separated from one another by the mediastinum. None of the structures of the mediastinum are rigid, and in the anterior chest, under the sternum, the two pleural cavities are nearly in contact with one another. This lack of rigidity of the mediastinal structures means that any pressure difference across the mediastinum will push the mediastinal structures in the direction of the lower pressure.

The pleural cavities are lined by a thin mesothelial membrane which covers the entire parietes and lung except in the region of the hilum and pulmonary ligaments. Beneath this membrane there is a network of capillaries. Under the visceral pleura there are more capillaries per square centimeter than under the parietal pleura. The visceral and parietal pleura are in intimate contact with one another, so the shape of the lung assumes the contour of the chest cavity. During expiration, as the diaphragm rises, the lungs are pushed out of the lower chest and the parietal pleura over the diaphragm is in direct contact with that over the chest wall and mediastinum.

To serve its function the chest cavity must be kept free of air and fluid. This is accomplished by a fine balance of forces across the capillaries under the mesothelial linings of the visceral and parietal pleura (see pp. 83–88).

THE UPPER AIRWAYS

The airways provide a path for air to enter and leave the lungs. During quiet breathing air enters through the nose, where it winds its way through the maze of turbinates. This circuitous route permits the air to be filtered, warmed, and moisturized. However, these filters and moisturizers have such a high resistance that during hyperventilation the forces required to move air are too great, so that the open mouth rather than the nose is used and the air is only partially warmed and moisturized.

The larynx is the guarded entrance to the trachea. The larynx permits air to enter but keeps foreign matter out of the trachea; it directs food and fluid into the esophagus. It can be closed off completely, can withstand the high pressures created in the trachea during cough, and it also can precisely regulate its size to permit phonation.

THE TRACHEA, BRONCHI, AND LUNGS

The function of the lungs and trachea is controlled by the geometry of their various anatomical partitions. Ten percent of the lung volume is made up of conducting airways and connective tissue; the other 90% is the respiratory portion of the lung—the alveolo-capillary networks and the transitory area where the alveoli connect to the conduction airways. The 90% of the total lung devoted to the transitory and respiratory areas is subdivided so that 54% is air in the alveoli, 29% is air in the transitory ducts, and only 7% is tissue and blood vessels. Fifty percent of the volume of the tissue and blood vessels in the respiratory and transitory regions consists of blood in alveolar capillaries, 15% of capillary endothelium, 14% of alveolar epithelium, and 21% of interstitial tissue. Thus, of the total lung volume, 77% is blood and air in the transitory and respiratory regions of the lung. In effect this is an efficient system in which the majority of volume is occupied in the exchange of gases.

The conducting zone requires a complex, compact set of airways to move air to and from the respiratory zone. The largest of these, the trachea, is 10 to 12 cm. in length and 13 to 22 mm. in diameter. It is not circular, having a bigger lateral dimension than anteroposterior dimension. Anteriorly and laterally it is supported by heavy, cartilaginous rings and smooth muscle, while posteriorly it lacks the cartilaginous component. The discontinuous, rigid support permits the trachea to be flexed and elongated, and the muscular support allows its lumen to be diminished in size. The bifurcation of the trachea is the first of 17 to 27 branchings (the average number of branchings is 23). The branches are not always equal in size; for example, the right main-stem bronchus is 12 to 16 mm. in diameter, while the left is 10 to 14 mm. The combined cross-sectional area of each pair of bronchi is greater than the parent bronchi by about six-fifths, so the aggregate cross-sectional area of the bronchial tree increases as the tree is descended.

The principal bronchi, like the trachea, have large, cartilaginous plates, considerable smooth muscle between cartilages, and abundant mucous glands. As the cartilaginous bronchi decrease in size, the glands decrease in number and the smooth muscle becomes first circular and then helical inside the cartilage. This arrangement permits longitudinal shortening as well as changes in diameter of the bronchi. These cartilaginous bronchi have a definite connective sheath which separates them

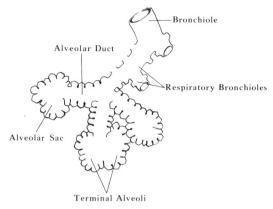

Fig. 1-3. The terminal respiratory unit starts with the bronchioles, defined as bronchi of less than 1 mm. in diameter. The bronchioles branch into a number of respiratory bronchioles, which have occasional alveoli. The respiratory bronchioles branch into alveolar ducts and terminate in alveolar sacs. Along the walls of each of these ducts are alcoves—the alveoli. (Reproduced from Peter Gray, *Encyclopedia of Biological Sciences.* By permission of Reinhold Book Corporation, a subsidiary of Chapman-Reinhold, Inc., New York, 1961.)

from the parenchyma. The final, terminal cartilaginous bronchi of about 1 mm. in diameter are reached in the eighth to thirteenth generation.

Bronchioles are bronchi less than 1 mm. in diameter. Bronchioles have no cartilage or loose connective sheath and have the greatest relative amount of smooth muscle. The generation after the bronchioles is the respiratory bronchioles, which have three or more divisions. The respiratory bronchioles have occasional alveolar outpouchings (Fig. 1-3). Alveolar ducts are the last division, and they may be pictured as hallways with many alcoves opening off them, which are the alveolar sacs.

The surface of the alveolus has a complete epithelial lining, the cells of which are thought to have a very active metabolism and to be the site of manufacture of alveolar surfactant. Air can pass from one alveolar duct to an adjacent one through pores between alveoli. This allows a lobule with a blocked duct to be filled from an adjacent alveolus. Between the air in the alveolus and the blood in the alveolar capillary are (1) fluid lining the alveolus, (2) alveolar epithelium, (3) basement membrane, (4) connective tissue layer, (5) basement membrane of the capillary, and (6) capillary endothelium. The distance occupied by these layers is 0.7 μ. Around all these alveoli and the conducting airways is a complex net of elastic and collaginous fibers. They permit stretch, prevent overdistension, and supply part of the recoil force of the lung.

During a deep inspiration the large bronchi change very little in either length or diameter, but the smaller bronchi increase in diameter by a factor of 1.3 to 2 and in length by 1.2 to 2. Since the smaller bronchi contain less than 10% of the total lung volume, their change in diameter contributes little to the change in total volume.

Most of the change in volume during respiration occurs in the alveoli. It is at the surface of the alveoli that gas exchange takes place, so the important dimension of the alveoli is their surface area. The surface-to-volume ratio of alveoli is the same as a closed sphere, 4.8 to 1, even though they are shaped more like an open cup. The best estimate is that there are 24 million alveoli in an infant's lung at birth; by 8 years of age, these have increased to 300 million. Alveoli are about 200 to 300 μ in diameter, and each has 1,800 capillary segments running over it. This gives the astronomical number of 280 billion alveolar capillaries. The area of gas–tissue interface is at least 70 to 80 square meters, but, since the capillaries make ripples in the alveolar surfaces, it may be more nearly 90 to 100 square meters.

A system as complex and as delicate as the gas exchange apparatus is an easy prey to injury by infection, accidental trauma, and noxious fumes. It also has limited durability and suffers structural deterioration as it ages. The surprising fact is not its vulnerability but its durability. All abnormal respiratory states are not the result of structural change; some are due to changes in environment, others to changes in function. However, most disease states are associated with some structural change in the airways, lungs, or chest cage.

2. BLOOD GASES AND ACID-BASE BALANCE

ONE of the principal functions of the blood is to provide a connecting link between the lungs and the metabolic furnaces. The propelling force to move the blood between tissues and the lungs is provided by the heart, and the conduits are provided by the vascular system. At the two ends of this conduit system are a pulmonary capillary bed connected to a gas exchange ventilating system, the lungs, and a systemic capillary bed connected to a myriad of metabolic factories in the various organ systems. A precise measure of the effectiveness of the coordination of the needs of the consumers, the metabolic factories, with the effectiveness of the ventilating and transport system, the heart and lungs, is found in a study of the blood. Since a study of the gas content of blood is the ultimate measure of the effectiveness of pulmonary function, any discussion of pulmonary physiology must presuppose an understanding of the physiology of the blood.

Each minute that the body is at rest the blood must transport 250 cc. of oxygen to the tissues and return 200 cc. of carbon dioxide to the lungs. With strenuous exercise, ten times as much must be transported. According to Henry's law (see Appendix, p. 323), the amount of gas dissolved in a liquid is equal to the Bunsen solubility coefficient times the partial pressure. The solubility coefficient for oxygen in blood is 24 cc. of oxygen per liter per atmosphere of pressure; for carbon dioxide it is 480 cc. of carbon dioxide per liter per atmosphere. The partial pressure of oxygen in arterial blood is 95 mm. Hg and that of carbon dioxide in the venous blood is 46 mm. Hg. If all the oxygen were

9

extracted in the tissues and all of the carbon dioxide excreted in the lungs, each liter of blood could carry in solution only

$$\frac{95 \times 24}{760} = 3.0 \text{ cc. of } O_2 \text{ per liter}$$

and

$$\frac{46 \times 480}{760} = 29 \text{ cc. of } CO_2 \text{ per liter}$$

The tissues cannot extract all the oxygen from the blood, nor can the lungs extract all the carbon dioxide. At rest the venous blood has an oxygen partial pressure of 35 mm. Hg, or 1.1 cc. of oxygen per liter dissolved in the blood. Arterial blood has a finely regulated partial pressure of carbon dioxide (40 mm. Hg); it therefore has 25 cc. of carbon dioxide dissolved in a liter. Thus, one liter of blood can transport per minute in simple solution 3.0–1.1, or 1.9 cc. of oxygen, and 29–25, or 4 cc. of carbon dioxide. To provide 250 cc. of oxygen and excrete 200 cc. of carbon dioxide would require a cardiac output at rest of 125 liters per minute and ten times this, or 1,250 liters per minute, with exercise. This is forty to fifty times the capacity of the heart. This problem in evolution was solved by the development of hemoglobin, described by Peters and Van Slyke* as follows:

At some epoch in animal development . . . there appeared an extraordinary substance in the circulating fluid that enabled the latter to take up from air a hundredfold the amount of oxygen which could be absorbed by simple solution and yet hold the vital gas so loosely that the oxygen-thirsty tissues could, if they needed, take it all as it passed through their capillaries. At the same time this substance furnished alkali to combine with all the carbonic acid that could be liberated in periods of most vigorous activity, yet so controlled the combination that when blood reached the lungs the surplus CO_2 was free to escape instantly into the atmosphere. That substance was hemoglobin.

HEMOGLOBIN AND OXYGEN

THE CHEMICAL COMPOSITION AND NATURE OF HEMOGLOBIN

Hemoglobin is a conjugated protein of molecular weight 67,000, and it is made up of a globin and four active iron-porphyrin, or heme, groups. The iron-containing heme groups give the red color to the hemoglobin

---

*J. P. Peters and D. D. Van Slyke, *Quantitative Clinical Chemistry*. Vol. 1, *Interpretations*. Baltimore: Williams & Wilkins, 1932. P. 518.

molecule. Each one of these heme groups can react with one molecule of oxygen, or each molecule of hemoglobin can combine with four molecules of oxygen. Hemoglobin from even a normal individual is a mixture of hemoglobins, the variations being in the globin fraction. The different types of hemoglobin differ only by the nature of the subunits or polypeptides. These variations in polypeptides seriously affect both the physical and chemical nature of a particular hemoglobin. X-ray crystallography has shown the molecule to be formed by a twisting and folding of its polypeptide chains. These folds exclude water from the interior of the molecule but leave a large number of charged amino acid chains on the surface of the molecule which can react with water, salts, carbon dioxide, and other proteins.

The iron of hemoglobin must be in the Fe^{++} state to combine with oxygen. The combination of oxygen with hemoglobin is in a uniquely balanced equilibrium which permits the acquisition of oxygen in the lungs and its release in the tissue.

THE OXYGEN-HEMOGLOBIN DISSOCIATION CURVE

Before discussing the oxygen-hemoglobin dissociation curve, it is important to define the terminology. Oxygen is carried in the blood in two states: dissolved in the fluid medium of the blood and in chemical combination with hemoglobin. The solubility of oxygen in the blood at any body temperature is a constant. According to Henry's law, the amount of oxygen dissolved in the blood depends on the partial pressure of oxygen in the blood. This is designated by the term *oxygen tension,* abbreviated as pO_2, and is expressed as oxygen tension, or pO_2, in millimeters of mercury (mm. Hg). This partial pressure of oxygen also determines the amount of oxygen that will combine with hemoglobin. If the pO_2 is high enough, all of the heme groups will contain oxygen and the hemoglobin will be fully saturated with oxygen.

The maximum number of cubic centimeters of oxygen that 100 ml. of blood can hold in chemical combination is called the *oxygen capacity.* The oxygen capacity is obviously a measure of the amount of hemoglobin, and thus is another method of expressing the hemoglobin concentration of blood. (Each 1.34 cc. of oxygen can combine with 1 gram of hemoglobin.) The hemoglobin is expressed as grams per 100 ml. of blood, or grams percent, and the oxygen capacity as cubic centimeters of oxygen per 100 ml. of blood, or volumes percent. A sample of blood with a hemoglobin of 15 grams percent would have an oxygen capacity of 20 volumes percent.

The term which defines the actual number of cubic centimeters of oxygen present in a given sample of blood is called the *oxygen content.*

The oxygen content is expressed in volumes percent. The *oxygen satura-tion* is the percent of the hemoglobin available for combination with oxygen which has combined with oxygen. The percent saturation is obtained by dividing the oxygen content by the oxygen capacity:

$$\text{Percent saturation} = \frac{\text{oxygen content (vol. percent)}}{\text{oxygen capacity (vol. percent)}}$$

The unique quality of hemoglobin is its ability to reversibly combine with oxygen. This reaction is controlled by the partial pressure of oxygen, pO_2, in the blood. Since the reaction of hemoglobin with oxygen is a reversible reaction, one would anticipate that it would be covered by the mass-action law, as is myoglobin.

$$MbO_2 \rightleftarrows Mb + O_2$$

If this is so, then, using the value 3.3 for K, the dissociation constant, the following equation should apply:

$$\frac{Mb + pO_2}{MbO_2} = K = 3.3$$

Figure 2-1 shows the oxygen saturations for various oxygen tensions of myoglobin which follow the mass-action law. If the values for myoglobin saturation are calculated from the mass-action law and plotted with per-cent saturation on the vertical axis and pO_2 is plotted on the horizontal axis, a rectangular hyperbola is described. This is a curve that can be de-scribed algebraically by the equation above. If the dissociation curve of hemoglobin were the same as that of myoglobin, oxygen would be held by chemical bond until pO_2 was nearly zero. Over the range of difference in pO_2 between arterial and venous blood (95 to 35 mm. Hg), hemo-globin saturation would change only 7%.

Fortunately, hemoglobin does not obey the mass-action law; rather, the curve is skewed (Fig. 2-2), and has no known mathematical descrip-tion. This skewing is believed to result from the interaction of the four heme groups in the hemoglobin molecule. Between pO_2 of 95 and 35 mm. Hg the skewing allows 38% rather than 5 to 7% of the carrying capacity for oxygen to be used. Note further that between a pO_2 of 50 and 10 mm. Hg, 70% of the combined oxygen can be released, while a pO_2 of 60 mm. Hg permits oxygenation of 90% of the hemoglobin.

The curve is flat at the top, and the saturation varies less than 10% when the partial pressure of oxygen varies between 60 and 110 mm. Hg.

Thus, in the lungs a large drop in oxygen tension may occur with only a small drop in arterial oxygen saturation. It is for this reason that man can survive at high altitudes or with pulmonary or cardiac disease. On the venous side of the circuit the sharp break in the dissociation curve

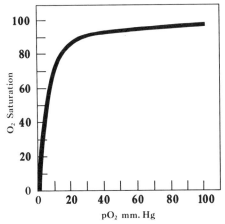

Fig. 2-1. Myoglobin dissociation curve. This curve plots the mass-action law of the equation $(Mb + pO_2)/MbO_2 = 3.3$. Note that at pO_2 of only 10 mm. Hg, 75% of the myoglobin is saturated with oxygen, and so the pO_2 has to fall below this before myoglobin will give up its oxygen.

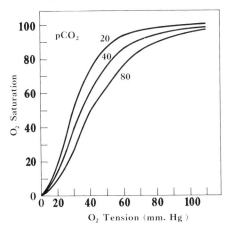

Fig. 2-2. Hemoglobin dissociation curves. The center of the three curves is the oxygen dissociation curve for hemoglobin at a pCO_2 of 40 mm. Hg. Note that between an oxygen tension, pO_2, of 95 and 35 mm. Hg, 70% of the oxygen combined with hemoglobin is released, while at a pO_2 of 60 mm. Hg, 90% of hemoglobin is saturated with oxygen. A fall in pCO_2 to 20 mm. Hg shifts the curve to the left, making hemoglobin more avidly acquire oxygen. A rise in pCO_2 to 80 mm. Hg shifts the curve to the right and diminishes the amount of oxygen combined with hemoglobin at any pO_2 level.

allows 25% of the oxygen to be released from the hemoglobin at a partial pressure of oxygen of 40 mm. Hg, thus making oxygen available to the tissues.

Since myoglobin would not release the oxygen to the tissues until the partial pressure of oxygen was nearly zero, it is a poor donor but an excellent recipient of oxygen from hemoglobin. Its oxygen dissociation curve is as precisely suited to its task as the dissociation curve of hemoglobin is for transporting oxygen between tissues and lungs. By removing oxygen from the extracellular fluid, the myoglobin lowers the partial pressure of oxygen in the tissues and the hemoglobin in its turn can release more oxygen. In the lungs, where the oxygen tension in the pulmonary capillaries is high, desaturated hemoglobin which has an avid appetite for oxygen quickly replenishes itself with oxygen.

pH AND HEMOGLOBIN DISSOCIATION (BOHR EFFECT)

The reaction between hemoglobin and oxygen is affected by the pH of the blood. When the pH falls, making the blood more acid, the hemoglobin dissociation curve shifts to the right (see Fig. 2-2). This means that when the pH falls, at any given pO_2 the amount of oxygen combined with hemoglobin will be less than when the pH is normal. In the tissue capillaries the pH is lower than in the lungs due to the presence of acid waste products, principally carbon dioxide. This permits the hemoglobin to release more oxygen at any given pO_2. Recent work has shown that the flat part of the oxygen dissociation curve does not change with a fall in pH. Hemoglobin is thus able to release more oxygen at the low pH and oxygen tension encountered in the tissues, but an alteration in pH does not affect its ability to combine with oxygen at the level of pO_2 encountered in the lungs. The pH, or Bohr, effect gives an added edge in time of need. In strenuous exercise or when a disease prevents normal oxygenation, the alteration in pH due to lactic acid entering the blood can substantially increase the available amount of oxygen without markedly lowering the tissue pO_2.

TEMPERATURE EFFECT ON THE OXYGEN
DISSOCIATION CURVE

As the temperature falls for any given pO_2, the affinity of hemoglobin for oxygen and the amount of oxygen dissolved increases. This is of minor importance over the temperature range encountered in health and disease but is important in conditions of induced hypothermia. If the temperature is also lowered 10°C., the shift of the hemoglobin curve prevents the release of oxygen until the pO_2 of tissues is very low. In a hypothermic patient high arterial and venous oxygen saturations may not be a sign of good tissue oxygenation. The tissues may be starved for oxygen because the hemoglobin cannot release oxygen to the tissues until the tissue pO_2 is dangerously low. During fast warming the shift of the dissociation curve back to the right results in the release by hemoglobin of more oxygen than can be dissolved in plasma, and microbubbles can form in the blood (see Appendix, p. 323). The stress of hypothermia is greatest during cooling and rewarming. Careful consideration of the solubility of oxygen and carbon dioxide in blood and the shift of the dissociation curve will make it clear that an extreme temperature difference between blood entering and blood leaving the warming or cooling chamber is dangerous. The maximum safe difference on warming is 8°C. During cooling, more extreme changes are allowable.

VARIATIONS IN HEMOGLOBIN CONCENTRATION

There is a significant diurnal variation of hemoglobin concentration (oxygen capacity) of the blood. This may be as much as 1.4 grams percent of hemoglobin, or two volumes percent in oxygen capacity. Brief vigorous exercise can cause a rise of 20% in the hemoglobin concentration. Prolongation of exertion does not lead to any further increase in concentration but rather to a partial return to resting level. Rest returns the hemoglobin to normal in approximately one hour. The increase in hemoglobin concentration with exercise increases the oxygen and carbon dioxide carrying capacity of the blood when it is most needed and represents a useful adaptation.

Exposure to low oxygen pressure, whether due to reduction of the percentage of oxygen in the atmosphere or to lowering of the total atmospheric pressure, results in an increase in the hemoglobin concentration of the blood. The acute rise may be similar to the response to exercise, but chronic exposure leads to stimulation of the bone marrow and a rise in the total hemoglobin available. Presumably, the same mechanism operates in conditions in which arterial oxygen saturation is diminished, either due to a shunt or to pulmonary disease. The low arterial pO_2 stimulates the bone marrow.

CARBON MONOXIDE

The carbon monoxide dissociation curve of hemoglobin has exactly the same shape as the oxygen dissociation curve. However, carbon monoxide has an affinity for hemoglobin two hundred times that of oxygen. At sea level in the absence of oxygen, at a pCO of only 0.5 mm. Hg or a concentration of only 0.07%, hemoglobin will be fully saturated with carbon monoxide. When oxygen is present, competition takes place between carbon monoxide and oxygen for hemoglobin. The amount of hemoglobin combined with oxygen and carbon monoxide will depend on the partial pressure of each gas. For this reason the administration of 100% oxygen speeds the release of carbon monoxide by hemoglobin. Since it takes time for enough carbon monoxide to get into the blood to saturate all the hemoglobin, the tolerable limits of carbon monoxide exposure depend on the duration of exposure as well as the carbon monoxide concentration in the air.

CARBON DIOXIDE AND CARBONIC ACID

The lungs, in addition to being the flue through which oxygen is drawn into the metabolic furnaces, are the smokestack that vents the waste product, carbon dioxide. Carbon dioxide is hydrated to carbonic acid in the tissues, and this waste acid is excreted by the lungs in amounts of 13,000 to 20,000 mEq of carbonic acid per day. The kidneys during the same period excrete only 40 to 80 mEq of acid. The lungs, in addition to being quantitatively more important than the kidneys in acid-base balance, are able to respond much more rapidly to sudden changes in acid production.

Since blood is easily removed for chemical analysis, it has been used to measure acid-base balance to assess whether the pulmonary, renal, and other metabolic processes are functioning effectively. Investigators interested in acid-base balance often are more interested in one than in another of the controllers of acid-base balance or only in the blood itself. This diversity of approach has led to terminologies to describe acid-base balance that can be bewildering, and recent controversy over these semantics has further served to confuse the issue. Unfortunately, new names will never substitute for understanding, nor will they make incomplete measurements more precise. However, the reader inevitably will get caught in the semantic argument when pursuing the current literature. The author has his prejudices in these arguments, but he will attempt to deal fairly with the terms preferred by others.

ANIONS AND CATIONS, ACIDS AND BASES, ACIDOSIS AND ALKALOSIS

Some atoms can donate an electron from their outer shell, and others are able to accept such a donated electron. An atom that lacks an electron in its outer shell has a positive charge and in an electrical field will migrate toward the negative pole, or cathode. Such an atom is, therefore, called a *cation*. Conversely, an atom with an extra electron has a negative charge and will migrate toward the positive pole, or anode, and so is called an *anion*.

Some compounds, when dissolved in water, are completely dissociated into negatively and positively charged ions. Since such a solution can conduct an electrical current, it is called an *electrolyte solution*. Sodium chloride (NaCl) and hydrochloric acid (HCl), a strong electrolyte and a strong acid, dissociate almost completely in water. Other compounds, such as carbonic acid, which is a weak acid, only partially dissociate when dissolved in water.

A compound capable of donating a free proton (a hydrogen ion) is an *acid*, while a compound capable of accepting a proton is a *base*. By these definitions, some of the acids present in blood are H_2SO_4, H_3PO_4, and H_2CO_3, and some of the bases are HCO_3^- and $H_2PO_4^-$. The clinical definition which labels Na^+, K^+, and Ca^{++} as bases is not valid in this terminology since they cannot accept a hydrogen ion. Acidosis, then, is an accumulation in the body of an excess of acid (hydrogen ions or proton donors), and alkalosis is an accumulation of an excess of bases (compounds capable of accepting hydrogen ions).

HYDROGEN ION CONCENTRATION AND PH

Any acid (HA) in aqueous solution will dissociate to varying degrees into its component ions:

$$HA \rightleftharpoons H^+ + A^-$$

The measure of the strength of the acid is the degree to which the reaction goes to the right to make available free hydrogen ions. The acidity of a solution is defined by the concentration of hydrogen ions in the solution. This is called the hydrogen ion concentration, written $[H^+]$. The weak acid, water, dissociates also to give

$$H_2O \leftrightarrows [H^+] + [OH^-]$$

In distilled water, $[H^+] \times [OH^-] = 10^{-14}$, there are 10^{-7} hydrogen ions and 10^{-7} hydroxyl ions per H_2O atom in water. Thus, a neutral aqueous solution will have 10^{-7} hydrogen ions (protons) and 10^{-7} hydroxyl ions (proton acceptors).

To avoid dealing with such small numbers (and because the electrodes used in measuring pH give a reading which is logarithmically proportional to the ratio of hydrogen ion concentrations in two different solutions), the term *pH* has been introduced. It is the negative logarithm of the hydrogen ion concentration. A neutral aqueous solution would be one with equal amounts of hydrogen and hydroxyl ions and would have a pH of 7. Since, as the negative logarithm increases, the quantity decreases, any rise in pH will represent a fall in hydrogen ion concentration and any fall in pH a rise in hydrogen ion concentration. This is one area of confusion since, unfortunately, most clinicians are not accustomed to dealing with exponential functions, much less negative exponential functions. (Considerable present controversy rages around whether one should deal with them.)

The pH of blood is slightly alkaline, or 7.4, in the normal individual. When the pH falls to 7.1, the hydrogen ion concentration is doubled.

$$pH\ 7.4 - 7.1 = 0.3$$
$$antilog\ 0.3 = 2, so\ [H^+]\ is\ doubled$$

This can be illustrated another way by converting log 7.4 and 7.1 to express $[H^+]$ in nanomols, or 10^{-9} mols:

$$[antilog\ (9 - 7.4)] \times 10^{-9} = [H^+] \times 10^{-9}$$
$$[antilog\ 1.6] \times 10^{-9} = 40 \times 10^{-9}$$

$$[antilog\ (9 - 7.1)] \times 10^{-9} = [H^+] \times 10^{-9}$$
$$[antilog\ 1.9] \times 10^{-9} = 80 \times 10^{-9}$$

Thus, a change in pH of 0.3 doubles hydrogen ion concentration. To make clear the absolute amount of change, Table 2-1 compares change in pH with change in hydrogen ion concentration expressed as nanomols (nM).

The concentration of hydrogen ions in body fluids is controlled by the buffers. Quantitatively the most important of these are carbonic acid and bicarbonate. At the hydrogen ion concentration in body fluids, carbonic acid, which is a weak acid, is not completely dissociated. Some of it exists as hydrogen and bicarbonate ions, most as undissociated carbonic acid. In addition to the bicarbonate ions, HCO_3^-, present as a result of dissociation of carbonic acid, H_2CO_3, there are other bicarbonate ions present from dissociation of the salt sodium bicarbonate, which is almost completely dissociated in body fluids. The body fluids thus have carbonic acid, which is capable of giving up protons, and bicarbonate ions from the dissociation of sodium bicarbonate, which are capable of accepting protons. Since carbonic acid can neutralize bases and salts of bicarbonate can neutralize acids, the body fluids which contain both of these compounds must have a hydrogen ion concentration that is the result of an interaction between carbonic acid and salts of bicarbonate. The equilibrium equation for all such solutions of acids and their salts has been described by Henderson.

Table 2-1. Change in Hydrogen Ion Concentration for Any Given Change in pH

[H+] (nM/L.)[a]		pH
130		6.89
120		6.92
110		6.96
100		7.00
90	Twice normal	7.05
80		7.10
70		7.15
60		7.22
50		7.30
45		7.35
42	Normal	7.38
40		7.40
35		7.45
30	One-half normal	7.52
20		7.70
10		8.00

[a]Hydrogen ion concentration is given in units of nanomols, or mols $\times 10^{-9}$. A negative pH of 7 equals the negative logarithm of 10^{-7} times logarithm of zero, or 1×10^{-7} mols, or 100 nanomols, a more convenient term in decimal expression. Note that a change of only 0.3 pH units doubles or halves hydrogen ion concentration.

THE HENDERSON AND HENDERSON-HASSELBACH EQUATIONS

Henderson showed that the hydrogen ion concentration is proportional to the ratio of carbonic acid to salts of bicarbonate. The exact relationship is described by the Henderson equation, which is derived from the fundamental mass-action law. A weak acid such as carbonic acid, when dissolved in water, partially dissociates:

$$K[H_2CO_3] = [H^+] + [HCO_3^-]$$

The degree of dissociation depends on the strength of the acid and is a function of the dissociation constant, K. If no salt of a base, such as sodium bicarbonate, is present, hydrogen ions will be equal in number to bicarbonate ions. If a salt is present, more bicarbonate ions will be present than hydrogen ions.

The salts of weak acids, such as sodium bicarbonate, are almost completely dissociated in solution, so that most bicarbonate ions derived from the salts exist free as base ions in solution. The factor defining this dissociation is called γ and varies from 0.6 to 0.9. In a near-neutral solution such as body fluids, almost all of the base ions in a mixture of a weak acid with its salt will be made of the ions of the basic salt. The equation can, therefore, be written:

$$K_1 [H_2CO_3] = [H^+] \times [HCO_3^-]$$

K_1 stands for a constant for the combined dissociation constants γ of $BHCO_3$ plus K for H_2CO_3. K_1 is designated the apparent dissociation constant. The Henderson equation for carbonic acid can then be written:

$$[H^+] = K_1 \frac{[H_2CO_3]}{[HCO_3^-]}$$

This is the basic equation which defines the hydrogen ion concentration in any solution containing a weak acid and its salt. When this equilibrium is defined in terms of pH rather than hydrogen ion concentration, it becomes more complicated both in name and form. Hasselbach modified Henderson's basic equation, converting hydrogen ion concentration and K_1 to the negative logarithms pH and pK_1. The Henderson-Hasselbach equation is an algebraic conversion of Henderson's fundamental equation to one expressing hydrogen ion concentration as the negative logarithm, or pH. This is derived as follows:

$$pH = - \log [H^+] = - \log K_1 - \log \frac{[Ha]}{[Ba]}$$

The negative log of K_1 has been designated pK_1, and the negative log [Ha]/[Ba] is the positive logarithm of its reciprocal, or log [Ba]/[Ha]. The equation is, therefore, written:

$$pH = pK_1 + \log \frac{[Ba]}{[Ha]}$$

For the special case of carbonic acid and bicarbonate, the equation reads

$$pH = pK_1 + \log \frac{[BHCO_3]}{[H_2CO_3]}$$

The value for pK_1 in serum is 6.1.

Since carbonic acid is formed by the solution of carbon dioxide in water, the concentration of carbonic acid is a direct result of the amount of dissolved carbon dioxide and, thus, the partial pressure of carbon dioxide. The amount of dissolved carbon dioxide is a function of its partial pressure times the solubility coefficient (see the introduction to this chapter).

Partial pressure of carbon dioxide times the solubility coefficient gives the number of cubic centimeters of dissolved carbon dioxide per liter of solution. Since 1 mM of gas occupies 22.26 cc., each cubic centimeter of gas represents 0.04 mM of carbon dioxide. The combined constant for the solubility coefficient plus the conversion of cubic centimeters to millimols is called α and is 0.0301. Using this constant, the Henderson-Hasselbach equation for this particular buffer becomes

$$pH = 6.1 + \log \frac{[BHCO_3]}{0.0301 \; pCO_2}$$

At the normal pH of body fluids, 7.4, there are twenty times as many bicarbonate ions as carbonic acid molecules. The ratio in whole blood is sixteen to one, because the pH of red cells is more acid than that of plasma. Thus, if there is a millimol increase in carbonic acid there will have to be a twentyfold increase in bicarbonate ions to maintain the same pH. For example, if the pCO_2 increases from 40 to 60 mm. Hg, which would be an increase of $20 \times 0.0301 = 0.6$ of carbonic acid, a 12 mM increase in bicarbonate ions will be required to maintain the same pH. On the other hand, a fall of 5 mEq in bicarbonate ions will require a 0.4 mM fall in carbonic acid, or a fall of 13 mm. Hg in pCO_2, to maintain the same pH.

It is impossible to measure directly bicarbonate ion concentration. However, the measurement of the total amount of carbon dioxide (TCO_2) present both as the base and the acid is possible. Because bicarbonate ion concentration cannot be measured, it is necessary for practical purposes to rearrange the equation to cover this situation.

Since $\qquad\qquad [BHCO_3] = [TCO_2] - [H_2CO_3]$

and $\qquad\qquad [H_2CO_3] = 0.0301 \; pCO_2$

then $\qquad\qquad pH = pK_1 + \log \dfrac{[TCO_2] - 0.0301 \; pCO_2}{0.0301 \; pCO_2}$

From this basic equation if any two of the three values, pH, TCO_2, or

pCO_2, are known, the bicarbonate and the remaining measurable values can be calculated.

ROLE OF CARBON DIOXIDE AND HEMOGLOBIN IN
THE CONTROL OF ACID-BASE BALANCE

As stated in the introduction, the partial pressure of carbon dioxide in venous blood is 46 mm. Hg, and that of arterial blood, 40 mm. Hg. This difference of 6 mm. Hg would result in each liter of blood picking up and transporting only 4 cc., or 0.2 mM, of carbon dioxide from the tissues for excretion by the lungs. In fact, each liter transports 50 cc., or 2.2 mM, of carbon dioxide. This large amount of carbon dioxide can be transported because carbon dioxide formed in the tissues is hydrated to carbonic acid. This is a slow reaction, but is speeded 13,000 times by the enzyme carbonic anhydrase which is present in the red cells and other tissue cells. The carbonic acid formed by the hydration of carbon dioxide then partially dissociates into hydrogen and bicarbonate ions. The hydrogen and bicarbonate ions react with the various protein buffers and the major buffer hemoglobin to neutralize the hydrogen ions and permit more dissociation. The 2.2 mM of carbon dioxide carried to the lungs for excretion by each liter of blood are partitioned between the various forms of carbon dioxide compounds—0.2 mM (4 cc.) as carbon dioxide and carbonic acid, 1.4 mM (31 cc.) as bicarbonate ions, and 0.6 mM (15 cc.) in a reversible combination with hemoglobin (Table 2-2).

The conversion of 1.4 mM of carbonic acid results in 1.4 mM per liter of free hydrogen ions, and the combination of carbon dioxide with hemoglobin releases 0.6 mM per liter of hydrogen ions. These two reactions leave 2 mM per liter of hydrogen ions that must be neutralized. If this acid were left unbuffered, there would be a severe change in pH. The bicarbonate cannot contribute to this neutralizing of acid radicals

Table 2-2.   Whole-Blood Carbon Dioxide Distribution[a]

From	Arterial		Venous		Difference		Percent of Total Carried
	(mM/L.)	(ml.)	(mM/L.)	(ml.)	(mM/L.)	(ml.)	
Total CO_2	22.0	489.0	24.2	538.0	2.2	49.0	100
$CO_2 + H_2CO_3$	1.2	26.7	1.4	31.1	0.2	4.4	9
$HCO_3{}^-$	19.7	438.8	21.1	470.0	1.4	31.2	64
HbNHCOO$^-$	1.1	24.5	1.7	37.9	0.6	13.4	27

[a]This table lists the distribution of carbon dioxide among the various chemical buffers in venous and arterial blood. The majority of the carbon dioxide is transported as bicarbonate and in chemical combination with hemoglobin.

formed from carbonic acid, since each molecule of carbonic acid will give one hydrogen ion and one bicarbonate ion.

To increase the bicarbonate ions 1.4 mM, it is necessary to neutralize the hydrogen ions from both carbonic acid and carbamino carbon dioxide by some other means. The principal source for the buffering of these hydrogen ions is the hemoglobin molecule. Hemoglobin is an effective buffer because the molecule contains large numbers of terminal carboxyl (acid groups COOH) and amino (basic HN_2) groups as well as imidazole groups. At the neutral point hemoglobin can be depicted as in Figure 2-3A; the hydrogen ions are added to free carboxyl and nitrogen groups, as depicted in Figure 2-3B. In this manner hemoglobin can take up and neutralize hydrogen ions.

An *oxy*hemoglobin-acid titration curve can be constructed, and it will show that each millimol of oxyhemoglobin can neutralize 0.22 mM of acid. The normal hemoglobin concentration is 9 mM per liter, or 1.98 mM of acid can be neutralized in one liter of blood. This would allow the uptake of 2.2 mM or 49 cc. of carbon dioxide by the blood with a change of pH from 7.40 to 7.32, a difference of 0.08. Actual measurement of the pH of venous and arterial blood shows they differ by only 0.03 pH units. Oxyhemoglobin cannot account for the entire buffering.

The titration curve of reduced hemoglobin is different from the titra-

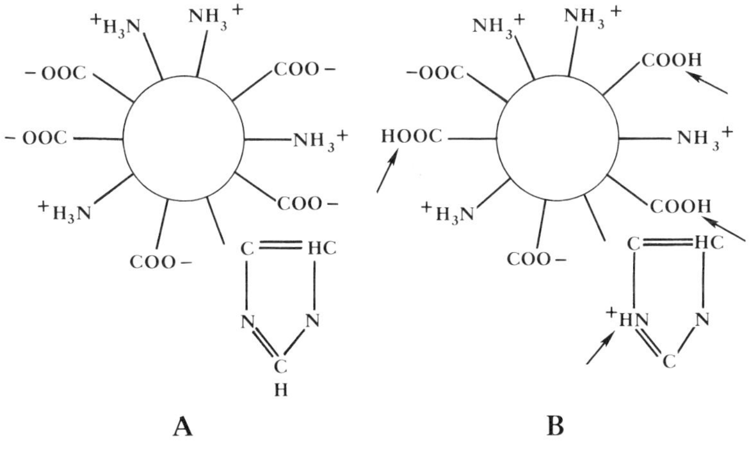

Fig. 2-3. The hemoglobin molecule. (A) The form of hemoglobin molecule at neutral pH. When carbon dioxide is added to the blood, it is hydrated to carbonic acid by carbonic anhydrase in the tissues and hydrogen ions are added to the free carboxyl (COO^-) and nitrogen groups, as depicted in (B), leaving bicarbonate ions free.

tion curve of oxyhemoglobin. Most of the additional acceptors of hydrogen ions in venous blood (the middle line) are supplied when hemoglobin releases oxygen. When oxygen is removed from hemoglobin, the spatial arrangement within the molecule is changed, resulting in new hydrogen acceptors. The rearrangement is called the *Haldane effect,* and it acts for carbon dioxide as the Bohr effect does for oxygen (see p. 14). A fall in pH (rise in hydrogen ion concentration) makes hemoglobin release oxygen and at the same time causes it to accept hydrogen ions more readily. This effect is due to the coordinate linkage of the heme ion to the imidazole group. When oxygen is present, the spatial arrangement is altered, making fewer hydrogen ion acceptors available, and vice versa.

This increase in the ability of reduced hemoglobin to accept hydrogen ions permits most of the neutralization of hydrogen ions produced by reaction of other buffers with carbonic acid to take place without any change in pH. Without the Haldane effect the pH difference between arterial and venous blood would be 0.08 to 0.09 of a pH unit, whereas this unique quality of hemoglobin reduces the arterial-venous difference in pH to 0.03. This reaction between hemoglobin and hydrogen ions leads to other shifts, the principal among these being the chloride shift.

When carbonic acid is formed from carbon dioxide and water by the carbonic anhydrase in the red cells, the hydrogen ions are fixed by the hemoglobin. A net negative charge results from unpaired bicarbonate ions left in the red cells. The bicarbonate ion concentration in the red cells exceeds that in the plasma. Since the positive ions cannot cross the cell membrane, the chloride ions, therefore, move into the red cells and the bicarbonate ions out, so the ratio of bicarbonate to chloride ions in the cells and plasma is kept relatively the same and electrical neutrality is restored. At the lungs this process is reversed.

THE CARBON DIOXIDE ABSORPTION CURVE

From these data it is possible to construct a carbon dioxide absorption curve for blood (Fig. 2-4), just as an oxygen absorption curve for blood was drawn in Figure 2-2. You will note that this is not an S-shaped curve like the one for oxyhemoglobin dissociation. Over the physiological range of pCO_2 there is virtually a straight-line relationship between pCO_2 and carbon dioxide content. Actually, the carbon dioxide dissociation curve is a family of lines, one for each oxygen saturation. The S-shaped curve for oxyhemoglobin dissociation as compared to the straight-line curve for carbon dioxide explains the presence of hypoxia without hypercapnia when ventilation-perfusion imbalance or shunts are

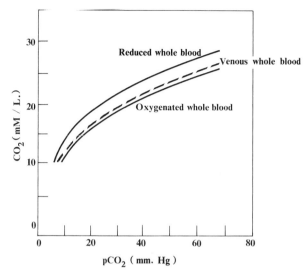

Fig. 2-4. Carbon dioxide dissociation curves. The carbon dioxide dissociation curve at body temperature is altered by the degree of oxygenation of hemoglobin, just as the carbon dioxide dissociation curve is altered by the acid-base balance of the blood. Note that in contrast to oxyhemoglobin curves, the carbon dioxide dissociation curves are nearly straight lines until pCO_2 falls to 10 mm. Hg. Over the range of pCO_2 encountered in patients, the increments in total carbon dioxide for a given change in pCO_2 are the same.

present. (See Analysis of Abnormalities in Blood Gases, pp. 37–38, and Chapter 7, "Coordination of Ventilation and Perfusion.")

TEMPERATURE EFFECTS ON THE CARBON DIOXIDE
ABSORPTION CURVE OF BLOOD

Temperature affects the carbon dioxide absorption curve of blood just as it does the absorption curve of oxygen. When the temperature falls, the amount of carbon dioxide dissolved increases for any given pCO_2; that is, the value for K rises from 0.0301 at 38° to 0.0362 at 30°C. (see Appendix, p. 323).

If the amount of dissolved carbon dioxide rises, the proportion of the total carbon dioxide present as carbonic acid also will rise, because the percent of total carbon dioxide dissolved at any given pCO_2 is greater by a factor equivalent to the change in K. The ratio of carbonic acid to bicarbonate ions is changed by this change in solubility. The pH is actually altered very little, because the pK_1 changes in the opposite direction. Many fancy calculations have been devised to correct total carbon dioxide content and blood pH for temperature changes. All leave much to be desired in the accuracy of prediction, and it is probably just as accurate to report values at the temperature at which they were measured.

DISTURBANCES IN ACID-BASE BALANCE

Hemoglobin supplies the body with a unique and useful method of transporting carbon dioxide without significant alterations in pH. The ability to alter the pCO_2 of arterial blood from the normal by hyper- or hypoventilation further enhances this mechanism. Analysis of the hydrogen ion concentrations (or pH), carbon dioxide content, and pCO_2 permits interpretation of the types of acid-base disturbances occurring in the body. The levels of pH, pCO_2, and bicarbonate ion concentration in the blood are indications of the other changes in the body, and their proper determination depends on an understanding of how the blood changes are related to changes in renal, pulmonary, and metabolic functions.

The formation of carbonic acid is not the only source of hydrogen ions; many other metabolic intermediary or end-products also release hydrogen ions. One of the most important of these reactions is the formation of lactic acid during anaerobic metabolism. The hydrogen ion dissociates from lactic acid:

$$\text{Lactic acid} \rightleftarrows \text{lactate} + \text{H}^+$$

The hydrogen ions are then neutralized by the various buffers, principally bicarbonate. If lactate or any of the other metabolic end-products, such as phosphates, sulfate, or acetoacetic acid, are produced in excess or are removed or metabolized ineffectively, alterations in acid-base balance will occur. These acid metabolites are called *fixed acids,* in contrast to carbonic acid, the mobile acid excreted by the lung. Some of the fixed acids may be burned to carbon dioxide and water, as lactic acid is during the recovery from exercise or as are the keto-acids on administration of insulin to a diabetic. If they cannot be burned to carbon dioxide and water, the kidney must excrete them. The kidney excretes only 40 to 80 mEq of acid per day. The rest of the acid load is converted to carbon dioxide and excreted by the lungs. If the kidneys fail to excrete the acid load that cannot be burned or if the metabolic pathways are blocked, as in diabetes or shock, fixed acids will accumulate in the body. Acidosis can also occur due to excess carbonic acid accumulation if the lungs are not fully effective in the elimination of all the carbon dioxide produced.

Just as excess amounts of acid can be accumulated, so also can excess amounts of alkali be present. This can result from the elimination of too much carbon dioxide by the lungs, from the accumulation of *fixed base* as the result of vomiting of hydrochloric acid from the stomach, or from the ingestion of excess alkali.

TERMINOLOGY OF ACID-BASE DISTURBANCES

The classification of these acid-base disturbances is a matter of considerable controversy. There are, in essence, two schools of thought: one describes each condition on the basis of the physiological disturbance initiating the abnormality, and the other advocates classifying in terms of the changes found on analysis of a blood sample. For a clinician, the physiological classification seems more useful.

Using the physiological language, *acidosis* is an abnormal condition which produces a depression of pH (increase in hydrogen ion concentration) if no secondary or compensatory change occurs. *Alkalosis* is an abnormal condition which causes an elevation of pH (decrease in hydrogen ion concentration) if no secondary or compensatory change occurs.

The next step in definition using the physiological classification is to define the primary causative factor or factors leading to the disturbance in acid-base balance. If there is a single causative etiological factor, the disturbance is called *simple.* If there is more than one primary etiological cause for the disorder, it is called *mixed.* There are two simple classes of primary etiological disturbances, *metabolic* and *respiratory.*

Metabolic disturbances are those in which the *primary* etiological factor involves a loss or gain of acid other than carbonic acid (such acid is called by some *fixed acid*) or a loss or gain of bicarbonate by the extracellular fluid. The term *primary* is the crux of this definition, since there can be a loss or gain of acid or bicarbonate secondary to changes in the excretion of carbon dioxide by the lungs.

Metabolic acidosis results from the primary accumulation in the extracellular fluid of acid other than carbonic acid or a loss of bicarbonate from the extracellular fluid. Clinical examples are the accumulation of keto-acids in diabetic acidosis, the accumulation of lactic acid in shock, and the loss of bicarbonate as a result of diarrhea or during perfusion with a pump oxygenator. In these conditions the blood bicarbonate will be depressed.

Metabolic alkalosis results from the primary loss of hydrogen ions, or gain of hydroxyl ions or exogenous bicarbonate in the extracellular fluid. This alkalosis can result from loss of hydrochloric acid from the stomach, movement of hydrogen ions into the cells in exchange for potassium ions, or preferential renal excretion of hydrogen ions when intracellular potassium is depleted. The blood bicarbonate will be elevated when the excess anions remaining as a result of loss of hydrogen ions react with metabolically produced carbonic acid to form bicarbonate. The increase in blood bicarbonate is the result of loss of acid, not a primary cause of the disturbance. Without readily available carbonic acid, no change in bicarbonate would result.

Respiratory acidosis is the acid-base disturbance produced by relative hypoventilation, or a primary reduction in alveolar ventilation relative to the existing level of carbon dioxide production. The simpler explanation, a condition in which carbon dioxide production exceeds excretion, is incomplete because a person with a fixed elevated pCO_2 is excreting as much carbon dioxide as he produces but his ventilation is inadequate to maintain a normal pCO_2. The blood pCO_2 level will be elevated in patients with respiratory acidosis.

Respiratory alkalosis is a condition in which hyperventilation results in a primary increase in alveolar ventilation relative to carbon dioxide production. The pCO_2 will be low.

Any primary disturbance in acid-base balance results in secondary or compensatory changes which serve to counteract the primary change and thus diminish the change in pH. In metabolic acidosis this change is a secondary increase in ventilation to lower the pCO_2 and thus restore blood pH toward normal. In respiratory acidosis there is increased excretion of chloride by the kidney, resulting in a rise of bicarbonate to restore pH toward normal. The compensatory decrease in pCO_2 with metabolic acidosis is secondary and does not represent a primary increase in alveolar ventilation relative to carbon dioxide production; rather, it is a secondary increase due to fall in pH. The increase in bicarbonate in respiratory acidosis is not a primary increase due to accumulation of excess base but rather a secondary one due to fall in pH as a result of rise in pCO_2. There are thus four primary types of disturbance, four compensated types, and four mixed types of acid-base disturbance for a total of twelve. These may be classified as shown in the list that follows.

PHYSIOLOGICAL CLASSIFICATION OF THE TWELVE
TYPES OF ACID-BASE DISTURBANCE

Simple
  Respiratory acidosis
  Metabolic acidosis
  Respiratory alkalosis
  Metabolic alkalosis

Simple Compensated
   Respiratory acidosis
   Metabolic acidosis
   Respiratory alkalosis
   Metabolic alkalosis

Mixed
   Respiratory and metabolic acidosis
   Respiratory and metabolic alkalosis

Complex Mixed
   Respiratory acidosis and metabolic alkalosis
   Respiratory alkalosis and metabolic acidosis

The clinician needs to have some method of determining the type of acid-base derangement and its primary or initiating cause. This requires proper interpretation of blood-gas determinations and of the clinical picture. Success in such an interpretation depends on narrowing the twelve choices down by properly using the available information. The most useful place to start is by interpreting the blood gases. Figure 2-5 gives a graphic demonstration of the various possible physiological disorders which can cause changes in pH, pCO_2, and bicarbonate ion concentration. These various changes cannot be distinguished without a study of all three determinants of acid-base balance.

The direction of change of pH defines whether acidosis or alkalosis is present. Then the various combinations of change in pCO_2 and bicarbonate lead one to the most likely primary cause. If pH is depressed and pCO_2 elevated, respiratory acidosis exists regardless of the level of bicarbonate ion concentration. Likewise, if pH and bicarbonate are depressed, metabolic acidosis exists regardless of the level of pCO_2. If pH and bicarbonate ion concentration are depressed and the pCO_2 elevated, mixed acidosis is present. This is a very common finding in the sick thoracic surgery patient. If pH is depressed and pCO_2 and bicarbonate ion concentration are elevated, compensated respiratory acidosis is present. If pH is normal or high while pCO_2 and bicarbonate ion concentration are elevated, the disturbance is compensated metabolic alkalosis rather than compensated respiratory acidosis. Likewise, in both compensated metabolic acidosis and compensated respiratory alkalosis, in which bicarbonate ion concentration and pCO_2 are depressed, the clue to differential diagnosis is the low pH in acidosis and elevated pH in alkalosis.

The other possibilities are apparent in Figure 2-5. Complex mixed disturbances such as respiratory acidosis and metabolic alkalosis are not diagramed because the differential diagnosis cannot be made from

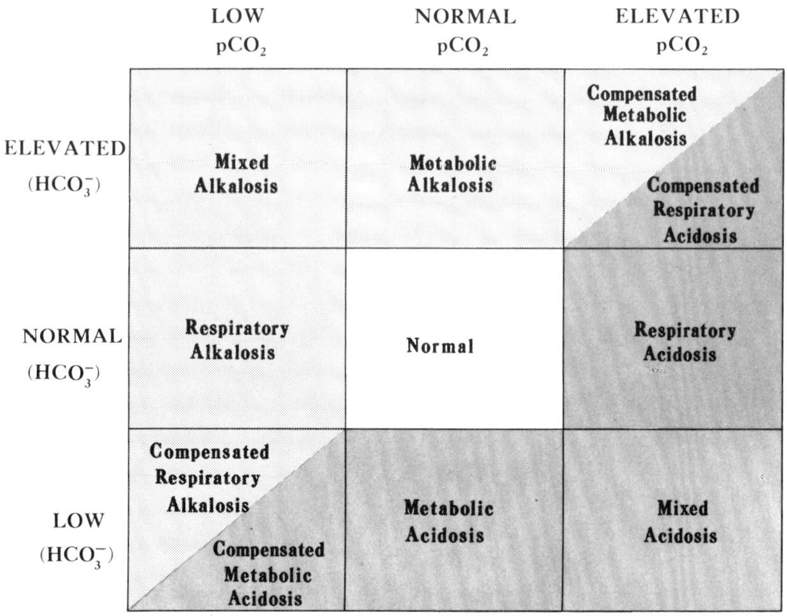

	LOW pCO_2	NORMAL pCO_2	ELEVATED pCO_2
ELEVATED (HCO_3^-)	Mixed Alkalosis	Metabolic Alkalosis	Compensated Metabolic Alkalosis Compensated Respiratory Acidosis
NORMAL (HCO_3^-)	Respiratory Alkalosis	Normal	Respiratory Acidosis
LOW (HCO_3^-)	Compensated Respiratory Alkalosis Compensated Metabolic Acidosis	Metabolic Acidosis	Mixed Acidosis

Fig. 2-5. Diagram for diagnosing type of acid-base disturbance. Light gray area represents pH above 7.4 (hydrogen ion concentration below 40 mM/L.). Dark gray area represents pH below 7.4 (hydrogen ion concentration above 40 mM/L.). The pCO_2 is represented on the horizontal axis, bicarbonate ion concentration on the vertical axis. Total carbon dioxide concentration, buffer base, or base excess can be substituted for bicarbonate ion concentration. To fit a physiological diagnosis to a blood acid-base determination, identify the pH level and then the square or triangle which fits the pCO_2 and bicarbonate ion concentration.

analysis of blood gases alone. These disturbances require careful analysis of the clinical picture as well as the blood gases.

Use of a system such as is shown in Figure 2-5 to analyze the blood-gas alterations allows one to predict what the primary disturbance or disturbances are and to deal with them directly. If the clinician is to use most profitably the classification of acid-base disturbances based on primary physiological disturbance, he must be able to interpret the laboratory determinations of changes in the acid-base factors in blood.

LABORATORY ASSESSMENT OF ACID-BASE BALANCE

Much of the controversy about terminology mentioned earlier arises when the acid-base abnormalities are described in terms of the state of the blood as revealed by chemical analysis. This conflict is exaggerated by the advocates of various methods for chemical analysis of blood. The methods of analysis all depend in part on the Henderson-Hasselbach equation. With proper calculations or nomograms, each chemical method of analysis can provide the calculated values available from any other method.

There are three principal chemical analytic methods in use today. One is the determination of total plasma CO_2 content, TCO_2, with the Van Slyke–Neill apparatus or one of the automated methods and the measurement of pH; from these two measurements the calculation of pCO_2 and bicarbonate ion concentration is made. Another is the determination, on whole blood with a Severinghaus glass electrode, of pH and pCO_2, and from these two measurements calculating the total carbon dioxide and bicarbonate ion concentrations. A third is the Astrup method of (1) determining the pH of whole blood as drawn from the patient; (2) determining the pH after equilibration with two gases of known partial pressure of carbon dioxide; (3) then, by simultaneous solution of three equations or using Astrup's diagram, calculating the patient's pCO_2, total carbon dioxide, and salts of bicarbonate.

Each of these methods is equally valid if carefully done. The determination of total carbon dioxide in venous blood alone, as is done in most clinical laboratories, is inadequate to make a precise diagnosis of changes in acid-base balance, since, as Figure 2-5 shows (p. 30), a rise or fall in total carbon dioxide can be associated with a number of defects. This determination is helpful only in nonrespiratory metabolic acidosis or alkalosis provided the clinician is confident there is no associated respiratory defect.

Singer and Hastings and, more recently, Astrup have introduced the concepts of whole-blood buffer base and base excess or deficit. They point out that the buffering capacity of blood is not defined by the ratio of bicarbonate to carbonic acid alone but is affected by the buffering capacity of hemoglobin and other proteins.

Singer and Hastings define whole-blood buffer base as the sum of the concentrations of all the buffer ions in whole blood expressed as milliequivalents per liter. Normally this concentration is 45 to 50 mEq per liter, most of which is contributed by bicarbonate and hemoglobin. They have constructed a nomogram which permits the calculation of whole-blood buffer base if the hematocrit or hemoglobin and any two of the four factors—pH, pCO_2, concentration of salts of bicarbonate, or total carbon dioxide concentration—are determined on a sample of blood. The deviation from normal is then calculated by difference.

Using their method and nomogram, Astrup and colleagues calculate the bicarbonate concentration that would be present if the pCO_2 were normal, or 40 mm. Hg. This is called the *standard bicarbonate,* or the bicarbonate present at a standard pCO_2. The normal value for standard bicarbonate is 24 mEq per liter. Any deviation above or below this value is called a *base excess* or *base deficit*.

These terms would be most useful if one could say ipso facto that if the standard bicarbonate is low (a base deficit), nonrespiratory metabolic acidosis exists; or, if the standard bicarbonate is high (a base excess), nonrespiratory metabolic alkalosis is present. This is not the case, however. If the kidney has retained base to compensate for a respiratory acidosis, the buffer base of Hastings would be increased and Astrup's nomogram would reveal a base excess or nonrespiratory metabolic alkalosis. These terms, then, do not relieve one (nor do their authors contend they do) of the necessity of using pH change to determine the primary cause of the change in the so-called base excess.

In addition to the limitations of definition, there are chemical differences depending on whether blood is equilibrated with various pCO_2 levels in vivo or in vitro. If a sample of blood is exposed in a tonometer to two partial pressures of pCO_2, as is done in the Astrup method, the calculated bicarbonate level, base excess, or buffer base is different from that of blood exposed to the same levels of pCO_2 in the patient's lungs. When blood is exposed to gas with an increased concentration of carbon dioxide, the pCO_2 of the blood rises and pH falls. Some of the carbonic acid added as a result of increased pCO_2 reacts with buffers of the blood, principally hemoglobin, and is converted to bicarbonate. In a tonometer the hydrogen and bicarbonate ions then distribute themselves in the water of blood cells and plasma.

The bicarbonate ions generated by an elevated alveolar pCO_2 are not confined to the water of the blood cells and plasma. They are distributed in a volume at least as large as the extracellular fluid. The excess hydrogen ions are distributed over the whole extracellular fluid volume, and some are buffered by the tissue buffers. Schwartz has studied the differences in bicarbonate levels when subjects breathe high concentrations of carbon dioxide or when blood is exposed in vitro to gas with an elevated pCO_2 (Fig. 2-6). At low pCO_2 levels the discrepancy is small, but it widens markedly at high pCO_2 levels. Using the Astrup method there would be an apparent base excess, signifying a mixed acidosis rather than a pure respiratory acidosis.

Schwartz has gone further and studied the hydrogen and bicarbonate ion concentrations that would be expected for any given change in alveolar and arterial pCO_2 both in chronic as well as acute exposure to increased concentrations of carbon dioxide. Figure 2-7A and B defines the 95% confidence limits for such changes. In a patient with elevated pCO_2, if the level of bicarbonate is below the levels predicted by these

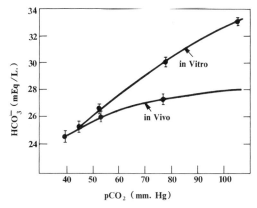

Fig. 2-6. Comparison of the in vitro and in vivo effects of alterations in pCO_2 on blood bicarbonate ion concentration in man. In vivo, when subjects breathe high concentrations of carbon dioxide, a given change in pCO_2 results in a much smaller change in bicarbonate ion concentration than the same change in vitro when blood is equilibrated with increased concentrations of carbon dioxide. The in vivo curve above 78 mm. Hg is an extrapolation. (Adapted from W. B. Schwartz, N. C. Brackett, Jr., and J. J. Cohen, Response of extracellular hydrogen ion concentration to graded degrees of chronic hypercapnia. *J. Clin. Invest.* 44:291, 1965, and from N. C. Brackett, Jr., J. J. Cohen, and W. B. Schwartz, Carbon dioxide titration curve of normal man: Effect of increasing degrees of acute hypercapnia on acid-base equilibrium. *New Eng. J. Med.* 272:6, 1965. Used by permission.)

graphs, then a complicating metabolic acidosis is present. For example, if a patient was known to have a pCO_2 of 60 mm. Hg for more than two days, the bicarbonate should be at least 29 mEq or else one should expect a complicating metabolic derangement.

It is important that the proponents of each of the various ways of interpreting acid-base disturbances understand enough of each other's terminology to communicate with one another and that they avoid being semantic isolationists. Figure 2-8 is a modification of the Siegaard-Andersen nomogram which permits a translation of any terminology to any other and the calculation of the total acid-base picture if any pair of factors is known. In addition, predicted changes in bicarbonate level for various acute or chronic levels of pCO_2 can be read from the columns surrounding the pCO_2 line.

ANALYSIS OF ABNORMALITIES IN BLOOD GASES

In this section the various combinations of alterations in pCO_2, oxygen saturation, or pO_2, will be analyzed. These changes can be the results of changes in ventilation, pulmonary circulation, diffusion, ventilation perfusion, and respiratory control as well as mechanical

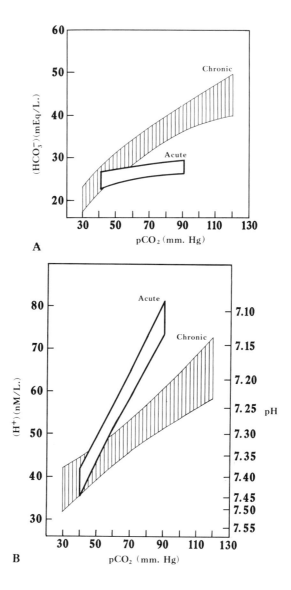

Fig. 2-7. The in vivo effects of acute and chronic hypercapnia (A) on the bicarbonate level and (B) on pH level, or hydrogen ion concentration of blood. The zones bounded by the lines represent the 95% confidence limits for normal subjects exposed to elevated concentrations of inspired carbon dioxide. With acute rises in pCO_2 the change in hydrogen ion concentration is larger and in bicarbonate ion concentration smaller than following chronic elevation of pCO_2, which permits the kidneys to conserve bicarbonate ion concentration and correct hydrogen ion concentration toward normal. The acute measurements were made in man and the chronic ones in dogs. (Adapted from W. B. Schwartz, N. C.

derangements. In this discussion pO_2, oxygen saturation, pH, pCO_2, and bicarbonate are used to define the concentrations of dissolved gases and the acid-base parameters of the arterial blood.

EXAMPLE I

Arterial Blood-Gas and Acid-Base Concentrations
Oxygen saturation 85%

pO_2	60 mm. Hg
pH	7.26
pCO_2	60 mm. Hg
HCO_3^-	26 mEq/L.

The determination of either the oxygen saturation or the pO_2 would provide the needed information. They are both depressed, showing incomplete oxygenation of the blood. The pCO_2 is also elevated and the pH depressed. Reference to the nomogram (Fig. 2-8) shows that the bicarbonate is within the normal range for a pCO_2 of 60 if the elevation of pCO_2 is acute. Only the clinical history can answer the question of whether this is an acute or chronic alteration. If it is acute, the acid-base picture is one of uncompensated acute respiratory acidosis. The low oxygen saturation and pO_2 show that as well as failing to eliminate adequate amounts of carbon dioxide, the patient is failing to acquire enough oxygen. The most likely cause for such an abnormality is acute ventilatory insufficiency. Since the arterial pCO_2 is above the normal venous pCO_2 of 46 mm. Hg, the venous pCO_2 must also be elevated.

If the history supports the fact that the condition in Example 1 is chronic, a complicating renal failure or other metabolic disorder is present. The bicarbonate ion concentration should be between 29 and 34 mEq in chronic hypercapnia of 60 mm. Hg. Ventilatory insufficiency is present, but a metabolic defect which prevents the conservation of bicarbonate is also present. Two of a number of the associated diseases could be renal insufficiency or diarrhea.

In this patient the oxygen saturation and pO_2 are in the normal range, the pCO_2 and bicarbonate are elevated, and the pH is moderately depressed. The elevation in pCO_2 signifies underventilation. Despite this, the oxygen saturation is normal. The only reasonable way of reconciling these differences is to assume that the patient is breathing an oxygen-

Brackett, Jr., and J. J. Cohen, Response of extracellular hydrogen ion concentration to graded degrees of chronic hypercapnia. *J. Clin. Invest.* 44:291, 1965, and from N. C. Brackett, Jr., J. J. Cohen, and W. B. Schwartz, Carbon dioxide titration curve of normal man: Effect of increasing degrees of acute hypercapnia on acid-base equilibrium. *New Eng. J. Med.* 272:6, 1965. Used by permission.)

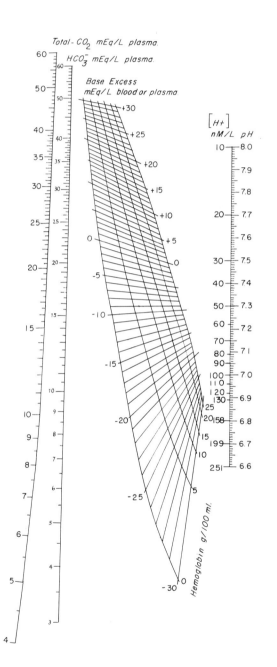

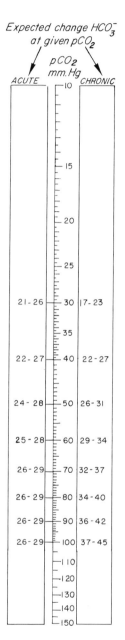

Expected change HCO₃⁻
at given pCO₂

EXAMPLE 2

Oxygen saturation 96%

pO_2	88 mm. Hg
pH	7.35
pCO_2	60 mm. Hg
$HCO_3{}^-$	32 mEq/L.

enriched gas mixture. The bicarbonate is elevated to the level predicted by the nomogram, showing that normal renal excretion of chloride has occurred with retention of bicarbonate to compensate for chronic hypercapnia and to bring pH up nearer normal than in Example 1.

The diagnosis, then, is chronic ventilatory insufficiency in a patient receiving oxygen therapy with good renal compensation. (This also could be acute respiratory acidosis complicating a metabolic alkalosis in a patient receiving oxygen treatment.)

EXAMPLE 3

Oxygen saturation 85%

pO_2	50 mm. Hg
pH	7.4
pCO_2	40 mm. Hg
$HCO_3{}^-$	24 mEq/L.

In this patient the oxygen saturation is depressed but the pCO_2, pH, and bicarbonate are normal. This must be a defect which affects oxygen acquisition but not carbon dioxide elimination. There are two explanations for this abnormality. The first is a diffusion defect of some kind. Carbon dioxide diffuses from the capillary to the alveolar air twenty times faster than oxygen, so any diffusion defect would lead to oxygen unsaturation without affecting carbon dioxide. (If oxygen in high concentrations is administered to a patient with a diffusion defect, the oxygen unsaturation can be largely corrected and is a good differential test [see Chapter 6, and Example 5, p. 39].)

Fig. 2-8. A modification of the Siegaard-Andersen nomogram permitting the translation of the terminology or the interpretation of any method of chemical determination of blood in the manner familiar to the user. If any two values, such as pCO_2 and pH, or pH and total carbon dioxide, are known, the other determinants of acid-base balance will be on a line connecting the two known values. When pCO_2 is either acutely or chronically altered, the change in bicarbonate ion concentration predicted by Schwartz is listed in the appropriate boxed columns on each side of the pCO_2 line. By comparing the bicarbonate ion concentration found in the patient, it is possible to determine whether the change in bicarbonate is the result of compensatory mechanisms due to alteration in pCO_2 or is a separate metabolic derangement.

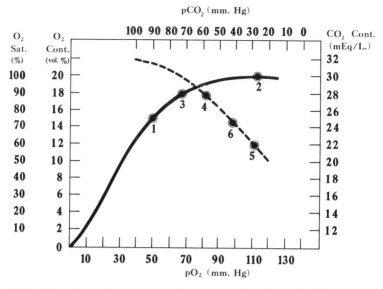

Fig. 2-9. The effect of the shape of oxygen and carbon dioxide dissociation curves on arterial gas contents. In this figure the oxygen dissociation curve (*solid line*) is plotted from bottom to top and left to right. The carbon dioxide dissociation curve is plotted reading from top to bottom and right to left. If blood from an underventilated alveolus has a pO_2 of 50 mm. Hg (point *1*), its oxygen content will be 16 volumes percent and oxygen saturation 80%. When this blood is mixed with an equal amount of blood with a pO_2 of 110 mm. Hg and an oxygen content of 20 volumes percent from a hyperventilated alveolus (point *2*), the arterial blood, a mixture of these, will have an oxygen content of 18 volumes percent, or 90% oxygen saturation (point *3*). Unless the arterial pCO_2 is elevated, the venous blood pCO_2 will not be above 55 mm. Hg. Its carbon dioxide content will be 27 mEq/L. (point *4*). If this blood is mixed with an equal amount of blood with a pCO_2 of 40 mm. Hg and a normal carbon dioxide content of 21 mEq (point *5*) which comes from a hyperventilated area of lung, the mixture will have a normal pCO_2 of 40 mm. Hg and a normal carbon dioxide content of 24 mEq (point *6*). The curved oxygen dissociation curve and straight-line carbon dioxide dissociation curve are the reasons patients with shunts or ventilation-perfusion abnormalities have normal levels of arterial pCO_2 and low levels of arterial pO_2 or oxygen saturation.

The other and more common explanation of the condition in Example 3 is a shunt in which some blood is not coming in contact with the alveolar air or some alveoli are poorly ventilated (Fig. 2-9). The explanation for this discrepancy lies in the shape of the two dissociation curves. The blood that perfuses the well-ventilated alveoli will be fully saturated, but hyperventilation to raise pO_2 further will not add more oxygen because the top of the oxygen dissociation curve is flat. Thus blood from the hyperventilated alveoli will have a normal oxygen content, but blood going by an unventilated or hypoventilated alveolus will not acquire a normal amount of oxygen and will have a low oxygen content. When the blood returning from these two types of alveoli is mixed, the result will be a low oxygen content and saturation. This is not the case for carbon dioxide. Blood perfusing the poorly ventilated area will have a high pCO_2, but blood perfusing the hyperventilated area will have a lower than normal pCO_2 since the carbon dioxide dissociation curve is straight, not S-shaped, over its physiological range. When blood with low carbon dioxide content is mixed with blood with a high carbon dioxide content, the result will be a normal carbon dioxide content. Thus hypoxia can exist without hypercapnia due to diffusion blocks, shunts, or ventilation-perfusion incoordination.

EXAMPLE 4

Oxygen saturation 97%

pO_2	100 mm. Hg
pH	7.31
pCO_2	30 mm. Hg
$HCO_3{}^-$	15 mEq/L.

This patient has high pO_2 and high normal oxygen saturation; the pCO_2 is low. This demonstrates that the patient is hyperventilating. The bicarbonate is low, as is the pH. The diagnosis is metabolic acidosis with partial respiratory compensation.

EXAMPLE 5

Oxygen saturation 97%

pO_2	100 mm. Hg
pH	7.45
pCO_2	30 mm. Hg
$HCO_3{}^-$	22 mEq/L.

In this instance the evidence for hyperventilation is the same as in Example 4. The pH, however, is alkaline, and the bicarbonate is within the range expected for a pCO_2 of 30 mm. Hg. This is, therefore, a respiratory alkalosis. This can occur with a central nervous system lesion or following the correction of metabolic acidosis.

EXAMPLE 6

Oxygen saturation 93%

pO_2	60 mm. Hg
pH	7.46
pCO_2	30 mm. Hg
$HCO_3{}^-$	20 mEq/L.

In this example the pCO_2 is again low, but the oxygen saturation and pO_2 are also depressed. The HCO_3^- is in the range expected for a pCO_2 of 30 mm. Hg. Thus there is definite respiratory alkalosis, or excess elimination of carbon dioxide, yet the oxygen saturation is low. This is a defect which interferes with oxygen acquisition. This picture is seen in a patient with a diffusing defect or at high altitudes, where the partial pressure of oxygen is diminished.

3. VENTILATION

THE air exchange system is a truly alternating flow system in which the same conducting airways are used for ingress and egress of air. This permits a maximum anatomical economy of space but imposes a more complicated system on the student than does the circulatory system, which is a continuous closed circuit of tubes with a unidirectional, phasic flow of blood. To permit an orderly and comprehensible exposition, the study of the transfer of gases from the atmosphere to the blood and then to the tissues and their return must be broken down somewhat arbitrarily into component parts. In this chapter the volume changes and distribution of gases in the various anatomical areas of the lung will be discussed.

THE UPPER AIRWAYS

Quiet breathing is usually nasal. The nasal passages filter and warm the inspired air; all particles over 4 μ in size are filtered out as the air is drawn over a moist surface of approximately 158 square centimeters in the small nasal volume of 8 cc. The nose offers considerable resistance to breathing, 1 cm. H_2O per liter per second, though there is wide individual variation in this resistance. During more marked ventilatory effort this high resistance in the nose forces the individual to use the alternative, low resistance, but less well filtered route—the mouth. The pharynx, larynx, and trachea complete the job of warming and moistening the air as well as afford further protection from foreign matter entering the smaller airways.

Although the temperature, humidity, and volume of inspired air can vary over a wide range, in environments that are tolerable to man the air is normally cooler than body temperature and not fully saturated with water vapor. The upper airways warm this air and add water vapor by convection and evaporation from the mucosal surfaces, so that air reaching the alveoli is at body temperature and fully saturated with water vapor. While most warming and addition of water vapor takes place in the upper airways, at extremes of temperature and at high rates of ventilation the process may be completed in the trachea. None of the exchange of heat or water takes place below the large bronchi.

Dry air has a specific heat of only 0.00026 kilocalorie per liter per degree centigrade. If inspired air is at 20°C. (70°F.) with a humidity of 50% (50% saturated with water vapor), the heat required to warm the air to 37°C. is just 0.0044 kilocalorie per liter. The heat required to raise the vapor pressure of water in one liter of air from 8 mm. Hg at 20°C. (50% humidity) to 47 mm. Hg or 37°C. (100% humidity) is 0.204 kilocalorie.

Thus the major heat loss in the respiratory tract is associated with the addition of moisture to the air. This is in turn dependent on the relative humidity and the temperature of the inspired air.

The body's addition of water vapor to inspired air leads to a water loss of between 250 to 300 ml. per day and a heat loss of 175 to 200 kilocalories, or approximately 10% of the total heat loss. With hyperventilation and/or fever, these losses of water and heat increase.

Expired gas as it emerges from the trachea is fully saturated with water vapor and is at body temperature. In extreme conditions it may be cooled in the upper airways, particularly in the nose, leading to condensation of water vapor and the drippy nose familiar to all on cold days.

COMPOSITION OF GASES IN THE RESPIRATORY TRACT AND BLOOD

The composition of inspired air is significantly altered by the addition of water vapor. The composition of inspired air at 20°C. with relative humidity of 50% at barometric pressure of 760 mm. Hg is approximately 1% water vapor (pH_2O, 8 mm. Hg), 21% oxygen (pO_2, 158 mm. Hg), and 78% nitrogen (pN_2, 594 mm. Hg). The air in the trachea at 37°C. and fully saturated will be 6.6% water vapor (pH_2O, 47 mm. Hg), leaving 93% rather than 99% to be divided between oxygen and nitrogen. This lowers the absolute oxygen percentage from 21% to 19.6% (pO_2, 149 mm. Hg) and the nitrogen to 74% (pN_2, 564 mm. Hg). The volume of the gas is increased about 9% and the partial pressure of oxygen is lowered 10 mm. by the addition of this water vapor. At an altitude of 6,500 feet, where the barometric pressure would be 596, inspired air at the same temperature (20°C.) and relative humidity (50%) would be 1.3% water vapor (pH_2O, 8 mm. Hg),

20.64% oxygen (pO$_2$, 123 mm. Hg) and 78% nitrogen (pN$_2$, 465 mm. Hg). In the trachea the composition would be 8% water vapor (pH$_2$O, 47 mm. Hg), 17.6% oxygen (pO$_2$, 105 mm. Hg), and 74% nitrogen (pN$_2$, 444 mm. Hg). The absolute pressure of water vapor is unchanged by the change in altitude because the amount of water vapor pressure is dependent on the temperature of the liquid, not the atmospheric pressure (see Appendix, p. 322). At sea level 6.5% of the air in the trachea is water vapor, while at an altitude of 6,500 feet, 8% is water vapor. This dilution of the inspired air with water vapor is an important factor in the fall in oxygen saturation with altitude, since the saturation of hemoglobin is related to the partial pressure of oxygen (see p. 11). Fever also leads to a rise in water vapor pressure and thus to dilution of inspired oxygen.

The warm gas saturated with water vapor in the trachea is further altered in the alveoli by the withdrawal of oxygen and addition of carbon dioxide. In the alveoli the oxygen concentration is lowered from 19.6% (pO$_2$, 149 mm. Hg) to 13.7% (pO$_2$, 104 mm. Hg), carbon dioxide concentration is raised from zero to 5% (pCO$_2$, 40 mm. Hg), and the nitrogen percentage is raised slightly to 75% (pN$_2$, 569 mm. Hg), since more oxygen is removed than carbon dioxide added.

The amount of oxygen removed depends on the oxygen demands of the individual and the ventilation. Man at rest consumes 250 cc. of oxygen per minute and excretes 200 cc. of carbon dioxide. This can be increased tenfold with strenuous exercise. The expired air is a mixture of air which has given up oxygen and gained carbon dioxide in the alveoli and air in the conducting portion of the respiratory tract which has not exchanged gases with the blood.

The level of pO$_2$ and pCO$_2$ in the alveolar air is determined by interaction between the amount of gas exchange in the alveoli and the production of carbon dioxide and consumption of oxygen by the tissues. The figures given in Table 3-1 for composition of venous blood represent only one example. The more active are the metabolic processes in the tissues, the more oxygen will be consumed and carbon dioxide produced. The systemic mixed venous pO$_2$ can be lowered and the pCO$_2$ elevated, thus increasing the transport capacity of each volume of blood that passes through the circulatory system. Unless some compromise is forced on the body, it attempts to keep the arterial pO$_2$ at about 100 mm. Hg and the pCO$_2$ at 40 mm. Hg. To accomplish this, fresh air must be continuously added to the alveoli and stale air removed at a rate to balance the continuous removal of oxygen and addition of carbon dioxide by the systemic venous blood. If the exchange of air to the alveoli removes more carbon dioxide than the tissues are producing and adds more

Table 3-1. Composition of Gases at Sea Level

Gas	Inspired Air 20°C. 50% Sat. H_2O Partial Pressure (mm. Hg)	Per cent	Moist Tracheal Air Partial Pressure (mm. Hg)	Per cent	Alveolar Air Partial Pressure (mm. Hg)	Per cent	Arterial Blood Partial Pressure (mm. Hg)	Per cent	Venous Blood Partial Pressure (mm. Hg)	Per cent	Expired Air Partial Pressure (mm. Hg)	Per cent
Oxygen	158	21	149	19.6	104	13.7	100	13	40	5.6	116	15.2
Carbon dioxide	0.3	0.04	0.3	0.04	40	5.3	40	5.3	46	6.5	29	4
Water	8	1	47	6.2	47	6.6	47	6.2	47	6.7	47	6.2
Nitrogen and rare gases	594	78	564	74	569	75	573	75	573	81	568	75
Total	760		760		760		760		706		760	

oxygen than the tissues are consuming (alveolar hyperventilation), the alveolar and arterial pO_2 will rise and the pCO_2 will fall. If the exchange of air in the alveoli removes less carbon dioxide and adds less oxygen than the metabolic rate of the tissue requires (alveolar hypoventilation), the alveolar and arterial pCO_2 will rise and the pO_2 will fall.

DEFINITION OF LUNG VOLUMES

In any respiratory cycle a volume of air is drawn into the lungs and a similar volume ejected. This is called the *tidal volume.* The absolute limit of the tidal volume is the *vital capacity*, the maximum amount of air which can be expired after a maximal inhalation. The vital capacity is divided into (1) the tidal volume; (2) the *inspiratory reserve volume*, the amount of additional air that can be inspired after a normal inspiration; and (3) the *expiratory reserve volume*, the amount of air that can be expired after a normal expiration.

At the end of a maximal expiration some air still remains in the lung. This is called the *residual volume.* At the end of a normal expiration the air remaining in the lung includes the expiratory reserve volume and the residual volume. This is called the *functional residual volume.* The sum of the residual volume and vital capacity is the *total lung volume.*

The normal values for these various volumes vary with age and size (Fig. 3-1). The vital capacity, residual volume, and total lung volume vary approximately as the cube of the body height. Vital capacity makes up approximately 75% of the total lung capacity. The vital capacity decreases in adults with age, and it is smaller in women than in men of comparable stature. A number of formulas have been worked out to predict vital capacity. A simple, rapid means of calculating the predicted vital capacity is:

Males: height (in cm.) $\times$ 25 cc.
Females: height (in cm.) $\times$ 20 cc.

MINUTE VENTILATION AND ALVEOLAR VENTILATION

The tidal volume times the number of breaths per minute defines the *minute ventilation.* In a normal person at rest this is 2.5 to 5 liters per minute per square meter of body surface area. Only part of an inspired volume reaches the alveoli. The last part remains in the conducting airway, where no gas exchange takes place. At the end of an expiration the conducting airways are filled with air that has been expelled from the alveoli. On the next inspiration the alveolar air in the airway will be

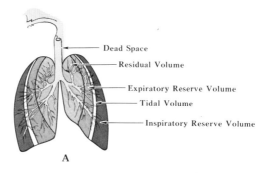

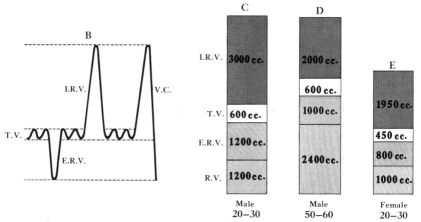

Fig. 3-1. The subdivision of lung volumes. (A) An anatomical depiction of the various subdivisions of lung volume. The residual volume includes 150 cc. which remain in anatomical dead space. The major reserve volume is the inspiratory reserve. (B) A typical spirometer tracing of lung volumes. (C, D, and E) The division of various lung volumes in young males, older males, and young females. *V.C.*, vital capacity; *R.V.*, residual volume; *E.R.V.*, expiratory reserve volume; *T.V.*, tidal volume; *I.R.V.*, inspiratory reserve volume.

drawn back into the alveoli before any fresh air can enter. The minute ventilation is, therefore, always greater than the *alveolar ventilation*.

The volume of the conducting airways is called the anatomical dead space. Just as the other volumes vary with the size and age of the individual, so does the dead space. It is approximately equal in cubic centimeters to the lean weight in pounds and increases slightly with age.

At the start of a normal inspiration the conducting airways contain air with a pO_2 of 100 and a pCO_2 of 40 mm. Hg (Fig. 3-2). The first 150 cc. of an inspiration will have this composition. Then subsequent

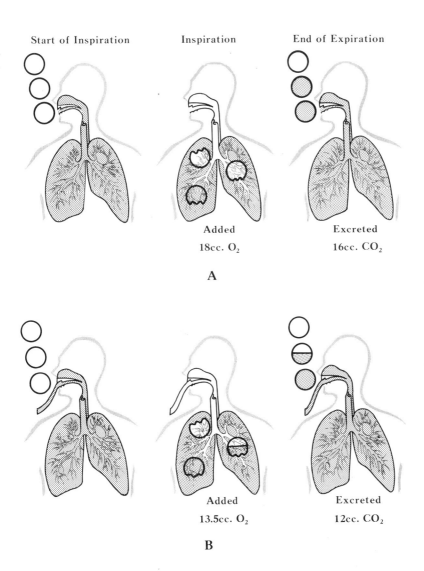

Start of Inspiration	Inspiration	End of Expiration
	Added	Excreted
	18cc. O_2	16cc. CO_2

A

	Added	Excreted
	13.5cc. O_2	12cc. CO_2

B

Fig. 3-2. The role of anatomical dead space. Each white circle represents 150 cc. of room air containing 31 cc. of oxygen and no carbon dioxide. If three aliquots of 150 cc. are inspired by a normal man, only two aliquots of room air reach the alveoli; the third aliquot remains in the dead space. After equilibration with alveolar air and the pulmonary capillary blood, the pO_2 of the inspired air is lowered from 150 to 98 mm. Hg, reducing the amount of oxygen in each aliquot to 22 cc. The pCO_2 rises from 0 to 40 mm. Hg, adding 8 cc. of carbon dioxide to each aliquot. During expiration, the first aliquot exhaled is the dead-space air, which has the same concentration as room air; the next two aliquots are alveolar air, and the dead space is now filled with alveolar air.

If the external dead space is increased by 75 cc. (B), only 275 cc. of room air are added to the alveolar air and only 275 cc. of alveolar air are expired, resulting in a decrease in oxygen acquisition to 13.5 cc. and in carbon dioxide excretion to 12 cc. per breath.

volumes drawn into the alveoli will have a pO_2 of 159 and a pCO_2 of 0 mm. Hg. The last 150 cc. of the inspiration remain in the conducting airways and are unchanged. The volume of fresh air drawn into the alveoli is equilibrated with the alveolar air and then expelled with a pO_2 of 104 and pCO_2 of 40 mm. Hg.

Each 150 cc. of air drawn into the alveoli after the dead space volume is washed out supply approximately 9 cc. of oxygen for exchange with the blood. Thus, in a breath of 450 cc. and with an anatomical dead space of 150 cc., 300 cc. of fresh air will reach the alveoli and 18 cc. of oxygen will be added.

In the same manner, air in the dead space prior to expiration has not equilibrated with alveolar air but remains the same as inspired air. Any subsequent expired volumes will have approximately 5 cc. more carbon dioxide per 100 cc. than on inspiration. In a breath of 450 cc. with 150 cc. of dead space, 300 cc. of alveolar air will be expelled, or 15 to 16 cc. of carbon dioxide.

The minute ventilation, the volume of the breaths times the rate per minute, does not define the exchange of oxygen and carbon dioxide. A minute ventilation of 6,000 cc. achieved by breathing 500 cc. per breath 12 times per minute in a patient with 150 cc. of dead space would provide an alveolar ventilation of 4,200 cc. and permit acquisition of 250 cc. of oxygen and excretion of 200 cc. of carbon dioxide. In the same subject a similar minute ventilation of 6,000 cc. per minute achieved by breathing 225 cc. per breath 24 times per minute would give an alveolar ventilation of 75 cc. per breath. The total alveolar ventilation would be 1,800 cc. The oxygen acquisition would be cut to 108 cc. and the carbon dioxide elimination to 90 cc.

THE EFFECT OF RESIDUAL VOLUME ON COMPOSITION OF ALVEOLAR AIR AND BLOOD GASES

Since the ventilation of the lungs is cyclical while the blood flow is continuous, the composition of alveolar air changes throughout the respiratory cycle. If an individual holds his breath, alveolar pO_2 falls and pCO_2 rises since the blood is constantly removing oxygen and adding carbon dioxide. Most of the breathing cycle simulates breath-holding. In a normal respiratory cycle, about 2 seconds are devoted to inspiration and 3 to expiration. During the first third of inspiration no fresh air is added to the alveolar air but the dead space is flushed; thus, only during 1.4 seconds out of 5 is fresh air being added to the residual volume.

If the residual volume were very small, the pO_2 would rise and pCO_2 fall to near to the inspired air values as soon as the dead space was flushed and inspired air brought into the alveoli. Then, until the next inspired air was brought in, the pCO_2 would rise and pO_2 fall to near to the venous levels. This would lead to wide fluctuations in the arterial blood gas levels.

In a normal young male with 6,000 cc. total lung volume, approximately 2,400 cc. of air remain in his lungs at the end of a normal expiration. To this is added 150 cc. of dead-space alveolar air and then 350 cc. of inspired air. During the simulated breath-holding prior to the addition of 350 cc. of fresh air, pO_2 drops to 98 mm. Hg and pCO_2 rises to nearly 41 mm. Hg. With inspiration, the alveolar air is then diluted with the 350 cc. of inspired air and the pO_2 acutely rises to over 101; it then falls slowly back to 98 while pCO_2 acutely falls to 38 to start a rise to 41 again (Fig. 3-3). Thus the residual air in the lungs damps the fluctuations in alveolar pCO_2 and pO_2 from nearly 40 mm. Hg to 2 to 3 mm. Hg.

The question then arises whether an increase in residual air above normal produces any respiratory disadvantage. If oxygen is being removed and carbon dioxide added to the alveoli by the ventilatory exchange at the same rate they are being removed and added to the blood, the volume of the total gas is immaterial provided mixing is complete. If a small fire in a box consumed 250 cc. of oxygen and produced 200 cc. of carbon dioxide per minute, the concentrations of these gases would remain unchanged if 250 cc. of oxygen were added and 200 cc. of carbon dioxide absorbed per minute. The same would be true if the fire were in a large, airtight room, provided there was rapid, complete, and uniform distribution of the exchanged gases.

If for some reason it is advisable to change the concentration of inspired gas (for instance, to induce anesthesia with an inhalation anesthetic or to give oxygen therapy), the volume of residual air does assume importance. Under these circumstances one is attempting to alter acutely the composition of alveolar gas. If the distribution of gas is not uniform (as is often the case when the volume of residual air is increased), then some areas of the lung will be hyperventilated while other areas which are hypoventilated will simulate prolonged breath-holding. When this happens it is not the large volume of residual air that leads to difficulty, but the uneven mixture of gases.

If the residual air is 2,400 cc., as in a normal individual, each time a breath of 500 cc. of oxygen is taken, 150 cc. of dead-space air is returned to give an undiluted alveolar gas volume of 2,550 cc. to which 350 cc. of oxygen is added (Fig. 3-4). If the original alveolar oxygen concentration was 14% of 2,550 cc., 350 cc. of oxygen would be present in the alveolar gas. To this has been added another 350 cc. of pure

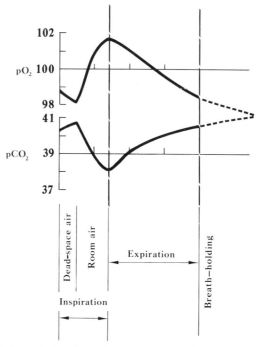

Fig. 3-3. Variation of alveolar pO_2 and pCO_2 during one breath. During the first portion of inspiration, as the dead-space air is brought back into the alveoli, there is a continued fall in pO_2 and rise in pCO_2. Then, as fresh room air is drawn into the alveoli during the remainder of inspiration, the pO_2 rises and pCO_2 falls. During expiration pO_2 falls and pCO_2 rises until completion of the washout of dead space on the next inspiration. If the subject holds his breath (*dotted lines*), the pCO_2 continues to rise and pO_2 to fall. The rates of rise and fall slowly level off as the alveolar pO_2 and pCO_2 approach the levels of pCO_2 and pO_2 in venous blood.

oxygen to raise the total amount of oxygen in the alveoli to 700 cc. and thus increase the oxygen concentration to 24% (700 cc./2,900 cc.). On the next inspiration 350 cc. more of oxygen is added, bringing the total to 1,050 cc. of oxygen (neglecting oxygen consumption for the moment) and the concentration to 40%, and so on.

If the functional residual volume is increased to 3,400 cc., on inspiration the undiluted alveolar gas volume will be 3,550 and the total volume 3,900 cc.; 350 cc. of oxygen will be added to the 14% of 3,550, or 500 cc., of alveolar oxygen to give a total of 850 cc. of oxygen and a concentration of 22%. The next breath would add 350 cc. of oxygen to 22% of 3,550, or 781 cc., to give a total of 1,131 cc. of oxygen, or a rise to 29% in alveolar oxygen concentration.

Thus, in this example the increase in residual air of 1,000 cc. has slowed the washout of nitrogen and its replacement of oxygen. The

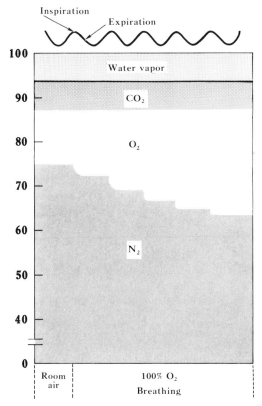

Fig. 3-4. The effect of successive breaths of pure oxygen on the composition of alveolar air. During room-air breathing, alveolar air contains 5.6% carbon dioxide, 6.6% water vapor, 13% oxygen, and 75% nitrogen. With each successive breath the nitrogen is diluted by the inspired oxygen. The oxygen concentration rises at a progressively slower rate with each breath because the percentage of oxygen in each given volume of alveolar air is steadily rising and so the diluting effect of 100% oxygen is less.

same relative deficit will occur for any new gas to be substituted for an original gas. When an anesthetic gas is added, the concentration can, *with care,* be increased at first above the final desired level, thus speeding up this process. Likewise, slow, deep breaths will increase alveolar ventilation and speed up the washing out of alveolar gas with the new gas.

THE ASSESSMENT OF ADEQUACY OF VENTILATION

The respiratory rate provides a rough estimate of the adequacy of ventilation. If the rate is slowed, presumably the volume of gas moved in and out of the lungs each minute, the minute ventilation, is decreased. If the rate is up, the minute ventilation is presumably increased. Some assessment of the amount of air moved, as well as the rate, however, is also necessary to assess the adequacy of ventilation. If the rate and tidal volume are known, the minute ventilation can be calculated. Since only fresh air which reaches the alveoli will function in the exchange of air, a measure of the minute ventilatory volume tells only how much air is being moved in and out of the respiratory apparatus per minute. Much of this volume ventilates dead space and does not reach the alveoli. If the respiratory rate is multiplied by the estimated dead-space volume for the individual in question and the product subtracted from the minute ventilatory volume, the amount of alveolar ventilation can be estimated. For example, the alveolar ventilation in a man with 150 cc. dead space who breathes 15 times per minute and has a minute ventilatory volume of 7,500 cc. would be:

$$7,500 \text{ cc.} - 15 \times 150 \text{ cc.} = 5,250 \text{ cc.}$$

This is roughly estimated by the clinician when he assesses the depth of respiration as well as the rate.

The alveolar ventilation is not a measure of the adequacy of ventilation since it signifies only how much newly inspired air is exchanged with the air in the alveoli. The amount of alveolar ventilation needed will depend on the size of the individual and his level of activity. Nomograms have been made to permit estimation of the amount of alveolar ventilation needed at rest and with various degrees of fever for patients of differing body size. However, nomograms can hardly do more than crudely estimate these needs, since the amount of alveolar ventilation needed for any level of activity will also be affected by the efficiency of the respiratory apparatus.

If ventilation and perfusion are poorly coordinated, more alveolar ventilation will be required per unit of gas exchange. If the alveolar membrane is damaged, diffusion will require a larger pressure gradient for oxygen and hence more ventilation. If the mechanical efficiency of the lungs and chest wall is so damaged that more effort is needed to ventilate the lungs, more alveolar ventilation will be required to exchange the added oxygen burned and carbon dioxide produced by the less efficient respiratory machine.

The only accurate way of determining the adequacy of alveolar ventilation to the needs of the individual is by determining the level of the arterial blood pCO_2 and pO_2 or by deriving these values from allied blood determinations such as oxygen saturation, total carbon dioxide content, and pH. At sea level in the normal man the regulatory system of the respiratory center maintains the pO_2 at about 100 and the pCO_2 at 40 mm. Hg. If the values vary from these norms, the alveolar ventilation is inappropriate to the needs of the individual. Because of the shape of the oxygen dissociation curve and the possibility of altering the concentration by inhalation of oxygen, the level of the arterial blood pCO_2 is a better indicator of the adequacy of alveolar ventilation than is the pO_2.

If the lungs and chest wall are in good condition, derangements of blood-gas levels due to alveolar hypoventilation are the result of neuromuscular dysfunction. Deficiencies in ventilation which lead to inadequate alveolar ventilation are much more commonly the result of complex defects in the mechanics of the pump (the chest wall), the exchange organ (the lung), the perfusion apparatus (the cardiovascular system), or in the coordination of the complex. These derangements may diminish the amount of ventilation reaching the alveoli or may increase the amount of alveolar ventilation needed to supply the oxygen used and eliminate the carbon dioxide produced.

The assessment of the adequacy of the ventilatory reserve represents the most commonly used clinical pulmonary function test. The simplest such test is done with a spirometer. The subdivisions of the lung volumes and the vital capacity can be measured from the spirograph tracing (see Fig. 3-1). The most useful of these static measurements is the vital capacity.

In an adult male a total vital capacity of 1.5 to 2 liters represents a severe restriction. Such marked restriction usually is the result of pleural or chest wall disease, such as fibrothorax or kyphoscoliosis. On the other hand, a patient may have a reasonably normal vital capacity but severe functional disability due to mechanical derangements of the lung.

A decrease in vital capacity only identifies restriction of volume but does not evaluate the speed with which volume can be changed. For this reason it has been found to be more useful to determine the timed vital capacity. This measurement not only evaluates the total volume but also indicates the ability to move this volume in and out. Using a spirometer with a fast driven kymograph, a patient is taught to take in a maximum breath and to blow it out as fast and hard as possible. Normal young adults can expel 83% of the vital capacity in the first second, the lower limit of normal being 75%. This time increases with age so that at age 70 the mean value has fallen to 75% and the lower limit of normal to 65%. A person with timed vital capacity prolonged beyond these norms has some obstruction to expiration. An obstructive defect such as is seen in asthma may be reversed by bronchodilators. In obstructive emphysema the defect is irreversible. These mechanical derangements are usually far more debilitating than simple restrictive decreases in vital capacity.

A related test of ventilatory function is the maximum breathing capacity (MBC). The MBC test is conducted by instructing the patient to breathe in and out as fast and as deeply as he can to move as much air as possible over a 15-second period. A longer period is fatiguing and leads to severe hypocapnia and dizziness associated with hypocapnia. The MBC decreases with age just as the timed vital capacity does. The commonest formulas for determining "predicted" MBC are:

Males: [86.5 — (0.522 × age in years)] × body surface area (M.^{2})
Females: [71.3 — (0.474 × age in years)] × body surface area (M.^{2})

From the MBC and the minute ventilation the *breathing reserve* (the difference between the resting minute ventilation and the MBC) can be calculated.

It is impossible to set the precise level at which a limitation of ventilatory ability contraindicates surgery. The type of deficit, the proposed surgery, and the likelihood that surgery will further decrease ventilatory function must all be considered. A patient with an obstructive ventilating pattern will usually fare less well than a patient who has merely restriction. This is because a normal individual has a large breathing reserve which is called on only for the most vigorous exercise. If the remaining volume has normal function (see Chapter 4), considerable restriction can be tolerated. On the other hand, if the mechanics are deranged at all volumes, respiratory efficiency is decreased. To walk 60 yards on the level requires an MBC of 20 to 40 liters per minute. If a patient's MBC falls below 35 liters per minute, he will evidence severe dyspnea on exertion preoperatively; thoracotomy will be hazardous. Following pneumonectomy the permanent average decrease in MBC is 20%. However, in the immediate postoperative period thoracotomy alone reduces MBC by 50%, and it takes six weeks for the maximum recovery to occur.

Simple tests of ventilatory function differentiate the overly disabled from the near normal, but there is a large gray zone in which there are poor differentiations. It is in the borderline patients that as complete an understanding as possible of the total disturbance in pulmonary function is necessary to predict the outcome of a chosen therapeutic course.

4. MECHANICAL PROPERTIES OF THE RESPIRATORY SYSTEM

THERAPY of respiratory disease is largely mechanical in nature. The physician is most likely to find that the respiratory difficulties his patients suffer are mechanical in nature. The respiratory complications which follow surgery or trauma are usually the result of altered respiratory mechanics. Successful treatment depends on how successful one is in restoring mechanics toward normal.

Galen in A.D. 170, Leonardo da Vinci in 1543, and Borelli in 1680 explained that it was the weight of the atmosphere that pushed air into the lungs when the volume of the chest was increased by expansion of the thorax. This apparently simple fundamental concept, that air is pushed into the lungs when atmospheric pressure exceeds intrapulmonary pressure and is pushed out of the lungs when intrapulmonary pressure exceeds atmospheric pressure, is often lost when the term *negative pressure* is introduced with reference to intrapulmonary pressure. The pressures involved in respiration are never below zero but are only below ambient atmospheric pressure; there is always a positive pressure to push air in and out of the lungs.

While the basic principle underlying ventilation of the lungs seems straightforward, to ventilate and perfuse 300 million alveoli requires the development, operation, and maintenance of a complex machine. This machine develops in utero and continues to develop during early life, but simultaneously it also slowly deteriorates from its inception.

The principles underlying the operation of this machine are given in the Appendix. The engineering mechanics of the respiratory system involve flow into and out of a complex of tubes and air sacs, not a familiar field for fluid flow engineers. Because of its complexity, mechanical analysis may require the use of electrical analogs, the only practical way of completely describing the respiratory system. To date electrical analogs have been invaluable in much of the mechanical analysis of the lungs. Since the description of the system involves many terms not necessarily familiar to the reader, a summary of these follows.

F = force	R = resistance
P = pressure	M = mass
C = compliance	I = inertance
V = volume change	r = radius
$\dot{V}$ = flow rate	Z = impedance
$\ddot{V}$ = rate of change of flow	f = frequency

Anatomical sites are identified by subscripts in parentheses.

(pl) = pleura	(rc) = rib cage
(aw) = airway	(ab) = abdomen
(alv) = alveolus	(di) = diaphragm
(bs) = body surface	(cw) = chest wall (rc + ab + di)
(usually at	(l) = lung
atmospheric	(rs) = respiratory system (cw + l)
pressure)	

Subscripts outside parentheses represent the state of the system or the type of physical force.

st = static	el = elastic
app = applied	in = inertial
res = resistive	m = maximum

The equivalent values in an electric circuit are: pressure = voltage; compliance = capacitance; resistance = resistance; inertance = inductance; volume = charge; and flow = current.

THE PULMONARY MACHINE

Any machine must obey Newton's first law of motion that force applied to a body is met by an equal and opposite force. The lungs can be characterized as a reciprocating bellows pump in which the chest wall acts as the outer layer of the bellows, to which the energy source of the muscles is applied. Intimately applied to this outer layer of the bellows is the lung itself, which contains the chamber: the 300 million alveoli and their connecting ducts. The major portions of the connecting ducts are within the bellows chamber and so are subjected to pressure variations created by the bellows. The various parts of the machine, in this case the chest wall, lungs, and their contents, are the bodies on which a force is applied by the energy source, the muscles. The opposing forces are developed as a result of the motion started by the energy source. They are the forces related to position, velocity, and acceleration. In the pulmonary machine the opposing forces due to position are those due to the compressibility of air and to the elasticity or compliance of the lung and chest wall. The opposing force due to velocity is frictional resistance to air flow and tissue movement. The opposing force due to acceleration is the inertia of the chest wall and of the lungs and their contents.

These opposing forces can be represented, as shown in Figure 4-1, by a mass which is attached to a fixed wall by a spring and which can slide along a lubricated surface. The force necessary to stretch the spring is related to the compliance. The force to overcome the friction between the two lubricated surfaces is that opposed by resistance and is equal to the resistance times velocity. The force to provide the acceleration is opposed by the inertia and is equal to the mass times the rate of change of velocity.

A more accurate mechanical analog of the respiratory system is a bellows pump, as shown in Figure 4-2A and B, in which the force ap-

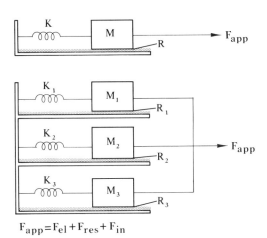

$$F_{app} = F_{el} + F_{res} + F_{in}$$

Fig. 4-1. Mechanical analogy of the respiratory system. (Top) Simple system: A mass, M, which can slide along the surface is restrained by an attached spring, K. The mass has inertia, the spring has elasticity (its reciprocal is compliance), and friction as the mass slides is equivalent to resistance, R.

(Bottom) A number of these systems are attached in parallel, just as the various components in the lung can be. The force that must be applied to set the system in motion, F_{app}, equals the sum of the force to stretch the spring, F_{el}, the force to overcome friction, F_{res}, and the force to overcome inertia, F_{in}.

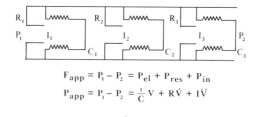

$$F_{app} = P_1 - P_2 = P_{el} + P_{res} + P_{in}$$

$$P_{app} = P_1 - P_2 = \frac{1}{C} V + R\dot{V} + I\ddot{V}$$

A

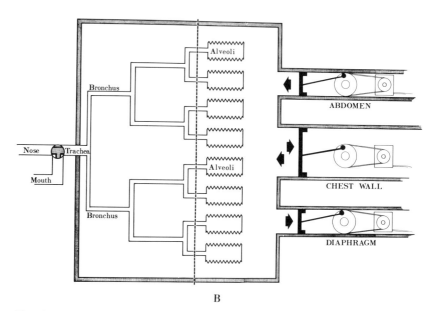

B

Fig. 4-2. (A) A volume-pressure analog of the respiratory system. In this instance force is measured as pressure applied, P_{app}, which is the difference in pressure across the system, $P_1 - P_2$. Each set of bellows represents a component of the respiratory system and has compliance, resistance, and inertance in it. The first component is the airway system, the second is lung tissue, and the third is the chest wall. The forces opposing the applied pressure can be expressed as in the first equation as P_{el}, pressure needed to stretch the bellows; P_{res}, pressure needed to overcome resistance; and P_{in}, pressure to overcome inertance. In the second equation these opposing forces are expressed as functions of volume change and the elastic, resistive, and inertial properties of the system. $P_{el} = 1/C \times V$. $C =$ compliance of the system; $V =$ volume change; $P_{res} = R$, resistance, times first derivative of volume or flow, $\dot{V}$; $P_{in} =$ the second derivative of volume, $\ddot{V}$, times inertia.

(B) A more complete mechanical analog of the respiratory system. Air can enter through the nose, which is the high-resistance orifice, or the mouth, which is the low-resistance orifice; it then progresses through multiple branches to the bellows, which are the alveoli. The many millions of alveoli cannot be drawn individually; the dashed line is to represent this incompleteness. The system is driven by the three piston pumps: the chest wall, which is bidirectional; the diaphragms, which are inspiratory only; and the abdominal muscles, which are expiratory only.

plied (F_{app}) is the pressure (P_{app}) across the bellows and the opposing forces are the compliance (P_{el}) related to the elastic recoil of the bellows, the resistance (P_{res}) related to the orifice of the opening, and the inertance (P_{in}) related to the mass of the bellows and air.

$$P_{app} = P_{el} + P_{res} + P_{in}$$

The bellows pump is a three-dimensional machine. Measures of change of motion must be changed from linear to three-dimensional terms: volume, flow, and rate of change of air flow. In terms of dimensions, they are liters, liters per second, and liters per second per second. The pressure applied in this second-order machine (see Appendix, p. 341) can be expressed algebraically:

$$P_{app} = \frac{1}{C} V + R\dot{V} + M\ddot{V}$$

In this equation C is constant for the compliance of the system, or the reciprocal of its elasticity, R is the constant for resistance, and M is the mass. V is volume change, $\dot{V}$ flow rate, and $\ddot{V}$ the rate of change of flow. The amount of motion of this machine is the result of the inter-action between the force applied by the energy sources, or the muscles, and the inherent compliance, resistance, and mass of the lungs and chest wall.

It is apparent that the rib cage and lungs are not simple machines with one compliant element, one resistive element, one inert element, and one energy source. In fact, the pulmonary machine is made of many resistance, compliance, and inertance components arranged in series and in parallel. Figure 4-2B roughly depicts this as a pressure-volume machine. In this bellows-pump diagram, the depiction is incomplete because it is hard to illustrate such items as the elasticity and inertia of the gas, the lung, and the chest wall. The symbolism used in an electronic diagram is more useful in depicting the pulmonary machine

THE ENERGY SOURCES

The energy sources, or motors, to drive the pulmonary machine and develop the forces or pressures to move it are the muscles of respiration. As pointed out in Chapter 1, there is still controversy about the exact function of individual groups of muscles. The external intercostal muscles, particularly those attached to the fifth through the ninth ribs, contract and lift the chest on inspiration. If the external intercostals are paralyzed,

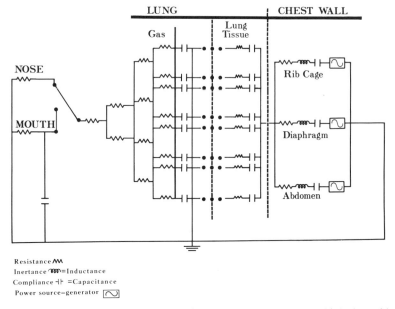

Resistance
Inertance =Inductance
Compliance =Capacitance
Power source—generator

Fig. 4-3. Electrical analog of the respiratory system. It is a multiple branching system, as shown in the mechanical analog, Figure 4-2B. Each bronchus has resistance and gas has compressibility, represented by the first set of capacitors as one follows the circuit from mouth toward lungs. The three dots depict the continued branching into millions of alveoli. The lung tissue has both resistance to motion and elasticity, represented by resistor and capacitor. No inductance is shown in the lung part of the circuit, because the inertance is so slight. The power source, or generators, come from the muscles of respiration, and all of these are attached to systems that have resistance, elasticity, and mass to give them some inertia.

exercise tolerance is only slightly affected; however, binding of the fifth to ninth ribs decreases maximum ventilation by 20 to 30%. The external intercostal muscles also act to stiffen the intercostal spaces so that they do not collapse during inspiration. The internal intercostals aid in pulling the rib cage down during expiration and also prevent bulging of the intercostal spaces. The intercostal muscles are most obviously designed to aid the motion of the chest wall, but they are only a small group among all the muscles active in ventilation.

All the muscle groups which fix the spine attach to the ribs posteriorly and have as part of their function the mechanical control of chest cage motion. They may move parts of the chest wall in or out, up or down, or fix in position a region of the chest cage to allow pivoting of the ribs or to prevent collapse when other muscles are brought into play.

In many of the analyses of the function of the muscles of respiration, the motion of the diaphragm and the role of the abdominal muscles have been separated from the other groups. The ease of assessing diaphragmatic motion has led to overemphasis on the importance of the diaphragm and belittling of the change in volume of the bony thorax exclusive of diaphragmatic motion. Recent work shows that 60 to 65% of the volume change in the chest is due to chest wall motion alone.

Contraction of the diaphragm, causing descent of the dome, acts like a piston. In addition to pulling the diaphragmatic dome down, the diaphragmatic contraction flares the lower rib cage out. In its descent the diaphragm pushes the abdominal contents down. The abdominal muscles diminish intraperitoneal volume as well as pull the rib cage down, thus opposing descent of the diaphragm; they are, for these reasons, muscles of expiration. Abdominal muscles take little part in respiration until ventilation gets up to higher levels, in the region of 40 liters per minute. Above this ventilatory rate they become increasingly active in aiding exhalation. During straining, coughing, and expulsive efforts, all of the muscles of the rib cage and abdomen are very active. The abdominal muscles are particularly important in forced exhalation. A horn player could not perform without abdominal muscles to aid in the expulsion of air. During expulsive efforts the maximal abdominal pressure can reach 400 cm. H_2O. Usually the diaphragm is fixed, preventing transmission of all of this pressure to the chest. Therefore the pleural pressure reaches only 200 cm. H_2O, and transdiaphragmatic pressure is 200 cm. H_2O.

Quiet inspiration and expiration are not an alternating contraction of inspiratory and expiratory muscles. Inspiration is the result of active contraction of the inspiratory muscles of the rib cage and diaphragm. During the early part of expiration the inspiratory muscles continue to contract, opposing the elastic recoil of the lungs and chest wall. In quiet expiration the expiratory muscles do not contract, and expulsion of air depends on the elastic recoil of the lungs and chest wall. The continued activity of the inspiratory muscles during expiration lets the system down gently, retarding the elastic recoil; as a result, expiration time is almost twice as long as inspiration time. As ventilation increases, the inspiratory muscles act for shorter and shorter periods during the expiratory phase and the expiratory muscles become increasingly active.

The force developed by the various respiratory muscles cannot be measured directly. The amount of force generated by the muscles which act to stretch or compress the lungs can be determined by measuring the intrapleural pressure. The level of pleural pressure is determined by the interaction of the forces acting on the lung and chest wall. Unless there are severe mechanical derangements of the chest wall or dense adhesions between the pleural surfaces, the pleural pressures in both hemithoraxes are nearly equal and uniform throughout. The hydrostatic pressure does cause pleural pressure in dependent areas to be slightly higher.

Intrapleural pressure can be measured either by direct needle puncture of the pleural cavity or from a well-functioning chest drainage tube. Gaining access to the pleural cavity in this manner is not without risk and discomfort. To avoid this risk, pleural pressure is usually measured from a catheter with a balloon on the end placed in the midesophagus. The intraesophageal pressure is used as a close approximation of pleural pressure. This is most valid as a means of measuring changes in pleural pressure, but the values obtained may be somewhat less negative than those of the true pleural pressure. The intraesophageal pressure recordings also have a superimposed pressure variation as a result of the myocardial pressure pulse.

The alterations in intrapleural pressure induced by muscle contraction lead to alterations in intraalveolar pressure. When no air is flowing, the difference between intraalveolar pressure and intrapleural pressure is that required to stretch the lung. At midposition the lung is stretched by a force of 5 cm. H_2O and, if the volume is unchanged, will remain 5 cm. H_2O.

With the airway obstructed so that no flow is possible and so that the volume cannot change except by gas compression, a well-trained man for short periods can, by maximum contraction of the inspiratory muscles, create a negative intraalveolar pressure of 100 to 140 cm. H_2O (Müller maneuver) and can, by a maximum contraction of the expiratory muscles, create a positive pressure of 160 to 190 cm. H_2O (Valsalva maneuver). In women and children somewhat lower pressures can be generated, such as -85 cm. H_2O on inspiration and $+110$ cm. H_2O on expiration.

If air is flowing into or out of the lungs, the maximum range of pressure change is smaller. The pressure maximums depend on the rate of shortening and strength of the respiratory muscles, the size of the chest, and the resistance and compliance of both the lungs and chest wall. In healthy males at maximum rates of inspiratory and expiratory flow, the pleural pressure range is not greater than 35 cm. H_2O in each direction.

Since the effects of contraction of respiratory muscles on change in volume and pressure in the system are a function of the resistances and compliances of the system and their interactions, it would be helpful to study the elastic and resistive properties separately and then in combination.

THE ELASTIC COMPONENTS OF THE PUMP

The bellows pump can be studied under two different circumstances: (1) the dynamic state, in which the pressure across the system is oscillating and will cause air to flow in and out of the circuit; and (2) the static state, in which a given steady pressure is applied until the flow stops. The dynamic state is the normal operating mode of the pulmonary machine. To make any analysis of the forces required and the inherent physical characteristics of the pulmonary machine, measuring devices must be applied to the system. The actual pressure driving air into and out of the system is the difference between the alveolar and the atmospheric pressure $(P_{(bs)} - P_{(alv)})$. Since there is no direct way of measuring pressure in the alveoli, the driving force cannot be measured directly. In practice, the system must be analyzed from measurements of intrapleural pressure and pressures at accessible sites within the main air passages (Fig. 4-4). It is helpful to measure changes in volume and pressure in the machine when a steady rather than an oscillating force or pressure is

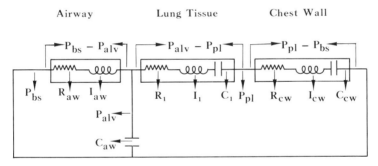

Resistance ᴧᴧ
Inertance ℓℓ = Inductance
Compliance ⊣⊢ = Capacitance

Fig. 4-4. Pressures in the respiratory system. This is a simplified electrical analog of the respiratory system in which the myriads of individual components are added so that each major area is represented as having one resistance, one compliance, and one inertance. Various pressures at different sites in the system are noted. For example, the pressure in the airways is the difference between alveolar pressure, P_{alv}, and pressure at the body surface, P_{bs}. The pressure across the lung tissue is the difference between alveolar (P_{alv}) and pleural pressure (P_{pl}) and P_{pl} minus P_{bs} equals pressure across the chest wall. Each subdivision has a compliance, resistance, and inertance. C_{aw} represents the compressibility of air and thus is represented as connected to ground since its degree depends on the difference between atmospheric and airway pressure. As noted in the text, the inertance can be ignored, since it is so small.

applied, because this permits recoil or elastic characteristics of the system to be separated from resistive and inertial components.

In the static condition, when the system has stopped moving, the system is left with an increased or decreased volume, depending on whether the pressure applied is above or below atmospheric pressure. When this system is at rest, the pressure in the alveolar space will be the same as that at the mouth ($P_{(aw)} = P_{(alv)}$). In fact, a valve must be turned so no air can enter or leave through the nose or mouth. At times of no flow, the air pressure throughout the tracheobronchial tree is uniform and resistance and inertance will have no effect on the system. Since pressure in the alveoli is the same as in the upper airways, pressure measured at the entrance to the airways gives the value for alveolar pressure. Since resistance and inertance have no effect at rest, pressure across the system is the result of elastic forces. The static pressure difference between the alveoli and the atmosphere will be the result of the elastic recoil of the entire pulmonary mechanism at that given volume. The difference between the pleural pressure and atmospheric pressure is that due to elastic recoil of the chest wall.

$$P_{(bs)} - P_{st(pl)} = P_{st(w)}$$

The difference between the airway pressure and the pleural pressure is that due to the elastic recoil of the lung.

$$P_{st(aw)} - P_{st(pl)} = P_{st(l)}$$

The pressure necessary to stretch the system and its parts to various volumes can be determined if airway pressure and pleural pressure are measured when no flow is occurring, as the system is inflated or deflated in a stepwise fashion. The pressure-volume relationship is nearly a straight line except at the extremes of the total lung capacity. The elasticity of a spring is measured by determining the force required to stretch it a given length and is expressed in grams per centimeter. In a pressure-volume system the elasticity or stiffness is measured as the added pressure required per unit increase in volume (centimeters of water pressure per liter). Physiologists have preferred to use the expression of pliability, or compliance, which is the reciprocal of stiffness. This is measured as the added volume required for a given increase in stretching pressure (liters per centimeter of water pressure).

The combined compliance of the chest wall and its cage is less than each part. Since the compliance is the reciprocal of stiffness, if the stiffness of the chest wall is added to that of the lungs, the combined stiffness will be greater and the compliance less. In other words, it takes more pressure to stretch the lungs and chest wall to a given volume than it does to stretch just the lungs or just the chest wall to the same volume. Expressed in mathematical terminology, compliance units connected in series are added as their reciprocal, so their sum is less than the smallest compliance (p. 347).

If two elastic units are connected in parallel rather than in series, the compliance of the parallel combination is the sum of the compliance of each element. The two lungs are connected in parallel, and each subsequent generation of branching represents increasing numbers of subdivisions of the lung connected in parallel. Therefore, if the upper and lower lobes are equally compliant, both lobes will have twice the compliance of one lobe, and if both lungs are equally compliant, they will have four times the compliance of one lobe (Fig. 4-5).

To measure the compliance of the respiratory system is more difficult than to describe the theoretical basis of such measurement. The elastic forces of the chest wall and lungs are in equilibrium at functional residual capacity. If the airways are completely opened and the muscles of the chest wall relaxed, the system will contain a volume equal to the functional residual capacity. In other words, at end-expiration the system is at rest.

To hold the lungs at a static volume other than functional residual capacity requires continued muscular effort, just as holding an unsupported arm in the outstretched position requires continued effort. The effort expended to support the arm in the outstretched position or the chest at other than the functional residual volume does no physical work since there is no motion. This does not mean that it requires no energy expenditure and does not lead to fatigue. If the outstretched arm is supported on a scale and the muscle relaxed, the weight registered will measure the force that was needed to support the arm in this outstretched position. If air is inspired or expired and then the airway blocked, the new volume will be trapped in the lungs. If the muscular effort is relaxed, the pressure in the blocked airways will measure the force necessary to maintain the system in the new position. The chest cage and lungs are, in effect, leaning on the airway obstruction, just as the arm leans on the scale. At this time of no flow, the pressure in the airway is uniform from alveolus to mouth, and only the force necessary to support the whole system at this new volume is measured. The pressure difference between the pleural space and the atmosphere is that necessary to stretch the chest wall, and the difference between the pleural and alveolar pressure is that necessary to stretch the lung.

$$P_{st(alv)} - P_{st(bs)} = P_{st(rs)}$$

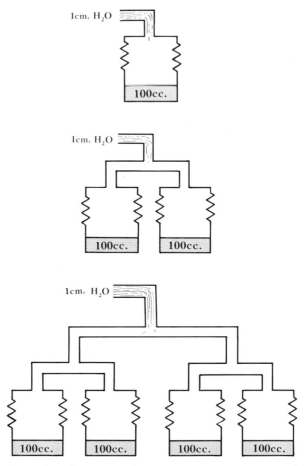

Fig. 4-5. Change in volume per unit change in pressure as increasing numbers of compliant units are connected in parallel. One centimeter of water pressure will increase the volume of a single unit 100 cc. If two such units are connected in parallel, each will increase its volume 100 cc. when 1 cm. is put across them, or a total increase of 200 cc. for the two together. If four are connected in parallel, the combination will accept 400 cc. from a forcing pressure of 1 cm. H_2O.

It is possible to determine the pressure necessary to expand the chest wall and lungs to different volumes throughout the vital capacity range. This can be done by measuring pressure in the subject's airway following inhalation of each of several increments of air while the subject's airway is obstructed and his muscular effort relaxed. The pressure in the airway will depend on the elastic recoil of the lungs and chest wall if relaxation is complete.

$$P_{st(aw)} - P_{(bs)} = P_{st(rs)} = P_{st(l)} + P_{st(cw)}$$

For the airway pressure to be equal to the pressure necessary to stretch the lungs and chest wall, no other force can be applied to the system. If some of the respiratory muscles are actively contracting, i.e., if the subject fails to relax completely, this force, expressed in pressure terms, must be added to or subtracted from the transthoracic pressure ($P_{st(aw)} - P_{(bs)}$), depending on whether it opposes the elastic recoil or acts to increase it. Unfortunately, since there is no practical way of measuring the force exerted by a respiratory muscle, there is no way of being sure that voluntary relaxation is complete and that true compliance is being measured. In a subject paralyzed with a muscle relaxant, the pressure necessary to hold the system at various volumes above residual volume can be measured, and the equilibrium is between the pressure applied by the equipment (equal to the airway pressure) and the recoil of the respiratory system. This pressure can be applied by raising the airway pressure above ambient barometric pressure, or, as in a Drinker respirator, by lowering the pressure at the body surface below the atmospheric pressure.

If the pressure necessary to maintain the lungs and chest wall at a given volume is plotted against the volume, the elasticity or compliance of the system over any given range can be determined. If the respiratory system becomes stiffer and requires more pressure to stretch it to a given size, the compliance will be less and the elastic recoil increased.

By measuring the difference between the pressure in the airway and the pressure in the pleura, one can determine the pressure needed to stretch the lung alone.

$$P_{st(aw)} - P_{st(pl)} = P_{st(l)}$$

The difference between the intrapleural pressure and the pressure at the body surface equals the pressure needed to stretch the chest wall alone.

$$P_{st(pl)} - P_{st(bs)} = P_{st(cw)}$$

Unless a patient is in a Drinker type of respirator, the pressure across the chest wall is equal to the absolute pleural pressure minus the barometric pressure, since all pressures are referred to atmospheric pressure.

$$P_{st(cw)} = P_{st(pl)}$$

During complete relaxation with airway wide open, the airway pressure equals the barometric pressure.

$$P_{st(aw)} = P_{st(bs)}$$

Since the difference between the mouth and pleural pressures is equivalent to the force stretching the lung when no air is flowing, the pressure difference between the mouth and chest wall equals the pressure necessary to stretch the lung. Since at end-expiration and end-inspiration there is no motion of the chest wall, the difference between the end-inspiratory and end-expiratory pleural pressures is the pressure needed to stretch the lung an amount equal to the tidal volume. This assumes equilibrium between mouth and airway pressures during the brief period of no flow between inspiration and expiration. Values for lung compliance measured in this manner do not agree with and are lower than compliance measured by step-and-pause inflations. This is probably because air continues to flow from areas of high pressure to areas of lower pressure as air redistributes itself among various alveoli. For this reason compliance measured in this manner has the contradictory name of "dynamic compliance." Some of the factors leading to these differences between "static" and "dynamic" lung compliance depend on the unique factors in the lung which determine its elasticity.

LUNG COMPLIANCE

The forces which lead to recoil of the lung and thus determine its compliance are complex and result from the tissue elements, the geometry of the air spaces, and the air–fluid interface in the alveoli. If the lungs are expanded in a stepwise fashion from the end-expiratory volume to maximum inflation and then allowed to deflate, the mean alveolar pressure at any given volume during inspiration will be higher than during expiration. Figure 4-6 shows a plot of pressure at moments of no flow as the volume is increased to maximum volume and then decreased to minimum volume. Less pressure is required during deflation to maintain the lung at a given volume.

If the lungs are inflated with a liquid such as plasma rather than with a gas, the amount of pressure needed to inflate the lungs to any given volume is less and there is no difference between the inflation and deflation pressure curves (see Fig. 4-6). When the lungs are inflated with liquid, they appear to obey Hooke's law for elastic bodies. For each unit of force applied, in this case for each centimeter of water pressure, a given volume expansion results until the elastic limit of the body is reached at which point the body will be deformed permanently or broken if further pressure is applied. The elements in the lung which are the major contributors to this tissue elasticity are the elastic and collagen fibers. These are arranged in a complex geometric pattern which might be likened to a knitted sweater made in three rather than two dimensions. Some of the elasticity is due to the geometry of the knit as well as

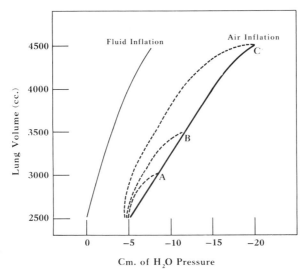

Fig. 4-6. Compliance curves of the lung. When the lungs are inflated with fluid rather than air, less pressure is required per unit of volume because there are no opposing surface forces when the air–fluid interface is absent. With air inflation it takes more pressure to inflate the lungs (*solid line*) than to deflate them (*dotted lines*). This difference is greater following maximum inflation volume, *C,* than with lesser inflations, volumes *A* and *B.*

to the recoil qualities of the fibers. Disruption of the continuity or arrangement of these fibers will result in loss of elastic recoil of the lung. Contraction of smooth muscle plays a role in altering the alveolar and smaller airway geometry, but this does not alter the pressure required to stretch the lungs with liquid. This means that smooth muscle tone has very little effect on the elastic recoil of the structural elements of the lung.

The Effect of Lung Surfactant on Compliance.   It is apparent from Figure 4-6 that the pressure required to stretch fluid-filled lungs to any given volume is less than one-half that required to stretch air-filled lungs to the same volume. This difference is the result of the surface tension at the air–fluid interface on the surfaces of the alveoli. The number of molecules in any given volume of gas is less than in a corresponding volume of water. This results in the gas molecules being farther apart than the molecules in the fluid medium. The attractive force between two molecules is a function of the mass divided by the square of the distance. At the surface of the liquid the attractive force on the molecules is greater on the liquid side than it is on the gas side. This greater force in the liquid pulls the molecules back into the liquid and shrinks the liquid surface to the smallest area that can be achieved by this attractive force.

The surface tension of a given liquid can be measured if a thin film of fluid is placed in a trough and a force applied to a crossbar which, as it is pulled, increases the surface area. For any given liquid, the further the bar is moved, the greater the force that will be necessary. This gives the dimension of surface tension, which is force per unit of length or dyne per centimeter. Water at 37°C. has a surface tension of 70 dynes per centimeter, and plasma and other body fluids, 50 dynes per centimeter. The surface tension of the alveoli is not the same as plasma, as the measured surface tension at the alveolar surface is less than 50 dynes per centimeter. Some other fluid must be on the pleural surface or the surface tension is being altered. The special nature of the surface tension of the alveoli can explain this discrepancy.

The alveoli are nearly spherical in shape, and so the effect of surface tension on alveolar pressure can best be explained by reviewing the physics of bubbles. In a bubble lined with water, which has a fixed surface tension, the size of the bubble will depend on the hydrostatic pressure of the gas in the bubble which is pushing against the confining force of surface tension. The amount of tension in the wall of a tube or sphere necessary to contain a given pressure is defined by Laplace's law (p. 335). For spheres, the equation is:

$$p = \frac{2\gamma}{r}$$

where γ = surface tension
  p = pressure
  r = radius of the sphere (see Fig. 4-10)

This equation states that as the radius decreases, the pressure in the bubble will rise. This means that the intraalveolar pressure in a small alveolus would be greater than the intraalveolar pressure in a large alveolus.

The alveoli are intimately interconnected and so would have to all be the same size or the higher pressure in the smaller alveoli would push air out of them into the larger ones. This would result in all small alveoli collapsing and all large alveoli overexpanding. All alveoli are not the same size, so there must be some property which prevents the small alveoli from emptying into the large ones. Studies of the recoil force of the lungs have led to the answer to this enigma. From the anatomical estimates of the size of the alveolar "bubbles" and the total number of such bubbles, the recoil force of the lung due to surface tension can be calculated. Assuming that the surface tension of the alveolar fluid is the same as that of plasma (50 dynes per centimeter), the calculated recoil force of surface tension is 20,000 dynes per square centimeter. Since 980 dynes are equivalent to 1 cm. H_2O pressure, the recoil force would be equal to $+20$ cm. H_2O.

This calculated value is five to ten times higher than that found at resting lung volumes but is very nearly that found when the lungs are fully inflated. These discrepancies led to the postulate that the surface tension of the alveolar lining fluid must be altered by a surface-active agent, a *surfactant*. A surfactant is a substance like detergents in soap, which act at the surface of a liquid to alter the attraction between molecules at the gas–liquid interface. Due to the nature of their molecular structure, surfactant molecules exert a smaller attractive force on liquid molecules than liquid molecules do on one another, and, since they are less strongly attracted by the liquid molecules, the surfactant molecules tend to accumulate at the surface. The diminished attraction between molecules at the surface due to the effect of the surfactant lowers the surface tension.

An ordinary surfactant such as a detergent would lower the surface tension of the fluid independently of the size of the bubble. This is not the case with pulmonary surfactant. At low alveolar volumes the surfactant depresses surface tension more than at high alveolar volumes. An oversimplified explanation for this effect is that there is more surfactant per unit of surface area when the bubble is small than when it is large. In the lungs the effect of surfactant is to keep the intraalveolar pressure uniform despite changes in the radius of alveoli.

The action of surfactant can then be summarized by saying that alveolar surface tension falls with a decrease in alveolar radius, so that alveolar pressure is nearly uniform regardless of size (Fig. 4-7). Thus, the surfactant stabilizes the lung so that small alveoli do not dump their air into large alveoli. At small lung volumes the surfactant is the most active; while at maximum inflation the effect of surfactant is minimal and the recoil due to surface forces is nearly equal to that of plasma.

The exact nature of pulmonary surfactant is not yet determined. Dipalmityl lecithin, which has been extracted from lungs, has many of the properties of lung surfactant. It is most likely that lung surfactant is a complex protein molecule with dipalmityl lecithin as its active prosthetic group. The present theory is that this substance is manufactured by the alveolar lining cells.

Surfactant is in an unstable equilibrium in the lung. It has been shown that if the surfactant film is kept at a constant area, i.e., in an alveolus of

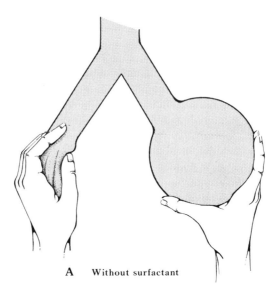

A Without surfactant

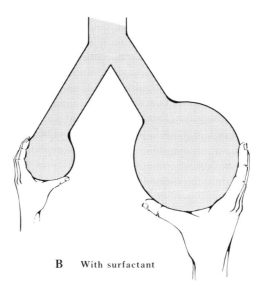

B With surfactant

Fig. 4-7. Surfactant effect. The Laplace formula states that for a substance with any given surface tension, as the radius of a bubble decreases, the pressure within the bubble will increase. Here the surface tension is represented by the size and strength of the right and left hands. If the hands are equal in strength, the left hand can squeeze the small sphere more effectively than the right can squeeze the large sphere. The left hand will squeeze all the air out of its sphere.

In (B) the hands are made proportional to the size of the bubbles. The smaller bubble has a smaller hand, so that the force exerted on the small bubble remains the same as the force on the large bubble. This is the role of surfactant, to decrease the surface tension as the bubble decreases in size, so that the small alveoli have a pressure in them no greater than that in the large alveoli.

nearly constant volume, the surface tension rises spontaneously from 10 to 15 dynes per centimeter to 30 dynes per centimeter. This is due to surfactant being desorbed or removed from the surface. As a result of this desorption, a greater force and thus a greater transpulmonary pressure is needed. If the transpulmonary pressure is maintained constant, the inactivation of surfactant would lead to eventual collapse of some alveolar units. Thus, a constant tidal volume will result in decrease in compliance and slow collapse of the lung. A single large inspiration, as in a yawn, will restore compliance to normal, and if these occur every ten minutes, compliance will remain normal. This is due to the fact that the yawn or deep breath, which requires a greater transpulmonary pressure, gives a force which exceeds the point at which the alveolar surface free energy is minimal; therefore, it recruits new surfactant material to line the alveolar surface and restore full surfactant effect.

This phenomenon explains the "hysteresis" of the lung (see Fig. 4-6). If the lung is maximally expanded, more surfactant is recruited to the surface and, during deflation, less pressure is needed. Normal quiet breathing is interrupted by deep breaths and yawns at intervals of two to ten minutes, and these apparently serve the useful purpose of regenerating the activity of the surfactant. When a patient is under anesthesia, unconscious, or being artificially ventilated, such spontaneous deep breaths cannot occur. This will result in a progressively smaller portion of the lungs being ventilated.

The loss of surfactant effect not only closes alveoli but also leads to transudation of fluid into the alveoli. Surfactant effect in diminishing the compressing force on the air bubble in the alveoli also lowers the sucking force on the pulmonary capillary. If surfactant is lost from the surface for any reason, the critical balance of pressures across the alveolar capillaries will be upset; fluid will escape into the alveoli and line the alveolar wall to cause a so-called hyaline membrane (see pp. 117–122).

It is apparent that artificial ventilation of the lungs at constant pressure, which leads to desorption of the surfactant, will result in progressive fall in compliance, collapse of alveolar units, and transudation of fluid into the alveoli. If occasional deep breaths are included in the cycle, this disastrous sequence can be prevented. The resorption of surfactant is also less likely to occur if artificial ventilation is carried out at constant volume rather than constant pressure; since, as surfactant is resorbed, more pressure is generated by the respirator to maintain the set volume and to set a limit on resorption. It is important to insure that anesthetized patients and patients being ventilated with a respirator have periodic hyperinflation.

A number of conditions can apparently result in loss of surfactant effect. It is not clear in all of these whether surfactant is absent from the lung or whether it may for some reason be desorbed from the surface. Critical experiments have not been designed to determine which is the case. Surfactant effect is altered with occlusion of the pulmonary circulation, 100% oxygen breathing for prolonged periods, occlusion of a major bronchus, and in the respiratory distress syndrome of newborns. Surfactant effect also may be altered following prolonged cardiopulmonary bypass, particularly if ventilation and perfusion of the lung has been interrupted during the time of bypass. In all of these conditions increased stiffness and progressive collapse of the lung will occur.

Surfactant, in addition to stabilizing the alveoli and preventing transudation of fluid, also lowers the force which must be exerted by the respiratory muscles to expand the lungs. If the tension in a normal alveolus is 5 to 7 dynes and the radius is 50 to 70 μ, it will take only 2 cm. H_2O to expand the alveolus. If surfactant is absent and effusion has partially filled the alveolus, decreasing its radius to 25 to 30 μ, the needed pressure may rise to 20 cm. H_2O, a tenfold increase in required transpulmonary pressure.

If an alveolus is completely collapsed, it takes a greater force to reopen it than it does to maintain an opened alveolus (Fig. 4-8). For example, if the pressures needed to reexpand a collapsed lung during thoracotomy are recorded, it will be found that they markedly exceed those used to ventilate the already aerated portions of the lungs. The greater pressure required to reaerate a collapsed alveolus is due to the geometry of the original bubble. A bubble must be started at the end of the tube, and, at the start, the radius of curvature is very large, so little pressure is needed; however, the radius rapidly decreases to the size of its duct. To further expand this minute bubble requires much greater pressure because of the increased surface tension of the small bubble and the relative ineffectiveness of surfactant as a result of its desorption from the surface. As the bubble enlarges, the increments of pressure required decrease. Thus, there is an opening pressure required to start reaeration of a collapsed alveolus which is considerably above normal intraalveolar pressures.

The Effect of Lung Structure on Compliance. In some diseases compliance is reduced due to fibrosis of interstitial areas of the lung leading to increased stiffness. In emphysema the opposite is true; the elastic and collagenous three-dimensional knit is disrupted, and the recoil force of the lung is thereby reduced. Blood volume and the amount of interstitial fluid can also affect lung stiffness. If the pulmonary blood volume is increased, the distended vessels are harder to distort and the lung

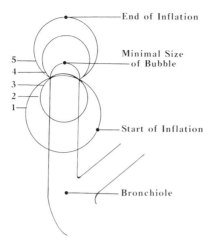

Fig. 4-8. Alveolar opening pressure. When an alveolus is completely collapsed, an increased pressure is required to reopen it. As the bubble at the air–surface interface starts to form (circle *1*), the radius is very large, so the tension of the wall is low. As the bubble continues to form, the radius gets progressively less (circle *2*), until it reaches a minimum of the size of a bronchiole (*3*). At this point the radius is very small and surface tension very high, requiring a large pressure to further increase alveolar volume. As the alveolus continues to expand, the radius of the bubble increases rapidly, and pressure necessary to expand it falls. Surfactant is not very effective in reducing surface tension in a collapsed alveolus, because it is resorbed from the surface.

becomes stiffer. This is particularly true if pulmonary venous pressure is elevated in association with increased blood volume. In mitral stenosis, in which blood volume, venous pressure, and interstitial fluid are all increased, the lung compliance is significantly decreased and more force is required to stretch the lung.

Other factors which can change the compliance of the lung are more clearly directly related to anatomical alterations. If a bronchus is occluded or a portion of lung removed, there will be a smaller number of alveolar units to be stretched. Since the force necessary to stretch each unit a given amount is nearly uniform, if there are fewer units, those present will have to be stretched further to accept the same volume (see Fig. 4-5). A patient with atelectasis or a patient who has had a pulmonary resection will require a greater than normal force to expand the intact lung, and thus more work will be required for a given ventilatory volume. It follows that the compliance of infants' and children's lungs should be less than that of adults, since there are fewer and smaller units present.

The actual volume of the lungs when the person is relaxed is determined not only by the compliance of the lungs. Since the chest wall has elastic recoil, just as the lungs do, the resting volume of each is determined by the net effect of the elastic recoil of the chest wall and the elastic recoil of the lung acting on one another.

THE COMPLIANCE OF THE CHEST CAGE

A number of elements determine the elastic recoil, or its reciprocal, the compliance, of the chest cage. These include the diameter and shape of the chest, the height of the individual, the mass of the musculature, the amount of body fat, the amount of abdominal fluid, and the integrity of the skeletal and muscular systems. Since the force to expand the rib cage of the chest comes from the respiratory muscles, it cannot be measured during spontaneous breathing. The force required can be measured only by determining pleural pressure during voluntary relaxation with the airway blocked or during artificial ventilation.

The Mass of the Chest Wall and Gravity. In individuals with heavy musculature, the increased mass of the respiratory and accessory respiratory muscles will lead to increased stiffness of the relaxed chest wall. A greater intrapleural and thus intraalveolar pressure would be needed to force air into such an individual during artificial ventilation, and greater muscle force may be needed during spontaneous breathing. The force to expand the chest is increased in an individual with a large, heavy, bony framework of the chest due to the increased mass of the bone. A woman with large breasts supported on the chest cage must lift their weight with respiration and so must exert more force. Likewise, an obese person needs to generate force to lift the added weight of fat with each respiration. Since these added burdens on the chest wall are hung on different portions of the chest, the effect of gravity on these masses is different in different postures (Fig. 4-9). The result is a difference in the force or pressure required to stretch the respiratory system in different postures as well as habitus.

Gravity effects were ignored in the discussion of lung compliance. The lungs are very light in weight, so the force necessary to stretch the lungs alone is not significantly altered with change in posture. However, the forces acting on the chest wall change with posture. Change in force on the chest wall stretches or compresses it, thus altering the pleural pressure and changing the stretch or compression force on the lung. The functional residual capacity or end-expiratory relaxed volume changes to return the system to equilibrium.

The difference in force of gravity on the rib cage can be measured by determining the static pressure in the pleura, $P_{st(pl)}$, at various lung volumes in various postures. The static pressure of the chest wall is maintained by the rib cage acting in parallel with the abdomen and the diaphragm. Since these elements are acting in parallel, the pressure across the rib cage must be equal to that contributed by the abdomen and the diaphragm.

$$P_{st(rc)} = P_{st(ab)} + P_{st(di)}$$

With change in posture the principal gravitational effect is that due to the weight of the fluid-filled abdomen. This acts like a bag of water in a partially distensible container; it pulls down on the diaphragm and rib cage in the upright posture and pushes them up in the supine position. The gravitational pull or push of this bag of fluid is counteracted by the elastic forces of the abdominal wall, the diaphragm, the rib cage, and the lungs.

In the erect posture at the resting volume (functional residual volume), the abdominal contents pull down on the diaphragm and rib cage with a force of 5 cm. H_2O and the rib cage pulls out with a force of 5 cm. H_2O. The resting volume is 55% of total lung capacity, and the residual volume is 20% of total lung capacity. At maximum expiration the pressure across the *relaxed* chest wall is +40 cm. H_2O, and at maximum inspiration the pressure across the relaxed chest wall is −40 cm. H_2O.

In the supine position at the relaxation volume, the pressure across the chest wall, $P_{st(cw)}$, is −1.5 cm. H_2O. The rib cage has moved outward and so pulls out with a force of only 1.5 cm. H_2O rather than 5 cm. The fluid in the abdomen pushes up with a pressure of 7 cm. H_2O, but this is counteracted by the diaphragm, which is stretched in this position and exerts a counterforce equal to 3.5 cm. H_2O. The abdominal wall is stretched by the fluid pressure and absorbs up to 2 cm. of the 7 cm. H_2O pressure. The resultant pressure across the chest wall drops, lowering the pressure acting to expand the lung, and the lung volume decreases. In the supine position, the relaxing volume is only 40% of total lung capacity and residual volume remains 20% of lung capacity. At maximum expiration the pressure across the relaxed chest wall, $P_{st(cw)}$, is +25 cm. H_2O and remains −40 cm. at maximum inspiration.

In the head-down position, the effects seen in the supine posture are exaggerated if the weight is supported on the shoulders. In the head-down position, if the weight is supported by the feet, the weight of the shoulder girdle pulling the chest outward begins to override the weight of the abdominal contents, and it acts to reexpand the chest. As one moves from the erect to the sitting posture, the abdominal contents are more supported and the relaxation position moves toward a lower lung volume. In the kneeling position the abdominal contents pull down on the dia-

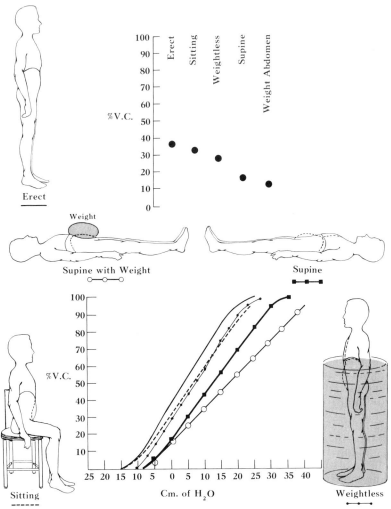

Fig. 4-9. The effect of position on total chest compliance and expiratory reserve volume. In the figures assuming different positions the dotted lines represent the position of the diaphragm, abdomen, and chest wall in the erect posture. The difference is the result of change of position. The values for change in expiratory reserve and total chest compliance were taken from a study of thirty individuals in our laboratories. The expiratory reserve volume is 40% of vital capacity in the erect position, in which there is the maximum effect of gravity pulling down on the diaphragms. Sitting supports some of this weight and diminishes expiratory reserve volume; supporting the trunk by submersion in water to the costal margin neutralizes the pull of the weight of the abdominal viscera (weightlessness). In the supine position and when a weight is added to the abdomen, the mass of the abdominal contents and weight push the diaphragms up, further reducing reserve capacity. With this low expiratory reserve capacity, some areas of lung may be hypoventilated.

In the bottom graph the changes in total chest compliance are plotted. The phragm and have an effect similar to that found in the erect posture. In the prone position the abdomen is supported and exerts less upward force on the diaphragm than it does in the supine position. In the weightless state, which can be simulated by immersion in water up to the top of the abdomen to minimize the gravitational effect on the abdomen, the conditions are between those in the upright and supine postures.

Height plays a significant role in the effect of gravity on the respiratory system. A tall individual will have a longer than average column of fluid pulling on the diaphragm and stretching the abdomen in the upright posture. For this reason tall individuals have a larger than average functional residual capacity in the upright posture but have no difference in the functional residual capacity in the supine position.

The Clinical Significance of Gravitational Effects.   The reduction in the functional residual volume in the supine posture enhances the likelihood of there being significant areas of the lung that will not be ventilated and that therefore will likely become atelectatic. Spasm of the abdominal muscles due to pain will prevent the dissipation into the elastic elements of the abdominal wall of any portion of the hydrostatic pressure generated by the weight of the abdominal contents. If none of the weight of the abdominal contents is absorbed by the elastic elements of the abdominal wall, all of the hydrostatic pressure will push up on the diaphragm. This will further reduce the functional residual capacity and increase the likelihood of underventilation of portions of the lung. One of the important reasons for promptly getting patients out of bed postoperatively is to counteract the combined effect of gravity and muscle spasm due to pain in reducing pulmonary aeration.

In the erect position, ascites acts to increase the force pulling down on the diaphragm and rib cage and increases the functional residual capacity. When the ascitic fluid distends the abdomen, thereby stretching the abdominal wall, the recoil of the stretched abdominal wall counteracts the added weight. In the supine posture, the weight of the ascitic fluid and the elastic recoil of the stretched abdomen act together to markedly elevate the diaphragm. Tilting the head down exaggerates this effect.

---

compliance decreases when an individual moves from the erect to sitting, supine, etc., just as the reserve volume does. In the weightless state the system is as compliant as in the erect position, and with weight on the abdomen the loss in compliance is proportionately much larger than the change in expiratory reserve volume. The fall in compliance and expiratory reserve volume in the supine position and with weight on the abdomen is one of the causes of intrapulmonary shunts in bedridden or obese patients and in those with abdominal distention.

Each inspiratory effort requires the lifting of this mass of fluid in the supine or head-down posture. In the upright posture during inspiration, the chest wall must oppose the force of the weight of fluid pulling down while the diaphragms are aided by this downward force. During expiration the chest wall is pulled down, but the abdominal muscles must support the fluid.

An obese individual has a mechanical situation qualitatively similar to ascites. In the upright posture, fat pulls down on chest wall and abdomen and must be lifted for all inspiratory efforts. If the intraabdominal fat is enough to stretch the abdomen, it will act like ascitic fluid. Each inspiratory effort requires the lifting of this weight, which then compresses the chest during expiration. It may be that partial submersion of the patient with ascites or marked obesity might lessen the work required to support the added weight of fat or fluid. (The whale, for instance, is aided during inspiration by its blubber, which is floated out by the buoyancy of the sea as air goes in.) In any case, the respiratory failure seen in markedly obese individuals or in those with massive ascites is the result of the reduction in lung volume, due to compression of the lung by the abdominal fat or fluid, and the increased force required of the respiratory muscles to lift the added weight hanging on the chest wall and abdomen. There is a definite mechanical advantage for these people in the upright or sitting posture, since the compression is less, even though the weight still must be lifted.

The Shape and Composition of the Chest Wall. In addition to the increase in weight and size in a large, heavy-boned, or muscular chest, such a chest is probably less elastic. This must be a surmise, because the muscular forces may be so applied as to stretch the muscular chest with ease. Anything which inhibits the motion of the chest wall, such as Marie-Strümpell arthritis, scarring of the chest wall after thoracotomy, or thoracoplasty, will increase the stiffness of the chest wall. If pain causes spasm of the muscles over an area of the chest and prevents its motion, compliance will be decreased by cutting down the number of parallel areas of chest wall that can be stretched.

In patients with chest deformities, such as pectus excavatum, pectus carinatum, or scoliosis, the mechanical properties of the chest wall may be seriously compromised. In these deformed patients, a decrease in chest wall compliance as measured by passive stretching may seriously underestimate the compromise of mechanical function of the chest wall. More serious than the decrease in compliance may be mechanical inefficiency of the respiratory muscles due to the altered geometry of the chest. If the functional mechanics of the chest wall could be more effectively measured, we might understand far more about the effect of scoliosis and congenital chest deformities on pulmonary function.

THE EFFECT OF AGE ON COMPLIANCE

Since size affects compliance of both lungs and chest wall and aging also causes changes in compliance, it is useful to bring together the changes that occur in normal individuals in the static properties of the respiratory system from fetal life until old age.

The transpulmonary pressure required in a child to inhale a normal tidal volume is much the same as that required in an adult. The child's tidal volume is smaller, but his lungs are stiffer; so the smaller tidal volume offsets the effect of the increased stiffness of the smaller lung. The child's muscles are small and the chest wall more pliable than an adult's, yet it must generate the same intrapleural pressures as those of a heavily muscled man.

The radius of the chest wall and the radius of curvature of the diaphragm are small in infants and children. Because of this small radius, a given tension created by the muscles of the chest wall results in a larger change in intrapleural pressure than the same tension would cause in a larger chest (Fig. 4-10). Therefore, although the muscles of infants and children are small, changes in intrapleural pressure can be created that are almost as great as those in adults. Since compliance is expressed as liters per centimeter of water pressure and the small radius of the child's chest results in larger pressure changes for a given volume change, the absolute compliance of the infant's and child's chest is much lower than that of the adult. The opposing effects of small radius and small tidal volume in infants and children result in the pleural pressures of infants and children being almost identical to those of adults. If compliance—the volume change for a given pressure change—is expressed as a percent of vital capacity rather than as an absolute figure, the values for adults and children are very similar. Using this relative terminology it has been found that the chest wall is more compliant for the first 12 to 24 months of life. This increased compliance of the infant chest wall explains the severe retraction that can be seen in this age group.

The mechanism by which a fetus can first fill its lungs with air and the subsequent changes with growth are an important series of events to understand if one is to be prepared to understand normal and abnormal respiratory mechanics in various age groups. Infants can develop a negative intrapleural pressure of minus 70 cm. H_2O despite their small muscles.

In the mature fetus the chest wall is very compliant, and its resting volume is that of nonaerated lung. This makes the pleural pressure atmospheric in the fetus. If the adult situation of negative intrapleural pressure prevailed in the fetus, fluid would be drawn into the lung during fetal life, and the lungs at birth would contain a considerable volume of fluid. Prior to aeration the lung has less recoil because there

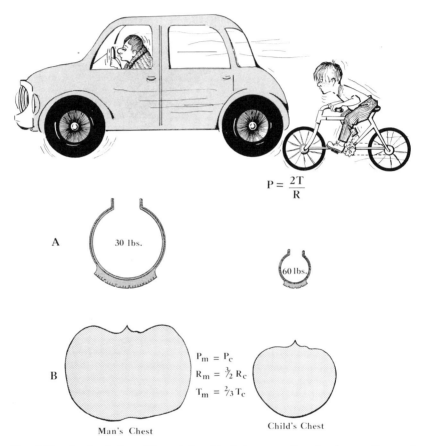

$$P = \frac{2T}{R}$$

A   30 lbs.

60 lbs.

B $P_m = P_c$
$R_m = \frac{3}{2} R_c$
$T_m = \frac{2}{3} T_c$

Man's Chest   Child's Chest

Fig. 4-10. Laplace's law: The relationship between surface tension, radius, and intraluminal pressure. A tire must have enough air pressure in it to maintain the wall rigid against the compressing force of the weight of the vehicle. The amount of inflation pressure needed is defined by Laplace's law, which states that the pressure equals surface tension divided by the radius. The tire of the car has a large radius, and so pressure to maintain a surface force to support the car is small, 30 pounds. The radius of the bicycle tire is small, so the pressure to support the bicycle and its rider is large, 50 to 60 pounds. The child's chest has a radius, R_c, which is two-thirds that of the man's, R_m, so to create the same pressure, P_m and P_c, within the chest the child needs to exert only two-thirds the force, T_c, with the muscles of the chest wall than is required by the man, T_m.

are no surface-active forces at the air–fluid interface; thus, the fetal fluid-filled lungs are more compliant than the infant's air-filled lungs.

At birth the fall in pulmonary capillary pressure leads to reabsorption of the small volume of fluid from the nearly collapsed alveoli, and a force must be supplied to open the collapsed alveoli and permit inhaled air to replace the fluid and create an air–fluid interface. These first breaths of an infant require pressures as great as 70 cm. H_2O below atmospheric pressure in the pleura to open the alveoli (see p. 74 and Fig. 4–8). When the air–fluid interface is established, it leads to some recoil of the lung due to surface tension. This recoil tends to pull in the chest wall. The chest wall opposes the inward pull that occurs after lung aeration, so the resting chest volume increases and a negative pleural pressure is established.

The compliance per unit volume of the chest wall in infants is particularly high. The compliance per unit volume of the lung, on the other hand, is the same as that of adults. During growth the compliance of the chest wall decreases markedly, and this decrease in the compliance of the chest with growth leads to increasing outward recoil of the chest, which produces a more negative pleural pressure. The negative pleural pressure stretches the lung to a greater volume, and the functional residual capacity is larger. The greater recoil of the chest wall enlarges the lung volume at which the recoil of the lung equals that of the chest. Throughout growth, as the radius of the chest grows, the respiratory musculature must increase to provide the needed force to supply the greater wall tension that results from the greater chest diameter. The effects of gravity are also increased with growth, since the weight of the abdomen and chest wall is small in infants and increases with age.

In middle and late adult life, the functional residual capacity increases further, but the resting pleural pressure does not increase. The late increase is due to decrease in the elastic recoil of the lungs as they age. The more compliant lungs are pulled to a greater volume by the unchanged elastic recoil of the chest wall.

PLEURAL SPACE AND COMPLIANCE

The pleural space is the place where mechanical forces of the chest wall are connected to the lung. The elastic recoil of the lungs and of the chest wall exert the opposing forces which lead to changes in pressure in the pleura. A normal subject at resting end-tidal lung volume, a state of relaxation, has a pleural pressure of −5 cm. H_2O. At this relaxation volume, the lung is stretched by an intraairway pressure ($P_{(aw)}$) equal to atmospheric pressure, which is 5 cm. H_2O higher than the pleural pressure ($P_{st(pl)}$). The lung volume is *greater* than it would be if there were no pressure stretching it. The chest wall is *smaller* due to the compression force resulting from the fact that the pressure on the body surface is 5 cm. H_2O greater than the pressure in the pleura. Thus, any leak or loss of integrity of the lung or chest wall would permit air to enter the chest.

If, during complete relaxation of respiratory muscles, air were allowed to enter the pleural cavity until the pleural pressure equalled the pressure at the body surface, the chest wall would be expanded and the lung would collapse. Air equivalent to 60% of vital capacity would enter the chest when pleural pressure equalled atmospheric pressure.

When the chest is widely opened, as during thoracotomy, pleural pressure is atmospheric. If under this condition the airway pressure is allowed to fall to atmospheric levels during expiration, the end-tidal volume of the lung will be less than it is when the chest wall is intact—unless a stretch force is continued at the end of expiration. Such a stretch force can be provided by maintaining airway pressure at 5 cm. above atmospheric pressure at the end of expiration.

Since lung volume is decreased when pleural pressure is allowed to fall to atmospheric pressure by air accumulating in the pleura, either due to open or closed pneumothorax, focal and even lobar atelectasis can occur. The decrease in lung volume lowers the volume of air in some of the alveoli enough so that the surface tension rises and forces the small amount of remaining air out of the alveoli and they collapse completely. The collapse of these alveoli requires the open alveoli to be stretched to a large volume with tidal exchange, and so the lung compliance falls. Since any accumulation of air or fluid in the pleural space will decrease the volume of the chest cavity occupied by the lung and indirectly will decrease the compliance of the lung, it is essential for the body to have a mechanism of removing air or fluid from the pleural cavity.

Since the visceral and parietal pleural surfaces, even at rest, are being pulled apart by a pressure of 5 cm. H_2O, this force might be expected to pull gas and fluid through the permeable pleural membranes (Fig. 4-11A). The total pressure of gases in the systemic venous blood is —73 cm. H_2O below atmosphere, so gas which is pulled from the alveoli through the visceral pleura by negative pleural pressure is reabsorbed into the blood in the venous capillaries of the parietal pleura. Until the pleural pressure reaches 73 cm. below atmospheric pressure, the pleura will be kept gas-free by the venous blood perfusing the parietal pleura.

If a closed pneumothorax occurs due to disruption of the chest wall or lung, the total gas pressure in the pneumothorax will be determined by the amount of air in the pleural space and by the elastic recoil of the

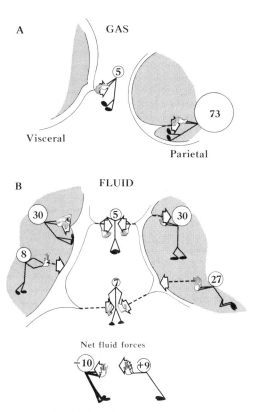

Fig. 4-11. Pleural space. (A) There is a pressure equivalent to 5 cm. H_2O, the negative pleural pressure, pulling air through the visceral pleura into the pleural space. Air is being pulled from the pleural space by a pressure of -73 cm. H_2O due to low partial pressure of gases in the systemic venous blood. This results in prompt absorption of air that leaks through the visceral pleural surface.

(B) The forces to maintain the pleural space free of fluid are more complex. The negative pleural pressure of -5 cm. H_2O (*top center*) and the colloidal oncotic pressure of proteins in the pleural fluid (*bottom center*), 7 cm. H_2O, are pulling fluid from both the visceral and parietal surfaces into the pleural space. On the parietal side, fluid is pulled into the parietal capillaries by a hydrostatic pressure in the capillaries of 30 cm. H_2O. This is opposed by an intravascular hydrostatic pressure of 27 cm. H_2O pushing fluid out of the capillaries, leaving a net force of 9 cm. which is allowing fluid to escape from the parietes into the pleural space. On the visceral side there is the same oncotic pressure of intravascular proteins pulling fluid into the surface capillaries, and this is opposed by a hydrostatic pressure of only 8 cm. H_2O. Thus there is a net resorptive force of 10 cm. H_2O in the visceral side. In addition, there are more visceral than parietal capillaries, so the resorptive area on the visceral surface exceeds the area on the parietes. If fluid accumulates in the costophrenic angle and pushes the lung up, reabsorption will be slow due to the limited area of lung in contact with the fluid.

lung and chest wall. Since the gas tensions in systemic venous blood are —73 cm. pressure, the tolerable limits of pleural pressure variation have little effect on the rate of absorption of the gas. The time needed to reabsorb the gas is mainly dependent on the relation between the volume of air in the pleural space and the surface area of the parietal pleura in contact with the gas in the pleural space. In other words, a large pneumothorax takes longer to reabsorb than a small one. Since gas is absorbed only through the parietal pleura by the force exerted that is due to the difference in pleural and venous blood parietal pressures, if the gas is kept well mixed by activity, the rate of reabsorption will increase. The concentration gradients for the various gases will also have some effect. For example, if the patient breathes 100% oxygen, washing out most of the nitrogen from the blood, this would speed the rate of reabsorption of nitrogen trapped in the chest.

The amount of fluid in the pleural cavity is controlled by a balance between the osmotic pressure of the colloids in the capillaries and the hydrostatic pressures in the capillaries (Fig. 4-11B). The pulmonary capillary hydrostatic pressure driving fluid out of the capillary is 8 cm. H_2O, to which must be added the negative hydrostatic pressure of 5 cm. H_2O in the pleural cavity plus the 7 cm. H_2O colloidal oncotic pressure of pleural fluid, which pulls fluid out of the capillaries. This total force of 20 cm. H_2O leading to the exit of fluid from the capillaries is opposed by the colloidal osmotic pressure of blood of 30 cm. H_2O. This leaves a net force of 10 cm. H_2O to reabsorb fluid from the pleura on the visceral side.

On the parietal side of the pleura, fluid is pushed into the pleural space by the mean capillary pressure in the systemic capillaries of 27 cm. H_2O. Fluid is also pulled in by the 7 cm. H_2O oncotic pressure of pleural fluid and the 5 cm. negative pleural pressure. The effusion pressure of 39 cm. H_2O is opposed by the pressure exerted by the colloidal osmotic pressure of the blood of 30 cm. H_2O. Thus, fluid leaves the parietal pleura under a pressure of 9 cm. H_2O and is absorbed by the visceral pleura by a force of 10 cm. H_2O. This net reabsorptive pressure of 1 cm. H_2O is adequate to keep the pleura free of fluid under normal circumstances because the visceral pleura is relatively more vascular than the parietal pleura; thus, its reabsorptive force acts over a greater area than does the net effusion force in the parietal pleura.

If the motion of the diaphragm is inhibited, there then may be a considerable area of parietal pleura which is not in contact with the visceral pleura. Under these circumstances any fluid which accumulates in the costophrenic angle, where there is little contact with the lung, is less likely to be absorbed. If the mean pulmonary capillary pressure increases, the balance is disturbed and effusion can result. An exudate with a high protein content or blood in the pleural cavity will also upset the balance and lead to effusion. The lymphatic system must then be called into play to remove protein and fluid.

Only the forces described above hold the lungs against the chest wall. There is no surface force of attraction. The often-used analogy of the visceral and parietal pleura being held together like two pieces of glass with a thin film of fluid between them is incorrect. There is a small film of fluid that acts as a lubricant so the two surfaces can slide across one another easily, but, since fluid can escape through the capillaries, the fluid can be increased if the force pulling the surfaces apart is raised. Thus, the force to pull the surfaces apart is equal to the force to increase transudation. One might say that the pleural surfaces are more like two sponges with millions of submicroscopic holes applied to one another than that they are like two plates of impermeable glass.

The very thin layer of liquid between the two pleural surfaces, in addition to being a lubricant, allows the surfaces to slide over one another as a means of getting synchronous and complete transmission of chest wall volume changes to the lung. This results in fairly uniform pressure throughout the pleural space. The force acting on the lung surface and the inner surface of the chest wall is much the same in different regions of the pleural cavities.

The balance of forces which acts to maintain the pleural space filled with lung rather than fluid or air is nicely summarized by Mead.*

What holds the lung against the chest wall? . . . occupancy of the chest cavity [is] a competition between solids, liquids and gases. The liquids are removed down to a vestige because the capillary pressure in the visceral pleura is considerably lower than its colloid osmotic pressure. . . . The gases are removed . . . because the total gas pressure in venous capillary blood is considerably less than atmospheric due to the relative capacity of the blood for carbon dioxide and oxygen. The lungs, chest wall, and diaphragm are then pressed into service by atmospheric pressure and occupy the space, as it were, by default.

The pleural space is well adapted to the function of providing an interface which allows the lung to respond to changes in the shape of the chest wall that result from forces developed by the respiratory muscles. If the lung could not move freely in the pleural space, the forces applied by the chest wall would be unevenly distributed to the lungs. Since the lungs and chest wall are in almost constant motion and

*J. Mead, Mechanical properties of lungs. *Physiol. Rev.* 41:306, 1961. Used with permission.

the shape of the chest wall constantly changes, it is essential that lungs be able to move freely in the chest. If the pleural space is obliterated, this motion is seriously inhibited. The construction of the pleural space and the forces which keep it air- and fluid-free do permit the lung and chest wall to be in almost constant motion. By studying the pleural pressures when the system is in motion, the dynamic properties of the lung can be determined.

DYNAMIC PROPERTIES OF THE LUNG

The elastic properties of the respiratory system, or the relation between the force applied and the change in volume of the system, covers only the first term of the equation of motion,

$$F_{app} = \frac{1}{C} V + R\dot{V} + I\ddot{V}$$

The system is dynamic and in almost continuous motion. To ascertain the proportion of the total force applied which is dissipated by the last two terms, the amount of force dissipated in stretching this system must be subtracted from the total force. If the total pressure across the system is known, then the pressure needed to overcome resistance and inertance equals this pressure minus the reciprocal of compliance times the change in volume.

$$P_{app} - \frac{1}{C} V = R\ddot{V} + I\ddot{V}$$

INERTANCE

The second of the two terms in the above equation, $I\ddot{V}$, which is the force necessary to overcome inertance, is of very little significance in the respiratory system. The inertant force is proportional to the mass times acceleration. The acceleration of the chest wall and lungs is very small—a fraction of to a few centimeters per second—so the term $\ddot{V}$ is very small. The term I is related to the mass, and for the lungs this is likewise small. For the chest wall I is significantly large. Despite the significant mass of the chest wall, the rate of acceleration is so slow that the accelerative force is still negligible. The total force needed to accelerate the respiratory system is less than 5% of the total pressure fluctuation in the system, or 0.01 cm. H_2O per liter per second per second.

Most of this small inertial force is not used to accelerate or decelerate the lungs or chest wall. The major portion of it is required in acceleration of the lightest element moving in the system, the air in the airways. The air reaches high enough velocities that $\ddot{V}$ becomes large enough to make acceleration of air require more force than is required for acceleration of the lungs and chest wall. Since, even considering the inertia of air, the force to overcome inertia in the system is only 5% of the total force, it is safe to ignore the inertia of the system and to analyze the respiratory system as if it had only compliance and resistance and no inertance.

RESISTANCE

For a volume-pressure system, resistance equals forcing pressure divided by rate of change of volume, or volume change per second, which is commonly called the flow rate. It is helpful to consider the relation between resistance, pressure, volume, and flow rate when resistance is fixed.

$$R = \frac{\Delta P}{\dot{V}}$$
$$\Delta P = R\dot{V}$$

Since forcing pressure equals resistance times flow rate, the faster the flow rate, the higher the required forcing pressure. Flow is volume divided by time.

$$\dot{V} = V/\text{sec}.$$

Since time is in the denominator of the dimensions of flow, to exchange a given tidal volume it will take less forcing pressure if the time allowed increases. More forcing pressure is needed if time decreases.

$$\Delta P = \frac{R\Delta V}{\text{sec}.}$$

Thus ΔP to overcome resistance is time dependent, while ΔP for compliance is independent of time. (When the system is not moving, the time for volume change becomes infinite and ΔP for resistance is zero, the static state.)

SOURCES OF RESISTANCE

There are three sources of resistance to be overcome in moving the respiratory system: tissue resistance in the chest wall, tissue resistance in the lungs, and resistance to air flowing into and out of the airways.

The tissue resistance of the chest wall has had very little study. It has been reported to make up as much as 20% of the total resistance of the system. It cannot be measured in the spontaneously breathing individual, because the force exerted by the various muscles cannot be measured. During artificial respiration in the completely relaxed subject, the difference between pleural and atmospheric pressure is the force applied to the chest wall. The part of this force required to stretch the chest wall to any given volume can be subtracted from the total transthoracic pressure, and the difference is the force required to overcome resistance to motion of the tissues of the chest wall. It is likely that in many conditions chest wall tissue resistances are increased. These conditions may include chest trauma, operative or accidental chest deformities, arthritis, heavy musculature, and obesity. The absolute effect on the chest wall resistance of alterations in its structure cannot be ascertained until new methods of measuring chest wall resistance are found.

Lung Tissue Resistance.   Resistance in the lung can be measured during spontaneous breathing by continuously recording the difference between mouth and pleural pressures and subtracting the pressure necessary to stretch the lung to get the pressure necessary to overcome resistance (Fig. 4-12). Pressure to overcome resistance varies throughout the respiratory cycle. Part of this variation is due to the change in flow rate during the respiratory cycle and part is the result of change in resistance. The resistance measured in this manner is resistance to airflow in the bronchi and to movement of lung tissue. To separate the portion due to lung tissue resistance from that due to the airways requires methods using gases of different density or the plethysmograph method. The latter can measure airway resistance only during panting ventilation. All these methods are rather unsatisfactory, and there have not been extensive measurements in disease states.

The measurements that have been made show that approximately 20% of the lung resistance is due to tissue, while 80% is due to airflow. The lung tissue resistance is approximately 0.2 cm. H_2O per liter per second. It is probable that diseases like pulmonary fibrosis, pulmonary congestion, and pulmonary inflammation all increase tissue resistance, though no adequate studies have been done to support this supposition.

Airway Resistance.   Resistance to flow of air constitutes the major resistive element in the lungs and is most subject to increase with disease. The anatomical configuration and dimensions of the airways control

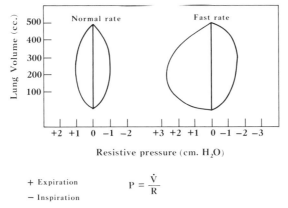

+ Expiration

− Inspiration

$$P = \frac{\dot{V}}{R}$$

Fig. 4-12. The effect of breathing rate on resistive pressure. At normal rate, about 1 cm. H_2O is required to overcome resistance. If R remains constant and $\dot{V}$, flow rate, increases (as flow rate must if volume is to be changed faster), P must increase and the resistive pressure loop fattens. It fattens more on expiration than on inspiration, because during inspiration the negative intrathoracic pressure pulls the bronchi open, while during expiration this force is less and the bronchi collapse.

the resistance to flow. Poiseuille's law (p. 327) states that the resistance is directly proportional to the length of the tube and inversely proportional to the fourth power of the radius. The distance to the alveoli in various parts of the lung is not uniform. Those closer to the hilum with short lengths of bronchi leading to them will have lower resistances than the more distant ones. Other than this effect, the length of the airways is not an important variant in affecting airway resistance. The length changes very little during the respiratory cycle and is little affected by disease.

The radius of bronchi is more important than length, not only because of the fourth-power effect, but also because bronchi can be markedly changed in diameter. Change in bronchomotor tone, inflammation, retained secretions, collapse or kinking, edema of bronchiolar tissues, compression, and fibrosis all can affect the bronchial radius. If some of the bronchi are occluded, the resistance will rise because there will be fewer tubes in parallel available. (Resistances in parallel add as their reciprocal, so the more parallel pathways available, the lower the resistance; see pp. 326–327).

The calculated resistance, or the quotient of pressure necessary to push air through the airways over flow rate, can be increased without change in airway size if there is turbulent flow. If flow is orderly or laminar, the pressure necessary to overcome a resistance is directly proportional to the flow rate. If there is turbulence present, the pressure required for the turbulent flow is proportional to the square of the flow rate. During quiet breathing, flow along the straight tubes is laminar. The only turbulence present is at the bends and bifurcations. As the airflow rate increases, turbulence becomes generalized in the larger straight bronchi, resulting in increased apparent resistance. In the small bronchioles, turbulence does not occur because the cross-sectional area of the tracheobronchial tree increases as it branches, so flow rates are less. In addition, the radii of the peripheral bronchi are small, and the Reynold's number remains below that which can cause turbulence (see p. 333).

The resistance in the airways is not evenly distributed along their course. During quiet breathing 50% of the total airway resistance is in the nares. With hyperventilation, turbulence increases so greatly in the nose that this means of breathing is abandoned. During mouth breathing, 25% of the total airway resistance is between the lips and upper cervical trachea. Seventy-five percent of the total resistance is located below the larynx, and the sites of this portion of the resistance have not been well identified. Probably little of the resistance is in the central large bronchi, but what proportion is in the small bronchi and what in the bronchioles and alveolar ducts is not known.

Passive Effects of Bronchial Size on Airway Resistance.   The diameter of the intrathoracic airways varies during each breathing cycle, because the distensible airways are subject to the changes in intrapulmonary pressure that occur during inspiration and expiration (Fig. 4-13). During inspiration the pressure in the airways is greater than that in the lung surrounding them; during expiration the opposite is true. As a result of the changes in transmural pressure across the elastic airways, the volume of air within the airways changes throughout the respiratory cycle. The end-inspiratory volume of the trachea is 102% of its end-expiratory volume, and the end-inspiratory volume of the 5 mm. bronchi is 145% and of the 2 mm. bronchi, 200% of the end-expiratory volume.

During breathing, when air is moving, the pressure is not uniform throughout the tracheobronchial tree because resistance to airflow dissipates some of the potential energy of pressure along the course of the airway. When an individual inspires, the most negative pressure in the air spaces of the lung is in the alveoli, and the pressure becomes progressively less negative in the bronchioles, bronchi, and trachea until, at the mouth, it is equal to atmospheric pressure. During inspiration the highest intraluminal pressure is in the trachea, so the passive distending force due to transmural pressure is greatest in the trachea and progressively less as one descends down the tracheobronchial tree. Despite a greater distending force on the trachea than on the small bronchi and bronchioles, the increase in lumen is greater in the smaller airways because the walls are more distensible than are the walls of the rigid trachea and large bronchi.

During expiration the intrapulmonary pressure must rise above atmospheric pressure to expel air from the lungs. This causes the pressure outside the tracheobronchial tree to be greater than that in the lumen, so the tracheobronchial tree is compressed. The transmural compressive pressure is greatest in the trachea and smallest in the bronchioles; however, the greatest decrease in lumen is in the flexible small airways, not the armored large bronchi and trachea. Expiratory force in normal

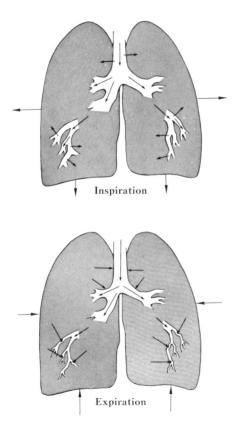

Fig. 4-13.   Effect of intrapleural pressure on airway size. During inspiration (top) the subatmospheric intrapleural pressure pulls air into the bronchi and also enlarges the lumen of the bronchi, reducing the resistance. During expiration (bottom) the expulsive force that pushes air out of the bronchi also collapses the bronchi, particularly if the pleural pressure rises above atmospheric pressure. The collapse is most marked in the small bronchi not protected by cartilage.

quiet breathing is supplied by the elastic recoil of the lungs, and this is so distributed as to minimize the compressive force on the small bronchi and bronchioles. If a greater force is required to expel air than can be provided by the elastic recoil of the lungs, then the expiratory muscles must create a positive intrapleural pressure. The positive intrapleural pressure increases the compressive force on the unsupported small bronchi and bronchioles and further narrows their lumina, increasing the resistance to airflow. An increase in pleural pressure can make the compressive force on the bronchi rise more rapidly than the pressure driving air along the bronchial lumen. As a result, there is a limit on expiratory flow rate which is set by these competing forces. The pulmonary function test, which measures the speed of expiration, or maximal expiratory flow rate, determines the interaction of the compression force and driving force. In normal individuals the maximum flow rate decreases steadily as the vital capacity is forceably expired, due to the escalating compression of the bronchi and bronchioles; this exhalation is exaggerated if compliance of the lung is diminished or airway resistance is increased.

Since transmural pressure alters bronchial diameter by changing the forces stretching the bronchi, an increase in functional residual capacity will increase bronchial diameters. In this way the position of respiration can alter the resistance to air flow. At normal position of respiration the chest wall muscles are presumably most efficient, and airway resistance is easily overcome by the recoil force of the lungs. With increase in airway resistance the elastic recoil force may not be great enough to expel all the air in the three seconds available for expiration. At the start of the next inspiration the functional residual capacity will be greater. By increasing the functional residual capacity the individual has greater elastic recoil, since recoil increases as lung volume increases. This increased recoil force can provide enough force to expel the tidal volume. The change in position of respiration with increased airway resistance requires more inspiratory muscular effort but diminishes muscular expiratory effort and, thus, the need to create a high intrapleural pressure which would tend to collapse the airways. Breathing is made easier by increasing functional residual volume, because the forces stretching the bronchi open will lower resistance and enhance the elastic recoil, decreasing the need for positive expiratory effort. If airway resistance is further escalated, the limits of increase in functional residual capacity are reached and positive pleural pressure may have to be created by the expiratory muscles as a means of creating added force to expel air even when the patient is at rest.

In patients whose lungs have become very compliant, such as those with emphyscma, there is very little elastic recoil to expel air. Most of these patients also have increased resistance in the bronchi due to chronic bronchitis. These patients have a greatly reduced maximum expiratory flow rate, because the lack of elastic recoil and increased resistance force them to push the air out of their lungs. They quickly reach the point at which the collapsing effect of positive intrapleural pressure exceeds the increase in driving pressure to push air out of the alveoli, and thus air is trapped in their lungs.

The compliance or static properties of the lungs have a profound effect on the airway resistance because of the distensible nature of the bronchi. To maintain the most favorable conditions, the individual with low compliance maintains an increased end-tidal volume to limit the collapse of the airways and breathes slowly to diminish the flow rate and thus the needed driving pressure. On the other hand, a person with decreased compliance takes rapid shallow breaths to decrease the volume to which the stiff lung must be stretched. The resultant increased airflow requires less added driving pressure than when compliance is normal, since airways are not compressed by a positive intrapleural pressure due to muscular effort. The added lung recoil alone is sufficient to push air out at the faster rate. This added pressure can be supplied by the recoil force of the stiff lung during expiration with less expenditure of energy. Thus, in lungs with abnormal elasticity or resistance the pattern of respiration chosen is the one that requires the minimum work or energy expenditure.

The aging process of the lungs includes a loss of elasticity, an increase in residual volume, and a decrease in maximum expiratory flow rate. The process can be accelerated by the quality of inhaled air. Even in young college students, smoking of a pack or more of cigarettes a day increases bronchial resistance enough so that maximum expiratory flow rate is diminished, presumably due to the chronic irritation. It is probable that the smog of our urban environment has a similarly deleterious effect.

All of these passive effects on bronchial size due to compression are exaggerated when resistance is elevated by contraction of bronchial smooth muscle.

The Effect of Bronchomotor Tone on Airway Resistance.   The effects of changes in bronchomotor tone on bronchial lumen size are not the same in different regions of the airways, due to the structure as well as the size of the various levels of airways. The trachea and large bronchi have cartilage rings which encircle two-thirds of the diameter. Smooth muscle is arranged in both transverse and longitudinal patterns, so these large bronchi can be narrowed and shortened moderately. The smaller bronchi have incomplete cartilaginous rings and somewhat more muscle. The bronchioles have no cartilage but relatively more smooth muscle, so they can be almost completely occluded. There are muscle sphincters about the alveolar ducts that can contract independently of those in the rest of the tracheobronchial tree. The nerve supply to the bronchial musculature is through the vagus nerves and the thoracic sympathetic chain. The sympathetic nerves supply the bronchial dilators, while the vagus nerves control the bronchioconstrictors.

Epinephrine, norepinephrine, and isoproterenol cause bronchodilation by stimulation of the sympathetic postganglionic receptors. Acetylcholine, pilocarpine, and anticholinesterases cause bronchoconstriction by stimulation of parasympathetic receptors. Atropine acts as a bronchodilator by inhibiting the bronchoconstrictive effects of parasympathetic receptors. Histamine constricts the alveolar ducts, and anything which liberates histamine will have the same effect.

Airways constrict in response to the inhalation of irritants such as cigarette smoke, exhaust fumes, and smog. These agents act on the subepithelial receptors of the vagus nerve, which are responsible for initiating the cough reflex. Cold air, perhaps in the same manner, constricts bronchi. Arterial hypoxemia and hypercapnia increase bronchomotor tone. These reflexes depend on an intact vagus nerve and can be reversed by the administration of atropine. Bronchoconstriction due to increase in arterial pCO_2 probably is mediated through medullary receptors and bronchoconstriction with hypoxemia through the carotid and aortic bodies, the same sensors as for ventilatory control. These reflexes may be the ones that cause bronchoconstriction in patients with pulmonary edema. Small pulmonary emboli can cause bronchoconstriction, as can complete occlusion of a pulmonary artery. When a large pulmonary artery is occluded, no carbon dioxide is excreted into the air ventilating that region of lung; the low alveolar pCO_2 leads to bronchoconstriction in that region of the lung and acts to diminish ventilation to unperfused areas of lung. This is a local response and is not affected by cutting the nerve supply to the lung.

Relaxation of bronchomotor tone occurs with hyperventilation and deep inspiration. Increase in systemic arterial blood pressure acts through the carotid sinus to relax bronchial smooth muscle.

The regulation of bronchial muscle tone profoundly affects the efficiency of the respiratory system, because it alters the resistance in the airways and can also affect the anatomical dead space, total lung volume, and compliance. Constriction of the terminal bronchioles, which increases airway resistance, decreases the total volume of the airways and thus the anatomical dead space. The greater resistance to airflow leads to an increase in end-tidal volume to enable elastic recoil to expel air more effectively, and thus the force to stretch the lung on inspiration must be increased. If the sphincters about the alveolar ducts are stimulated to contract, they act to expel air from the alveoli and decrease the number of ventilated alveoli and thus the lung compliance. When these various interacting alterations in mechanics occur, the central regulatory system apparently regulates the rate and tidal volume to provide the most efficient combination of airway resistance, anatomical dead space, and compliance.

It is apparent that resistance and compliance are related to one another and affect one another. These interrelationships are clarified when the impedance of the system is considered.

IMPEDANCE

The theoretical background for the concept of impedance is best developed in electronic circuits, though it is equally applicable to fluid flow and is a particularly useful concept if the tubes are flexible. For theoretical background of this concept see page 341; Figure 4-3 (p. 60) shows an example of the network. For consideration here we can either look at a single unit or consider the whole lungs as if they were such a single unit (Fig. 4-14A). Since the lungs have both resistance and compliance in them, they can be shown to behave like electrical circuits with resistance and capacitance. The simplest comparative model is one which depicts the lung as a single compliance unit and resistance unit in series.

When such a circuit is driven by alternating pressure or voltage, the resultant flow is dependent on the relative values of the compliance and resistance. Such a system will have a characteristic impedance. The value for this impedance during a given respiratory cycle can be found using Fourier analysis and calculating the ratio of peak pressure to peak flow of the first harmonic.

A system with both resistance and compliance is time-dependent. The peak of the pressure applied across the system will not occur at the same moment as peak flow. The phase angle, or time delay, between these two waves can also be measured by Fourier series analysis. If the phase angles between flow and pressure and impedance are known, compliance and resistance of the system can be calculated as follows. In a series resistance-capacitance circuit the trigonometric and geometric relationships between compliance, resistance, and inertance is as shown in Figure 4-14B. Theta equals the phase angle, Z impedance, R resistance, and $1/2\pi f C$ the compliant reactance. Using simple trigonometry,

$$\sin\theta = \frac{1/2\pi f C}{Z} \qquad Z = \frac{P_m}{F_m}$$

where $P_m =$ peak pressure
        $F_m =$ peak flow

Solving for C,

$$C = \frac{F_m}{2\pi f \sin\theta\ P_m} \qquad \cos\theta = \frac{R}{Z}$$

Solving for R,

$$R = \frac{P_m \cos\theta}{F_m}$$

Using this method, lung compliance and lung resistance can be determined from simple recordings of flow at the mouth and of transpulmonary pressure measured with an esophageal balloon. The results correlate well with conventional determinations of these values.

It is certainly inaccurate to consider that the lung is completely described by this simple electrical analogy. A glaring error is the fact that it ignores the elasticity of the bronchi and assumes that the lungs have fairly uniform compliances and resistances, or at least a uniform time constant. We know from studying the distribution of air within the lung that this is not the case. Further investigations will hopefully permit more accurate analogies; however, this simple analogy is useful for clinical measurements and reminds one that there is a lag between pressure and flow in the system. This lag is exaggerated if resistances increase and makes measurements of dynamic compliance of questionable value. The method presumably can also be used for measuring chest wall compliance and resistance in artificially ventilated patients.

The interaction of the variation in compliance and resistance (the variation in impedance) throughout anatomical regions of the lung alters the distribution of ventilation. This concept of unequal impedance to change in volume in various parts of the lung and its effect on the distribution of air within the lung is presented in Chapter 7.

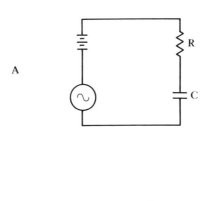

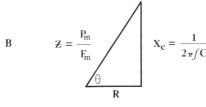

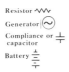

Fig. 4-14. (A) Simple electrical analog model of the lungs, as made up of a series circuit which has a single compliance and resistance in series and is driven by a generator. The battery represents the fact that the pleural pressure is biased negatively. (B) The relationship of impedance, resistance, and compliance. Theta represents the phase angle between flow and pressure, the hypotenuse impedance, the opposite side reactance, and the adjacent side resistance. If two quantities are known, such as phase angle and impedance, the others can be determined from trigonometric or geometric relationships.

Since the dynamic properties of the lung are dependent on the compliance and resistance of the system, the interaction of these two and also the rate at which the size of the lung is being changed—or, to state it another way, the effects of growth and activity level on dynamics—should be considered.

LUNG SIZE AND DYNAMIC PROPERTIES OF THE LUNG

In a child the size of the airways is smaller than in an adult, and so the resistance to airflow is increased just as the compliance is decreased. In discussing the relationship between lung size and the airway characteristics, the term for the reciprocal of resistance, *conductance*, is usually preferred. This is because the conductance increases as a direct linear function rather than as an inverse function of lung volume. The relation between airway conductance and lung volume in children varies during the growth period. As the child increases in size, the lung volume increases faster than the conductance, particularly between the ages of 8 and 14. There are no good anatomical studies to explain this discrepancy, but apparently the alveolar air spaces increase faster than the radius of the airways. After age 14 the radius of the airways, including the larynx, increases to exceed the ratio prior to age 8. These discrepancies may explain the quality of voice and also the physical limitations of prepubertal children. The small size of the airways in children also makes any bronchial inflammation or edema more hazardous than it is in adults. Since resistance increases as the fourth power of the decrease in radius, it takes only a small amount of inflammation to seriously compromise the lumen of the small bronchi of a child. It may be that the decrease in the severity of asthmatic attacks after the age of 14 can be attributed to the relative increase in size of the bronchi.

Pulmonary resection or ablation of lung by infection will decrease total airway conductance. However, the large inspiratory and expiratory reserve capacities of normal lungs permit extensive ablation without great disability. If the remaining lung is normal, the compliance and resistance of the various parts are unaltered, so that the integrity of mechanical function is preserved. Following pneumonectomy, patients with one normal lung can do all but the very heaviest exercise. If the lung mechanics are abnormal, as they are in emphysema, resection will be poorly tolerated.

DYNAMICS OF BREATHING WITH EXERCISE

Many patients with severe limitation of pulmonary function are well compensated at rest. When they must increase ventilation with exercise, the loss of the mechanical integrity of the lung becomes increasingly handicapping.

During normal breathing, inspiration takes one-third of the respiratory cycle, expiration two-thirds. Inspiratory flow takes one-third the time of expiratory flow, and, when graphed, its curve is dome-shaped. During expiration, flow is less symmetrical; peak flow occurs one-third of the way down the volume curve. This early peak of flow and falloff in the latter two-thirds of the cycle are the result of the narrowing of the airways, which decreases the effectiveness of the driving pressure during expiration. The recoil of the lungs and chest wall is slowed during the early part of expiration by continued contraction of the inspiratory muscles, or the peak flow would occur sooner. Thus, during normal quiet breathing expiration is passive, and no compressive force is applied to the bronchi.

With moderate exercise, respiratory rate is doubled and total ventilation is increased fivefold; inspiratory time equals expiratory time and flow resistance is halved by changing from nose to mouth breathing. Whereas quiet expiration is passive throughout, at the end of expiration during moderate exercise the expiratory muscles become active to maintain an adequate driving pressure for the increased flow rate. The increased tidal volume is achieved at the expense of inspiratory reserve; the functional residual capacity remains unchanged. During moderate exercise, the airway resistance is held at a minimum by calling on the inspiratory reserve only; since the increased lung volume tends to stretch the airways, the smaller lung volumes leading to maximum compression are avoided.

With heavy exercise, ventilation is increased tenfold, frequency trebled, and tidal volume is increased to one-half the vital capacity. To gain this increased tidal volume, some of the expiratory reserve must be used, and during the expiration pleural pressures are driven above atmospheric pressure by the expiratory muscles. This action of the expiratory muscles creates a high enough intrapleural pressure to compress the airways and thus limit expiratory flow rate. If mechanics are altered, either by an increase in resistance or by a decrease in compliance, expiratory flow will be limited at lower levels of ventilation and maximum ventilation will be decreased. Patients with decreased compliance or increased resistance usually have elevated residual volumes and functional residual capacities, since they are less able to empty their lungs. In such patients functional residual volume may increase with increased respiratory effort rather than decrease, as in the normal person, and thus endurance is limited.

Patients with poor lung mechanics should be encouraged to exercise regularly to keep the respiratory muscles in good condition. In the normal individual it is likely that the decrease in dyspnea with physical conditioning is due to increased strength of the respiratory muscles. Since patients with mechanical derangements of the lung must do more work per unit of ventilation, physical conditioning increases the strength of the muscles of respiration and makes them able to do such work more effectively. Just as conditioning of an athlete increases the amount of exertion that can be performed without uncomfortable dyspnea, so it can in the patient with respiratory disease. Conditioning provides a reserve ability which may enable patients to tolerate a disruption of function by trauma or infection that would cause respiratory failure in an unconditioned individual. The danger of poor physical conditioning is well illustrated by the frequency of serious postoperative respiratory difficulty in patients who have been at prolonged bed rest for tuberculosis without carefully graded preoperative exercise. One serious consequence of lack of respiratory muscle strength is an inability to cough effectively. If cough is not effective, accumulation of excretions will block the air passages and lead to increased resistance and decreased compliance.

THE MECHANICS OF COUGH

Cough requires maximum inspiration followed by maximum contraction of the expiratory muscles. This maximum muscular effort greatly alters the usual mechanics of airflow in the tracheobronchial tree. A cough is initiated by taking a deep breath, then closing the glottis to prevent escape of air while maximum compression of the lung is achieved by contracting all the expiratory muscles. This raises all pressures in the pleura and tracheobronchial tree to over 100 cm. H_2O. Since both pleural and alveolar pressures are raised, the disruptive force, or transmural force, in the alveoli is not significantly increased, so the alveoli are not subject to an excessive transmural force. When the glottis is suddenly opened, the pressure inside the trachea is immediately reduced, and the large transmural pressure narrows the cross-sectional area of the trachea to one-sixth its normal diameter. The flow rate during cough is increased sevenfold, to 7 liters per minute. Thus seven times as much air must flow through a tube one-sixth the size, and so the velocity of airflow in the trachea increases from the 660 cm. per second present during quiet breathing to 28,000 cm. per second at peak flow during cough. If the airway resistance is increased in the small bronchi or if lung compliance is decreased, cough will be less effective, because the added peripheral resistance will not permit the development of the high-flow velocity needed to sweep the foreign matter out of the tracheobronchial tree.

5. PULMONARY CIRCULATION

THE circulation is a closed circuit with the right heart, pulmonary vascular bed, left heart, and systemic vascular bed connected in series. This anatomical arrangement requires that the flow through the pulmonary and systemic circulations be equal. To maintain the integrity of the small pulmonary circulation, which contains 15% of the blood volume and has 70 square meters of capillary surface, requires a precise mechanism for regulating flow, pressure, and distribution of the circulation.

The basic principles of the relationship of flow to pressure outlined in the sections on fluid mechanics in Chapter 1 apply. However, the high flow required in this small vascular bed, the low hydrostatic pressures, and the delicate structure of its 70 square meters of capillary bed make this circulation particularly sensitive to cardiac dysfunction, shock, and other disease states which affect the integrity of the lung.

FUNCTIONAL ANATOMY

The lung has two circulations: the pulmonary, arising from the right heart; and the bronchial, arising from the aorta. Both the large pulmonary vessels and the microcirculation in the lungs differ significantly from the pattern seen in most areas of the systemic circulation.

THE PULMONARY ARTERIES AND VEINS

The main pulmonary artery is approximately equal in cross-sectional area to the aorta, but it branches sooner. After the major division into right and left pulmonary arteries, the vessels follow the branching of the bronchial tree; as they divide further, each follows an independent course without cross-connections to other branches. The tunica media of the main pulmonary artery is only one-half as thick as that of the aorta, and its elastic fibers are shorter and less orderly. This arrangement best suits the large pulmonary vessels for increasing volume capacity during surges in pressure; in addition, they may be able to actively constrict and thereby contribute to changes in pulmonary vascular resistance.

The pulmonary vascular bed does not contain an anatomical counter-part of the typical systemic arteriole. In the systemic bed the arteriole acts as an effective sphincter controlling flow to an area. It is 300 to 400 μ in diameter and has a heavy coat of circular smooth muscle and a high ratio of wall thickness to luminal diameter. The pulmonary vessels anatomically best suited for vasomotor control of the circulation are the large precapillary vessels that range from 100 to 1,000 μ in diameter. These vessels lie adjacent to the respiratory bronchioles and have a well-formed tunica media. The smaller arterioles, 50 μ in diam-eter, have very little muscle, but they take off at right angles to these large vessels and the muscle at these branchings may perhaps act as a sphincter. The 280 billion capillaries are 10 to 14 μ in length and only 7 to 9 μ in diameter. The red cells must squeeze through in single file. Since there is no muscle in the capillaries, any alteration in size depends on changes in the transmural pressure across the capillary wall. When the venous pressure rises, as in mitral stenosis, the capillary lumen can stretch to accommodate as many as three or four red cells abreast.

The venules corresponding in size to the precapillary vessels lie at the periphery of the lobules and have very little muscle. The rest of the venous system has less muscle than the arterial side of the circulation. Despite their small amount of muscle, the veins are capable of vaso-motor activity. As the veins enter the heart, a portion of cardiac muscle extends out into them, possibly acting as a sphincter.

BRONCHIAL ARTERIAL BLOOD SUPPLY TO THE LUNGS

The bronchial arteries are the nutrient arteries to the tracheobronchial tree and large pulmonary arteries and veins. Under normal conditions the pulmonary capillaries and alveoli are dependent for their nutrition on flow through the pulmonary vessels. The classical description of bronchial blood flow has return of blood from this circulation through the bronchial veins and then to the right atrium through the azygous system. These vessels are small and hard to identify. There are at least potential routes for return of blood from the bronchial arterial system through the pulmonary veins when bronchial blood flow is increased.

Within one to three days following ligation of the pulmonary artery, there is transient hemorrhagic collapse of many alveoli, presumably the result of ischemia. The alveoli recover later and after some months they may appear normal. This recovery is the result of new or expanded channels from the bronchial circulation which provide blood to these underperfused areas of lung. In patients with pulmonary blood flow decreased as a result of cyanotic heart disease or degenerative lung disease, a similar hypertrophy of the bronchial collateral circulation is seen.

The bronchial system also hypertrophies in an acute and chronic pulmonary infection or with pulmonary embolism. Whether these are all responses to decreased pulmonary flow is not certain. Chronic atelectasis without infection does not lead to increased bronchial flow, though it does diminish pulmonary flow and eliminates ventilation.

PULMONARY VASOMOTOR NERVES

Fibers from both the sympathetic and parasympathetic systems have been identified arising from the upper sympathetic chain and the vagus nerve and going to the pulmonary vascular tree. Both systems contribute vasoconstrictor and vasodilator fibers. The muscular arteries are more richly supplied than the corresponding veins. Stimulation of these vaso-motor nerves causes significant changes in the caliber of the vessels.

THE PUMP

Both the systemic and the pulmonary vascular tree have pumps at the inlet and outlet of their systems. If there are no shunts in this closed circuit, the two pumps must pump the same amount of blood. The amount of work required of the pumps depends on the blood flow rate, the impedance of the vascular bed, and the pressure required to fill the heart that drains the bed. Further, the energy cost of doing this work depends on the efficiency of the pump.

These pumps are phasic pumps, in which the flow and the pressure at the site of egress from the ventricles oscillate about a mean, or D.C., level. The phasic character of the flow and pressure waves generated by these pumps must not be ignored in studying the circulation. The relationship between the work the pump must do and the nature of the vascular bed is significantly affected by the pulsatile output. A simple example is the manner in which output is altered. The output can be increased by increasing the rate and/or the stroke volume. In most individuals stroke volume below a rate of 50 is too small to permit adequate output except at rest. Above a rate of 180, the pump becomes less efficient, because the limit of the rate of shortening of muscle is reached. By alteration in stroke volume and rate, the cardiac output per minute in a well-trained adult male can be increased from 5 to 6 liters at rest to 30 to 40 liters at maximum exercise level. Despite the fivefold increase in output, the pressures in the pulmonary artery and aorta rise very little. Since work is directly related to the product of pressure times flow, if flow can rise without a rise in pressure, the increments of work of the ventricle with increased flow are smaller. To accommodate the fivefold increase in flow without a corresponding increase in pressure means the impedance of the vascular bed must fall as flow increases. If the vascular tree is decreased in size and has a fixed impedance, when flow rises, pressure will also rise to escalate work per unit of flow.

The pressure differences in the two systems are an example of the effect described above. Despite the fact that flow through the systems is identical, pressures in the pulmonary circuit are about one-fifth to one-sixth those in the systemic circuit (Fig. 5-1). The nature of the pressure waves is also different. The right ventricular pulse lacks the higher frequency components of the left ventricular pulse. The initial acceleration is slower and the peak more rounded. The pulmonary artery pressure pulse wave has a mean pressure one-fifth to one-sixth that of the aorta. Systolic pressure is from 20 to 30 mm. Hg, diastolic is from 7 to 12 mm. Hg, and the mean pressure is 12 to 15 mm. Hg. Since it does less work, the right ventricle has a thinner wall and so is more easily filled. The

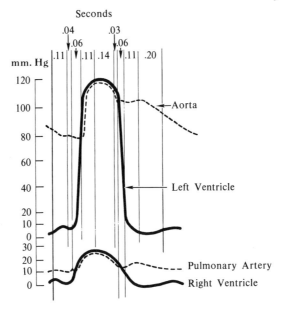

Fig. 5-1. The pulse curves of the right ventricle and pulmonary artery are less than one-fifth as great in magnitude as those of the left ventricle and aorta. The right ventricular pulse curve has a slower initial acceleration, and its peak is more rounded than that of the left ventricle.

filling of the right auricle is controlled more by posture, muscle activity, and the variations in intrapleural pressure than by pressure generated by the left ventricle. In contrast, the pressure head necessary to make blood flow into the left heart must be provided by the right ventricle.

The output of a ventricle is in part controlled by the pressure filling the ventricular cavity. The right atrial pressure, 3/2 or a mean of 2 mm. Hg, is lower than the left atrial pressure, 7/3 or a mean of 5 mm. Hg. If the impedance in the vascular bed rises or the stroke volume increases, the filling pressure may also be elevated. This is the so-called Starling law of the heart. One can plot the relation between output or stroke work and filling pressure. Sarnoff and others have shown that there is not a single Starling curve relating filling pressure to stroke work or cardiac output; rather, there is a family of curves. Some of the factors which modify the shape and position of curves describing this relationship are the administration of drugs, stimulation of cardiac nerves, release of catecholamines, cardiac disease, and changes in the bed draining the ventricle. An apparent fall in stroke work or output with increasing filling pressure can be shown to be the result of change in the relation between filling pressure and cardiac output, not a decreased output directly related to rising filling pressure.

The alteration of output by changes in filling pressure provides a primary control system to balance the output of the two ventricles. When the output of the right ventricle increases, the filling pressure of the left ventricle is elevated by the augmented blood flow, and this stimulates it to increase output. If the left ventricle is failing due to valve malfunction or myocardial disease, the slope and the position of the myocardial function curve are changed, so that the filling pressure required for an adequate cardiac output can rise to levels that compromise the integrity of the pulmonary circulation. Because of these relationships between vascular pressure and cardiac function, abnormality of myocardial function is the principle etiology of malfunction of the pulmonary circulation. If cardiac dysfunction persists for prolonged periods, structural changes in the pulmonary vasculature can ultimately prevent survival following successful correction of intracardiac defects. These abnormalities of the circulation can be understood only from an analysis of the factors which control the relationship between flow and pressure, which is the impedance, of the vascular bed.

RELATIONSHIP OF FLOW AND PRESSURE

The basic principles of fluid mechanics (Appendix, p. 324) define the ground rules for a description of flow-pressure relationships. In the pulmonary vasculature the pressures are low and flows high. Because of the high arterial pressures in the systemic circuit, great vein and right atrial pressures affect the driving pressure very little (Appendix, p. 324) and so can be disregarded in discussions of flow-pressure relations in this circuit. Since the pulmonary arterial pressure is low and the left atrial pressure is high, changes in left atrial pressure have significant effects on the driving pressure. It is therefore necessary to measure the pressure in the pulmonary artery and left atrium to study the pressure controlling flow in this smaller circuit. Filling pressure of the left heart, or mean pulmonary venous pressure, can be measured by introducing a catheter into the left atrium. A close approximation of this pressure can be obtained from a catheter wedged into a small branch of the pulmonary artery. Since the pulmonary arteries are end arteries, when the wedged catheter obstructs the lumen, the pressure measured is the downstream pressure, an approximation of pulmonary venous pressure. The pressure measured in this manner has been misnamed *pulmonary capillary wedge pressure.*

If the pressure across the vascular bed and the flow are known, the resistance can be calculated. The resistance equals the mean driving pressure over the mean flow. The resistance in the pulmonary bed can be calculated from the transpulmonary pressure and the cardiac output.

$$\frac{P}{\dot{V}} = R$$

$$\frac{15 - 5 \text{ mm. Hg}}{100 \text{ cc./sec.}} = 0.10 \text{ mm. Hg/cc./sec.}$$

The resistance of the bed can be related to its physical characteristics. Poiseuille's law states that $R = 8l\eta/\pi r^4$. The three variables controlling resistance are viscosity, η, length, l, and the fourth power of radius, r. These can be then divided into the viscosity factor, η, and the geometric factors, l and r.

VISCOSITY FACTOR

In simple fluids such as water, the viscosity of the fluid is unaffected by the velocity at which the fluid is flowing. Such a fluid is called a Newtonian fluid. The viscosity of blood is affected by the velocity of the flowing stream. As the flow velocity of blood increases up to the normal range of flow rates, the cells gather in the center of the stream due to the Bernoulli effect. (The cells along the walls move more slowly than those in the center, so the pressure on the lateral side of the cells is greater than that on the medial side and they are pushed toward the center.) The central grouping of the cells decreases the shear force along the wall and drops the apparent viscosity as the flow rate increases. Over the normal range of blood flow rates at normal hematocrit levels, viscosity changes are small, so anomalous viscosity has little effect on the resistance. This is not the case in disease states in which flow rate is decreased. In shock, for example, the decreased flow rate results in increased blood viscosity, which significantly increases the resistance and thus the driving pressure required for a given flow. This increase in viscosity as flow rate decreases acts to further compromise circulation in shock and may explain why in shock states agents which decrease blood viscosity help to increase flow.

The viscosity of blood is closely related to the hematocrit. As the hematocrit increases above normal, the viscosity rises, causing resistance to increase. To maintain the same flow, the driving pressure must be increased (Fig. 5-2). Individuals living at high altitudes who have developed high hematocrits have increased driving pressures across the lung, in large part due to the increased resistance associated with the rise in blood viscosity. In patients with cyanotic heart disease, the

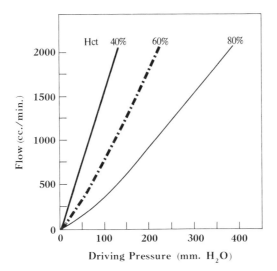

Fig. 5-2. The effect of hematocrit change on flow and pressure in the pulmonary circulation. When the hematocrit rises from 40 to 80%, there is a steady increase in the driving pressure needed. It is apparent from these graphs that in a patient with a hematocrit of 80%, the increased viscosity of the blood becomes an important factor in retarding flow. If such a patient has pulmonary vascular disease in addition, the high hematocrit adds to his difficulties. (From A. Roos, Poiseuille's law and its limitations in vascular systems [5th Conf. Res. in Emphysema, Aspen, Colo., 1962]. *Med. Thorac.* 19:224 [Karger, Basel/New York], 1962.)

elevated hematocrit acts to further burden an already compromised pulmonary circulation. In patients with shock due to dehydration or fluid loss, the low flow and high hematocrit combined can greatly increase the apparent viscosity of the blood.

GEOMETRIC FACTOR

The geometric factor is of far more physiological significance than the viscosity factor. The length of the vascular bed does increase slightly as the lung is inflated. However, these changes are of little significance compared to the possible changes in radius. Since resistance varies as the fourth power of the radius, small changes in this dimension have a large influence on resistance. Furthermore, the system is so constructed that many different forces result in large changes in individual vessel radius and, thus, the total cross-sectional area of the pulmonary vascular bed.

Intravascular Pressure and Vessel Radius. Since the vessels are distensible, a rise in transmural pressure (the difference between intravascular and perivascular pressures) will stretch the vessel (Fig. 5-3). The pressure distending the vessels can rise without an alteration in the driving pressure. If the normal mean pulmonary artery pressure of 15 mm. Hg and the normal mean left atrial pressure of 6 mm. Hg each rise 5 mm. Hg, the driving pressure will remain the same, 9 mm. Hg, but the transmural pressure will increase by 5 mm. Hg. This increment in transmural pressure distends the vessel, increasing the radius and, thus, the blood flow. If pulmonary artery pressure rises while left atrial pressure remains unchanged, both driving pressure and transmural pressure will increase. In this instance, flow will rise due to elevated driving pressure and lower resistance. If the driving pressure is increased by lowering left atrial pressure, the transmural distending pressure will be less, allowing collapse of the vessel and increase in resistance. The resultant flow in this case will depend on whether driving pressure or resistance rises faster.

Vasomotor Control of Vessel Size. The passive effects of changes in intravascular pressure depend on the distensibility of the vessels. The distensibility is altered by the vasomotor tone. Much of the vasomotor control may be by local reflex, although a significant amount results from activity of the vasomotor nerves. There is considerable evidence that the arterial and venous sides of the circulation can dilate and constrict independently. However, the precapillary vessels, not the arterioles or venules, are apparently the major site of alteration of vessel

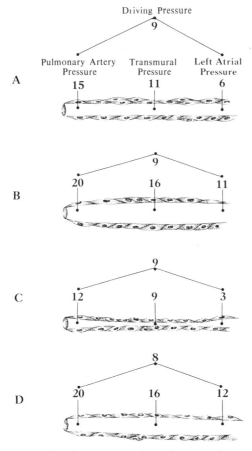

Fig. 5-3. The relationship between absolute intravascular pressures—driving pressure and transmural pressure—on the size of vessels and the resultant flow. These figures depict the results of changes in pulmonary artery and left atrial pressures on driving pressure (the difference between pulmonary artery and left atrial pressures) and on transmural pressure. In (A) the vessel is in the neutral state with a driving pressure of 9 mm. Hg and a transmural pressure of 11. In (B) the pulmonary artery pressure is raised from 15 to 20 and the left atrial pressure from 6 to 11; the driving pressure remains the same, but transmural pressure increases to 16, stretching the vessel and lowering the resistance. This results in increased flow, despite the same driving pressure. In (C) the driving pressure is 9 but pulmonary artery and left atrial pressures have each fallen by 3, dropping the transmural pressure to 9; this lets the vessel collapse and increases the resistance, causing flow to fall. In (D) pulmonary artery pressure remains 20, as in (A), but left atrial pressure has risen to 12, dropping the driving pressure to 8 but increasing the transmural pressure to 16. The flow may increase, decrease, or stay the same, depending on the balance between fall in resistance due to increased vessel diameter and decrease in driving pressure.

orifice by vasomotor activity. The great capacity of the pulmonary vascular bed to alter its cross-sectional area is illustrated by the response to exercise. If the resistance remained 0.09 mm. Hg per cubic centimeter per second, as blood flow increased from 6 liters per minute, or 100 cc. per second, to 30 liters per minute, or 500 cc. per second, mean pulmonary artery pressure would have to rise to 45 mm. Hg.

$$P = R \times \dot{V}$$
$$= 0.09 \times 500$$
$$= 45 \text{ mm. Hg}$$

Since mean pressure in both the left atrium and pulmonary artery rises very little with this increased flow, there must be a well-coordinated decrease in vascular muscle tone so the unchanged transmural pressure can distend the vessels. As illustrated in Figure 5-4, when there is complete relaxation of the vessel sphincters and maximum dilation, any further increase in flow is associated with an increase in pressure. When the system is fully dilated, it acts like a system with rigid tubes; resistance is fixed, so pressure rises as a linear function of flow rate increase. One of the early manifestations of pulmonary vascular disease or inability of the system to dilate is an increase in the pulmonary artery pressure with exercise.

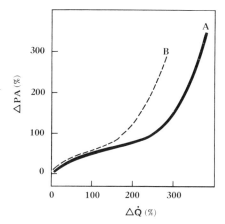

Fig. 5-4. Relationship between percent change in pulmonary artery pressure (vertical axis) and percent change in pulmonary artery flow (horizontal axis). In the normal situation (curve A), up to the point at which flow has increased 250%, flow rises much faster than pressure; then, when the bed is fully dilated, flow and pressure rise at the same rate. If the vascular bed is decreased by pulmonary resection or obliterative vascular disease, the point at which the bed is fully dilated will occur sooner and pressure will rise faster (curve B).

In addition to reflex vasomotor control of pulmonary vessel size resulting from reflex increase in cardiac output, there are drugs and chemical stimuli which can alter pulmonary vasomotor tone. Norepinephrine, epinephrine, serotonin, and angiotensin constrict the arterial side of the circulation. Serotonin, *E. coli* endotoxin, histamine, and alloxan constrict the veins. Acetylcholine and isoproterenol dilate constricted pulmonary arterioles. Since acetylcholine is destroyed during one circulation through the lungs, it has been used to determine the ability of the pulmonary arterioles to dilate in patients with pulmonary hypertension.

The most interesting of the chemical vasoactive stimuli are the gas concentrations in the alveoli and blood. Low alveolar concentrations of oxygen or high alveolar concentrations of carbon dioxide cause vasoconstriction. This is a local reflex that appears to limit blood flow to the poorly ventilated alveoli. In addition to the local effects, acute systemic hypoxia or hypercapnia causes reflex pulmonary vasoconstriction. Much controversy rages about the relative importance of change in alveolar gas concentrations versus change in systemic gas concentrations. Both can alter vasomotor tone, and their relative importance depends on the interaction of so many factors that different experimental designs can yield apparently paradoxical results.

Blood Volume as an Indicator of Alterations in Geometric Factor. Since the length of the pulmonary vessels can change very little, if the blood volume in the lungs increases, the cross-sectional area must increase. Normal blood volume in the lungs at rest is 750 to 900 cc.; 10% of this, or 75 cc., is in the capillaries, and one-half, or 375 cc., is in the pulmonary veins. The relatively large capacity of the venous bed permits it to serve as a reservoir for the left ventricle. Vasomotor change in the capacity of the venous bed can damp incoordination between right and left heart output. At rest in the upright posture, the apical regions of the pulmonary vascular bed have little blood in them and therefore have decreased perfusion. With exercise, as much as 600 cc. of blood can be pumped by the muscles of the legs into the lungs. This shift in blood from the systemic to the pulmonary bed provides blood to fill all the vessels, which dilate to allow increased flow without increased pressure. When a person lies down, or when a spaceman's g-suit is inflated, or if peripheral vasoconstriction takes place, blood is shifted from the systemic to the pulmonary circuit. This increase in lung blood volume fills the areas of the vascular bed that were relatively ischemic. At rest, in contrast to exercise, some of this blood may be stagnant and not associated with increased flow. In mitral stenosis or left ventricular failure the elevated intravascular pressure is associated with a markedly increased lung blood volume. In these patients the distension is such that more blood cannot be accommodated when the patient lies down or exercises, and so there is little shift from systemic to pulmonary beds. Just as position alters the distribution of blood between systemic and pulmonary vascular beds, it also affects distribution within the pulmonary bed.

POSITION IN CONTROL OF FLOW-PRESSURE RELATIONS

Position does not affect the driving pressures to various parts of the lung, but it does affect the transmural pressure and thus the distending force on the vessel walls (Fig. 5-5). Since in the upright posture the apices of the lung are higher than the outflow tract of the right ventricle, the pressure in the arterial vessels at the apices is less than that in the main pulmonary artery. The difference in pressure equals the gravitational force on the column of blood between the apex of the lung and the main pulmonary artery. Since the pulmonary veins are below the apices of the lung, on the venous side of the circulation the gravitational force acts to drive blood back into the heart and so lowers the venous pressure to a degree exactly equal to the lowered arterial pressure. As a result, the driving pressure is the same at the apices as it is at the level of the pulmonary artery, but the transmural or distending pressures are less.

At the base of the lungs the pressure relationships are the opposite of those at the apex. The hydrostatic pressure due to gravity is added to the main pulmonary artery pressure and the left auricular pressure. The driving pressure at the base is thus equal to that in the mid- and apical portions of the lung, but the distending pressure is greater. In the upright posture the effects of gravity on vessel distension cause progressively increased perfusion from the apices to the bases of the lungs. In the supine posture the gravitation effect causes more perfusion of the posterior portion of the lung, and in the lateral decubitus position the dependent lung receives increased perfusion.

To summarize the interrelationships between pressure, geometry, and flow: The difference between pressure generated by the right ventricle and that required to fill the left ventricle controls the driving pressure across the pulmonary vascular bed. Absolute levels of these same pressures determine the distending pressure resulting from cardiac function. Posture alters the effects of gravity on distending pressure in various parts of the lung and so affects the distribution of flow. Vasomotor tone determines what the cross-sectional area of the pulmonary vascular bed will be at any given distending pressure.

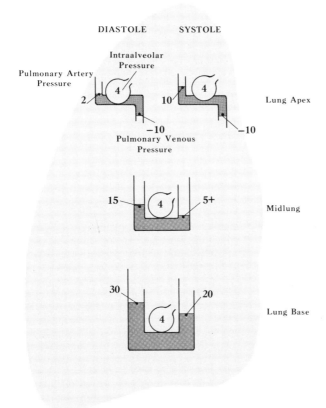

DIASTOLE   SYSTOLE

Intraalveolar
Pressure

Pulmonary Artery
Pressure

Pulmonary Venous
Pressure

Lung Apex

Midlung

Lung Base

Fig. 5-5. Effect of position on pressures and flow resistance in the pulmonary bed. In all areas of the lung the mean arteriovenous pressure difference is the same. When the individual is in the erect position, there is no effect of the hydrostatic column of blood at the midportion of the lung, since this portion of lung is at the level of the heart. The mean intravascular pressures are the same as the mean pressures for the entire system, and the size of the vessels depicted is the mean size due to transmural pressure. In the base of the lung a pressure equivalent to the hydrostatic pressure of the column of blood is added to the arterial and venous pressures. This results in greater transmural pressure, larger vessels, lower resistance, and therefore, increased flow, despite the same mean driving pressure.

In the apices of the lung the pressure due to the hydrostatic column of blood is subtracted from the pulmonary artery pressure, lowering it to less than alveolar pressure during diastole (left diagram) and flow stops. During systole pulmonary artery pressure rises above alveolar pressure and flow takes place. Throughout the cycle pulmonary venous pressure remains below alveolar pressure, so that when flow occurs, it is by the sluice mechanism (see Fig. 5-6). In the supine posture the anterior portions of the lung would be like the apices and the posterior portions like the bases. The pressure differences, however, would be smaller, and so the flow would be more uniform.

PULMONARY CAPILLARY CIRCULATION

FLOW

The capillary blood flow rate, like flow in any other segment of the vascular bed, is determined by the driving pressure across it and its cross-sectional area. The capillaries have no vasomotor mechanism, so the radius of the capillaries is actually the result of external forces acting on them. In the pulmonary capillaries these forces are different than in the systemic capillaries.

In the systemic circulation the precapillary vessels damp out pulsations and capillary flow and pressure are steady, so arterial pulse does not affect capillary flow. Because of the small capacity of the pulmonary arterial tree and the low resistance of the precapillary vessels, the pulse wave is transmitted to the pulmonary capillaries. Studies in human beings by the plethysmographic method of measuring pulmonary capillary flow have shown that there is a definite surge of flow during systole, though flow is continuous throughout the cardiac cycle in most areas of the lung. The surges in flow during systole are greater at the apices of the lungs, where the distending pressure during diastole may not open the capillary bed. Pulse transmission to the capillaries may be enhanced during exercise, when flow rate is increased. Along the course of the capillary the pulse wave is damped out, so that the only pulsations in the pulmonary venous bed are those reflected from the left atrium.

The size of pulmonary capillary is controlled by arterial, venous, and alveolar pressures. If the arterial pressure exceeds the alveolar and venous pressures, the capillary will open and blood will flow. However, the degree to which the capillary is opened depends on the venous and alveolar pressures as well as on the arterial pressure. If the venous pressure is greater than the alveolar pressure, the capillary will be opened; the force driving blood through the capillary will be the difference in pressure between the arteriole and venule. If the alveolar pressure exceeds the venous pressure, the alveolar pressure will collapse the venous end of the capillary. In this instance, flow is determined not by the difference between the arteriolar and venular pressures but rather by the difference between arteriolar and alveolar pressures. The point at which blood drains into the veins is like a sluice or waterfall; blood cascades into the low-pressure venule, past the constriction produced by the alveolar pressure on the venular end of the capillary. This type of variable transmural pressure acting to collapse capillaries is called a Starling resistor (Fig. 5-6). When a person is at rest, alveolar pressure in the apices of the lung exceeds both arteriolar and venular pressures during diastole. During systole, arteriolar pressure rises above alveolar pressure and the sluice opens.

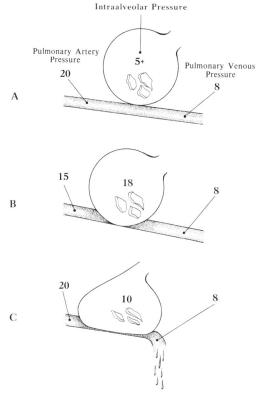

Fig. 5-6.   Starling resistors. (A) Both venous and arterial pressures are greater than intraalveolar pressure, so the driving pressure is the difference between pulmonary artery pressure and pulmonary venous pressure. (B) The intraalveolar pressure exceeds the pulmonary artery pressure, resulting in complete interruption of flow. (C) The intraalveolar pressure exceeds the venous pressure, and flow is like the flow over a waterfall.

CAPILLARY FLUID EXCHANGE

Actual measurement of alveolar pressure shows that the relationship between alveolar pressure and capillary pressure is not as simple as the above description makes it seem. The full force of the alveolar pressure is not transmitted to the capillaries which surround them. Since the transcapillary forces which control the geometry of the alveolar capillaries also control the exchange of fluid across the alveolo-capillary membrane, the effects of intra- and extracapillary pressures on fluid exchange and geometry are best discussed together.

Between the blood in the pulmonary capillary and the air in the alveolus are: (1) the endothelial lining of the capillaries, (2) the base-

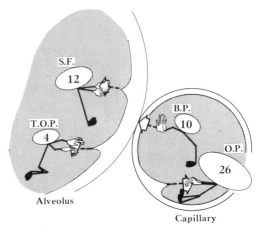

A   Normal

Fig. 5-7. The balance of pressure across the alveolo-capillary membrane. (A) Normal. The forces leading to egress of fluid from a capillary are: *S.F.*, pericapillary hydrostatic pressure of 12 cm. H_2O, most of which is an effect of surface tension at the air–fluid interface; *T.O.P.*, the oncotic pressure of the extravascular proteins, 4 cm. H_2O; and the mean capillary hydrostatic pressure, *B.P.*, 10 cm. H_2O. These forces favoring exudation are balanced by *O.P.*, the oncotic pressure of the plasma proteins, 26 to 30 cm. H_2O.

(B) Elevation of left atrial pressure. This upsets the balance, raising the capillary pressure (*B.P.*) from 12 to 25 cm. H_2O, so that fluid escapes. This will first be manifested in the dependent portions of the lung, where the effect of increased left heart pressure is added to the pressure resulting from the hydrostatic pressure of the column of blood (see Fig. 5-8). Because the filtration exceeds reabsorption, the surfactant is less effective.

(C) Loss of surfactant. The surface tension increases from 12 to 18 or 20 cm. H_2O, making the forces removing fluid from the capillary exceed the oncotic pressure of proteins, and fluid escapes into the alveolus.

(D) Hemodilution results in a fall in oncotic pressure from 26 to 23 cm. H_2O, due to decreased concentration of serum proteins, and effusion results.

ment membrane, (3) the alveolar epithelial lining, and (4) the film of fluid lining the alveolus. To maintain the functional integrity of this interface there must be no net exchange of fluid across it (Fig. 5-7). This requires a net force of zero across the membrane. The colloid osmotic pressure of the plasma proteins (oncotic pressure), which is 26 to 30 cm. H_2O, exerts a force to hold fluid in the capillary. Opposed to the oncotic pressure are the mean hydrostatic pressure in the capillary, 10 to 12 cm. H_2O, the colloid osmotic pressure of proteins in the extravascular space, 4 cm. H_2O, and the pericapillary hydrostatic pressure, -10 to -14 cm. H_2O. Since the oncotic pressure of intra- and extravascular proteins is quite constant, the pericapillary and intravascular

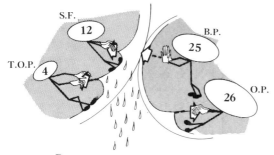

B Increased left atrial pressure

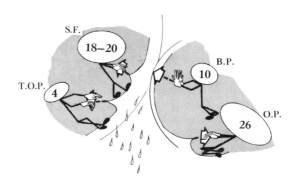

C Loss of surfactant

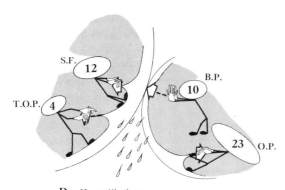

D Hemodilution

hydrostatic pressures are the variable forces which alter vessel geometry and fluid exchange across the capillary.

The negative pericapillary hydrostatic pressure results from the forces created at the air–fluid interface in the alveoli and is not the same as the alveolar pressure. The spheres of air contained by the alveoli are lined with a thin film of liquid, much like a soap bubble (see Surface Tension Statics of Lung, p. 00). The intramolecular forces in the film of fluid at the air–fluid interface which cause the film to compress the gas bubble create a negative force on the fluid, or capillary, side of the bubble. This negative pressure sucks in fluid from the capillary and opens its lumen. If this film was made up of body fluids without a surface-active compound, the pericapillary negative pressure would be 20 to 40 cm. H_2O instead of 10 to 14 cm. H_2O. The surfactant compound present in the alveolar lining diminishes the surface tension and thus the force sucking on the capillary membrane. To maintain an effective surfactant film on the alveolar surface and prevent fluid transudation, the alveoli must be perfused with blood and hyperinflated at regular intervals.

Lung inflation itself alters the forces on the capillary. As the alveolus expands, the air bubble gets larger, which should decrease the surface tension and thus the sucking force on the capillary. However, as the alveolar surface enlarges, the surfactant becomes less effective and surface tension remains the same despite the enlargement of the bubble. As a result, there is little change in the sucking effect of surface tension on the capillary during inflation of the lung. The intraalveolar pressure does rise somewhat and can decrease the size of the capillaries. However, the changes in pulmonary blood flow due to changes in intrathoracic pressure are more the result of changes in filling of the right heart than changes in capillary geometry. Only at very high lung volumes is the volume of blood in the lungs measurably decreased by compression of the vessels. In the range of normal tidal volume, the effect of lung inflation on capillary geometry and fluid exchange is minimal.

More commonly the loss of surfactant is the secondary, not the primary, cause of change in transcapillary pressure and associated changes in vessel geometry and exchange of fluid. The common primary cause of effusion of fluid out of the capillary is a rise in the mean intracapillary hydrostatic pressure. Fluid leaves the capillary at the arterial end, where hydrostatic pressure is highest; it is reabsorbed at the venous end, where hydrostatic pressure is low. Elevation in pulmonary artery pressure can increase hydrostatic pressure at the arterial end of the capillary while that at the venous end remains low, causing little alteration in mean capillary pressure. In some hyperkinetic states of the circulation, such as are present in patients with high-flow ventricular or atrial septal defects, the pressure at the arterial end of the capillary produces a rise in mean capillary pressure. In these conditions, fluid escape at the arterial end of the capillaries exceeds reabsorption at the venous end. In heart failure, escape of fluid from the capillaries results from an increase in mean capillary pressure, which is due to a modest rise in pulmonary arterial pressure and a more marked rise in pulmonary venous pressure.

Once fluid escapes into the alveoli, surface tension increases, due to a decrease in the size of the air bubble. At the same time, the surfactant also becomes less active, due to reabsorption from the surface. As a result, effusion initiated by a rise in intracapillary hydrostatic pressure is enhanced by the increase in surface tension due to fluid effusion. Since the sum of forces acting across the alveolo-capillary membrane is nearly zero, a small increase in intracapillary pressure can upset the balance and lead to effusion of fluid into the alveolus. However, the system is not as unstable as it might seem, because the amount of fluid that escapes from the capillary is not only dependent on elevation of pressure, but also on the duration of the elevation. Any given elevation in intracapillary pressure causes a certain amount of fluid to filter out per minute. If the elevation of pressure is small, the amount filtered out of the capillary per minute will be small, and vice versa.

In every individual fluid is constantly escaping from some pulmonary capillaries and being reabsorbed in others (Fig. 5-8). When a person lies on his back, intracapillary hydrostatic pressure in the posterior portions of the lung increases, due to the hydrostatic pressure exerted by the gravitational force of the column of blood in the vessels leading to the heart in its anterior position. In the lateral decubitus position the distance between the heart and the most dependent area of lung would be greater than in the supine position, and effusion would appear to be inevitable. In the portions of the lung above the heart the gravitational force of the column of blood in the vessels opposes the pressures developed by the heart, and fluid moves from the alveoli into the capillaries. Although in the dependent portions of the lungs some fluid does escape from the capillaries, no area of lung is dependent long enough for excessive effusion to accumulate, because the healthy individual, even in sleep, changes position frequently. The constant turning from one position to another assures that fluid which escapes when an area of the lung is dependent is reabsorbed when it becomes the superior portion of the lung. If a patient does not turn frequently, the dependent alveoli fill with fluid.

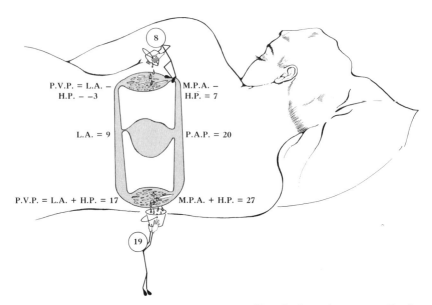

P.V.P. = L.A. –
H.P. – –3

M.P.A. –
H.P. = 7

L.A. = 9

P.A.P. = 20

P.V.P. = L.A. + H.P. = 17

M.P.A. + H.P. = 27

Fig. 5-8. Effect of position on pulmonary capillary hydrostatic pressure. In the lateral decubitus position, even with a normal left atrial pressure (L.A.) and pulmonary artery pressure (P.A.P.), the hydrostatic capillary pressure in the dependent areas of lung is increased due to the gravitational effect of the column of blood (H.P.) in the pulmonary arteries (M.P.A.) and pulmonary veins (P.V.P.) and fluid escapes from the capillaries into the interstitial spaces and the alveoli. In the superior lung, capillary hydrostatic pressure is decreased to 8 and fluid is removed from interstitial spaces and alveoli.

In addition to these hydrostatic and oncotic forces controlling fluid distribution in the lung, mention should be made of the lymphatic system, which reabsorbs both fluid and proteins escaping from the capillaries. The exact quantitative importance of the lymphatic system is not completely worked out.

ABNORMAL PULMONARY CIRCULATORY DYNAMICS

Most abnormalities of the pulmonary circulation are complex combinations of alterations in the circulatory dynamics. A description of some of the combinations which are associated with clinical entities will illustrate the mechanism of disease and the rationale of therapy.

PULMONARY EDEMA

Pulmonary edema results when the fine balance of pressures across the pulmonary capillaries is upset. The usual cause of the unbalance of forces about the capillary is a rise in mean intracapillary hydrostatic pressure. When the net pressure across the capillary favors escape of fluid into the alveoli, pulmonary edema does not occur instantaneously. The rapidity with which clinical pulmonary edema occurs depends on the level of increase in effusion pressure (Fig. 5-9). If the change in balance of pressures is small, it may take hours for significant edema to

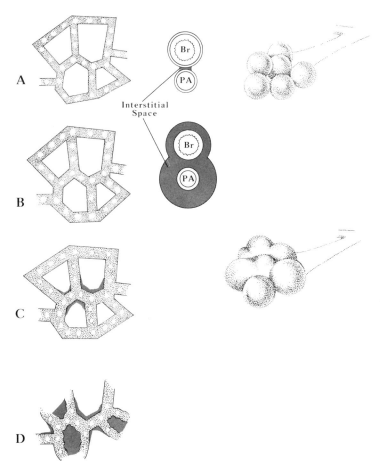

Fig. 5-9. The sequence of changes in effusion of fluid in the lungs. Fluid accumulation in the lungs is dependent on both the force and the time over which it acts. (A) Normal without effusion. (B) There is only an increase in interstitial fluid, first about the bronchioles (*Br*) and precapillary vessels (*PA*). (C) The tissues are distended; fluid starts to escape into the alveoli mostly at the corners, where curvature is greater and surface force larger. (D) Some alveoli have reached the point at which normal inflation pressure cannot maintain stability, and the alveoli collapse to a smaller volume. (From N. C. Straub, H. Nagano, and M. L. Pearce, Pulmonary edema in dogs, especially the sequence of fluid accumulation in lungs. *J. Appl. Physiol.* 22:237, 1967.)

occur. If the intracapillary hydrostatic pressure rises acutely to high levels, clinical pulmonary edema can occur in minutes.

The major force pulling fluid into the capillaries, the colloidal osmotic pressure of the plasma proteins, would have no effect without a semipermeable membrane to keep a concentration difference across the capillary wall. An overworked explanation for the occurrence of pulmonary edema is that there is an alteration in the permeability of this membrane. While occasionally pulmonary edema may result from an increased permeability of this membrane, most forms of pulmonary edema can be explained by a study of the balance of pressures across the capillary membrane.

An example of a type of pulmonary edema that has been erroneously attributed to altered capillary permeability is so-called neurogenic pulmonary edema. In this condition, rather than reflex alteration in the capillary permeability, there is acute systemic vasoconstriction resulting from central initiation of release of catecholamines and direct autonomic excitation. The increased systemic vascular tone increases right heart filling and thus right heart output; the left heart must therefore respond with a similar increase in output. Systemic vasoconstriction increases the impedance to blood flow in the systemic circuit and the force the left ventricle must generate to eject each cubic centimeter of blood. The combination of increase in volume to be ejected and force required per cubic centimeter of blood ejected requires an increase in left heart filling pressure, the pulmonary venous pressure. The rise in pulmonary venous pressure elevates the mean capillary pressure, so fluid escapes from the capillaries. If the function of the left ventricle is compromised by myocardial abnormality or coronary sclerosis, a lesser central nervous system stimulus can cause an excessive elevation in mean capillary pressure.

Once the chain of events is started, pulmonary vascular congestion and edema make the lungs stiff and may cause bronchoconstriction. These alterations in lung mechanics upset ventilation-perfusion coordination. This incoordination, plus alveolar edema, slow the exchange of gas across the alveolar membrane. The decrease in mechanical and gas exchange efficiency of the lung requires increased work to achieve the same oxygen and carbon dioxide transport. Hypoxemia often results, which further lowers the efficiency of the myocardium at the time the increased ventilatory work requires an increased cardiac output. Therapy for interrupting this interacting combination of factors which are worsening the pulmonary edema includes measures to relieve the patient of the work of ventilation, vasodilators to lower peripheral resistance, and inotropic agents such as digitalis to strengthen the myocardium.

The mechanism of production of pulmonary edema in patients with mitral stenosis is somewhat different from that of neurogenic pulmonary edema. In mitral stenosis obstruction is present proximal to the left ventricle. Anything which requires increased rate of flow through the fixed mitral valve orifice will require increased pressure. Tachycardia decreases the portion of the cardiac cycle devoted to diastole. This results in a decreased proportion of each minute for flow through the mitral valve. To merely maintain the same cardiac output, mitral flow rate will need to increase. The increased flow rate can be achieved only by increased left atrial pressure. If the tachycardia is associated with an increased cardiac output, the flow rate and thus the venous pressure will be increased, because both the time available is shorter and the volume that must pass through the valve is increased. These patients can develop massive pulmonary edema in only a few minutes. Often patients with mitral stenosis have reflex constriction of the precapillary vessels. This damps surges in flow and pressure due to changes in right heart output. The vasocontriction protects the capillaries from the right ventricular and pulmonary artery pressure surges, thus lessening the probabilities of pulmonary edema.

Patients with pulmonary edema feel better sitting bolt upright. In the upright posture the upper portions of the lung are protected from the total effect of elevated pulmonary venous pressure by the hydrostatic column of blood, i.e., by the distance from the venous end of the capillary to the left ventricle. The geometry of the pulmonary vascular bed is such that, in the supine position, a larger proportion of the pulmonary capillary and venous beds is at or below the level of the left ventricle than is the case in an upright posture. Thus people with left heart failure are orthopneic, or more comfortable in a sitting position, because the upper portions of the lung are protected by the gravitational force of the column of blood, which lowers mean capillary pressure in the apices and keeps them relatively free of edema.

The syndrome of paroxysmal nocturnal dyspnea illustrates an intriguing type of pulmonary edema that is related to posture. The supine posture leads to a shift of fluid from the systemic to the pulmonary circuit. In patients with elevated pulmonary venous pressure, the lungs have little further capacity to accept volume. In addition, the supine position removes the hydrostatic effect of the erect posture in protecting part of the lungs from the transudation of fluid into the alveoli and probably places a larger portion of the lung below the level of the heart than is the case in the upright posture. During the hours of sleep these two factors lead to progressive transudation of fluid into the dependent alveoli, until the patient awakes with the feeling of suffocation. The assumption of the upright posture diminishes venous return to the right heart and makes more use of the hydrostatic effect due to position to provide filling pressure to the left ventricle. This simple maneuver relieves the patient.

A sequence of events similar to that which leads to paroxysmal nocturnal edema can occur more slowly in the postoperative or unconscious patient. If a patient remains in the supine posture for a prolonged period, the pressure in the venous end of the capillaries in the posterior portions of the lung is elevated by the gravitational effect of the column of blood between the heart and the dependent lung. The net pressure forcing fluid from the capillaries is small, and over a short period little or no fluid escapes. However, if the patient is immobile for many hours or days, significant congestion will result in the dependent lung.

We have had one dramatic case which illustrates the dangers of remaining in one position (see Fig. 5-8, p. 122). A 13-year-old boy following repair of a ventriculo-atrial shunt persisted in lying in the right lateral decubitus position for the first four postoperative days. He developed cyanosis and dyspnea as a result of edema and congestion of the right lung. The edema cleared with ventilatory support and enforced turning from side to back to side. Frequent changes of position are essential to the preservation of the integrity of the alveolo-capillary gas exchange surface.

A special type of pulmonary edema, acute mountain sickness, is not associated with an increase in venous pressure. Before careful studies of patients with this syndrome were made, it was thought that the low inspired oxygen tension somehow led to increased permeability of the capillaries. In these patients both cardiac output and pulmonary artery pressure are elevated, a combination which increases the mean capillary pressure without increasing the pulmonary venous pressure. The elevation of mean capillary pressure causes transudation of fluid into the alveoli and severe dyspnea and cyanosis. When oxygen is administered or the patient is returned to sea level, cardiac output and pulmonary artery pressure fall and the patient promptly recovers.

It is probable that acute mountain sickness represents a prolonged inescapable stress. All individuals have a level of stress which if continued too long would elevate cardiac output and pulmonary artery and/ or venous pressure until mean capillary pressure is high enough to cause effusion. If the myocardium is weak, pulmonary edema may result from increased pulmonary venous pressure due to left heart failure. If the myocardium is strong, the mechanism of production of pulmonary edema will be that seen in mountain sickness.

Another mechanism for the production of pulmonary edema is the destruction or adsorption of surfactant from the alveolar surface (Fig. 5-7c, p. 119). The resultant increased surface tension sucks fluid in from the pulmonary capillaries and causes progressive pulmonary edema. This is the primary cause of fluid effusion into the alveoli in hyaline membrane disease, post-pump syndrome, oxygen toxicity, and ligation or embolic obstruction of the pulmonary artery. Secondary loss of the effectiveness of surfactant can follow alveolar effusion resulting from cardiac failure or failure to periodically regenerate surfactant by deep breathing.

To summarize, pulmonary edema results from the disturbance of the fine balance of forces across the capillary membrane. The initiating factors can be cardiac insufficiency, position, hyperkinetic pulmonary circulation, destruction of surfactant, severe hypoproteinemia, and uneven ventilation. In fact, in all clinical situations pulmonary edema is the result of a complex interaction of many, if not all, of these factors.

The treatment of pulmonary edema is both general and specific. The initiating cause must be identified and the abnormality corrected if possible. For example, in edema due to static position, frequent turning may suffice. In mitral stenosis slowing the heart rate may be critical. General treatment depends on inotropic agents to enhance cardiac function, sitting the patient up, and finally using artificial ventilation if lesser methods are ineffective. Artificial ventilation acts primarily by increasing oxygenation and removing respiratory work, which makes a small cardiac output adequate to the metabolic demands of the patient.

PULMONARY HYPERTENSION

Classification.   Pulmonary hypertension can have a number of initiating causes, but the clinical syndrome is always complex, the result of a number of changes in the character of the pulmonary circulation. One of the most difficult problems in cardiovascular and thoracic surgery is accurate assessment of the functional status of the pulmonary circulation, which is essential in predicting the likelihood of reversion to normal if the initiating cause for the hypertension is corrected.

The pulmonary vascular bed has a great reserve and can accommodate large increases in flow without increases in pressure. Two-thirds of the pulmonary vascular bed must be shut off to elevate pulmonary artery pressure at rest. If less than two-thirds of the vascular bed is shut off, pulmonary artery pressure will be elevated only when flow increases, as with exercise. There are five types of disturbance which can initiate elevation of pulmonary artery pressure.

Passive Pulmonary Hypertension.   Passive pulmonary hypertension is the result of malfunction of the left heart. If as a result of cardiac dysfunction the pulmonary venous pressure is elevated to maintain the same cardiac output, pulmonary arterial pressure must also rise to maintain an adequate driving pressure. The driving pressure may be less for any given flow when pulmonary venous pressure is elevated because of decreased vascular resistance as a result of vessel distension (see Fig. 5-3, p. 111).

Vasoconstrictive Pulmonary Hypertension.   The pulmonary vasomotor activity is a factor in all clinical conditions which result in pulmonary hypertension. To maintain the same pulmonary artery pressure as flow increases with increasing exercise requires vasodilation of the pulmonary vessels. In many patients with pulmonary hypertension, the critical prognostic problem is the relative contribution to the diminution in cross-sectional area of the pulmonary vascular bed due to reversible vasoconstriction versus irreversible organic obliteration.

Hyperkinetic Pulmonary Hypertension.   The term hyperkinetic pulmonary hypertension refers to those situations in which pulmonary blood flow is elevated, even at rest. Such situations include atrial and ventricular septal defects, patent ductus arteriosus, etc. This type of pulmonary hypertension comes about because the cross-sectional area of the pulmonary vascular tree has finite limits, and, therefore, if cardiac output is increased enough, pressure must rise to maintain flow.

There can be hyperkinetic pulmonary vascular flow without pulmonary hypertension if the added flow is accommodated by vasodilation of the vascular bed, and this does not result in an increased left heart filling pressure. If pulmonary vasodilation decreased resistance to one-third that at normal resting flow, a fivefold rise in flow from 100 to 500 cc. per second would require an increase in mean driving pressure from 12 to 20 mm. Hg.

At Cardiac Output 6 L./min. (100 cc./sec.)	At Cardiac Output 30 L./min. (500 cc./sec.)
$R = \dfrac{15 - 5}{100}$	$R = \dfrac{20 - 5}{500}$
$= 0.1$ mm. Hg/cc./sec.	$= 0.03$ mm. Hg/cc./sec.

If resistance fell by one-half instead of one-third, the mean driving pressure would need to rise to only 30 mm. Hg. Because of the ability of the normal pulmonary vascular bed to dilate, large shunts can be accommodated with only small elevations in driving pressure.

Obstructive Pulmonary Hypertension.   Obstructive pulmonary hypertension results from thrombosis or emboli blocking the pulmonary
vessels. Embolic obstructive pulmonary hypertension is presented in
the discussion of pulmonary emboli. In patients with long-standing
pulmonary vascular hypertension due to intracardiac shunts of valvular
heart disease, there is progressive medial and intimal thickening
and thrombosis of the small vessels. This can proceed to a point
at which so much of the pulmonary vascular bed is obliterated that
resistance in the pulmonary vascular bed exceeds that in the systemic
vascular bed and pulmonary artery pressure is greater than systemic
artery pressure. In patients with intracardiac shunts flow goes from right
to left rather than from left to right. Less severely affected patients with
shunts and obliterative disease may have left-to-right shunt at rest but
right-to-left or mixed shunt during exercise.

Obliterative Pulmonary Hypertension.   The label *obliterative pulmonary hypertension* covers all those disease states which result in loss
of pulmonary vessels by structural deterioration. As alveoli coalesce in
emphysema, the capillaries in the ruptured septa are destroyed. Athero-
sclerotic changes, either prematurely due to another cardiac or environmental stress on the pulmonary vasculature or simply as the result of the
"normal" aging process, can reduce the bed by obliterating larger vessels.

Clinical Syndromes Associated with Pulmonary Hypertension.   Many
authors list a sixth type of pulmonary hypertension, complex pulmonary hypertension, a combination of one or more of the five factors
listed above. Clinical pulmonary hypertension is always complex and
may have elements of all the five factors. An analysis of various clinical
states associated with pulmonary hypertension illustrates the critical
prognostic significance of determining which factors control the level of
pulmonary artery pressure.

Hypertension Initiated by Vasoconstriction.   The most extensively
studied type of vasospastic pulmonary hypertension is that seen in individuals living at or going to high altitudes, where the partial pressure
of oxygen is reduced. These studies have clarified the mechanism of
vasoactive pulmonary hypertension and so deserve a detailed discussion.
Young children who were born and raised at high altitudes have
pulmonary hypertension in the range of 58 to 32 mm. Hg, with a mean of
45 mm. Hg. This is a striking difference from children raised at sea
level, who have normal pressures by six months of age. Adults and older
children living at high altitudes have a lower but definitely elevated

pulmonary arterial pressure of 41 to 18 mm. Hg, with a mean of 28. In the adults, during exercise, when pulmonary blood flow is doubled, the pressure is also doubled. The breathing of 35% oxygen to restore normal oxygen tension or the infusion of acetylcholine reduces the resting pulmonary artery pressure to normal. After two years of living at sea level these same individuals have pulmonary artery pressures at rest that are nearly normal, but the pressures are still mildly elevated with exercise.

Anatomical studies of the lungs of people who have lived for prolonged periods at high altitudes show that their muscular pulmonary arteries extend more peripherally than is normal and that the amount of arterial muscle running along the alveolar ducts is increased. In those born and remaining at high altitudes it appears that the involution of the fetal characteristics of the pulmonary arteries and arterioles fails to occur during the first six months of life. This distinctive microscopic anatomy of people raised at high altitudes may be due to chronic vasoconstriction induced by anoxia. Regardless of the cause, this anatomical difference can account for the persistence of elevation of pulmonary artery pressure with exercise after descent to sea level. Persons acclimatized to high altitudes all have pulmonary hypertension and right ventricular hypertrophy. Whether the pattern returns to normal after prolonged periods at sea level is not known.

Studies of people living at high altitudes and those going to high altitudes show that there is considerable variation in individual response to the hypoxia. Some people develop mountain sickness, or Seroche, the result of poor acclimatization to altitude. (Brisket disease in cattle is similar.) These individuals have alveolar hypoventilation, easy fatigability, and respiratory distress with exertion. They develop severe hypoxemia, hypercapnia, polycythemia, and pulmonary hypertension.

A more acute manifestation of mountain sickness is seen in certain people who go to altitudes above 10,000 feet and, without acclimatization, undertake vigorous exercise such as skiing. (The same syndrome can occur without exercise.) It is more common in children but may be seen at any age. After 24 to 96 hours at high altitudes, these patients develop severe hypoxemia, pulmonary hypertension, and manifestations of shock and diffuse pulmonary edema. Unless they are removed to a lower altitude or are given oxygen, death can result. The best evidence suggests that the disease is initiated by a combination of pulmonary vasoconstriction and increased cardiac output. The theories to explain the mechanism of the development of pulmonary edema have been discussed in the section on pulmonary edema.

There is clear evidence now that, like hypoxia, acidemia can cause an increase in the pulmonary vascular resistance, which is dependent on the degree of hydrogen ion (pH) change, not on the level of the pCO_2. Alveolar hypoventilation with the consequent hypoxemia and hypercapnia can produce enough vasoconstriction and elevation of pulmonary artery pressure to cause the syndrome cor pulmonale. The most striking example of this is seen in patients with excessive obesity, the so-called Pickwickian syndrome. These patients have anatomically normal lungs but chronic hypoventilation and increased cardiac output. This combination of anoxia and hypercapnia leads to pulmonary vasoconstriction due to low pO_2 and elevated hydrogen ion concentration, or acidemia. The vasoconstriction and increased cardiac output can result in severe pulmonary hypertension and even cor pulmonale. Correction of the acidemia and hypoxemia will lower the pulmonary artery pressure.

During the immediate postoperative period following thoracotomy for either pulmonary resection or cardiac surgery, the pulmonary vascular resistance rises and leads to a rise in pulmonary artery pressure. The increased resistance is a vasospastic phenomenon and is more severe if hypoxemia or hypercapnia are allowed to develop. In areas of atelectasis there may be an associated transient obstructive element due to collapse of the capillary bed.

Loss of Lung Tissue.   A study of patients and animals who have had major pulmonary resections has permitted some quantitative study of the amount of lung which can be ablated before the development of pulmonary hypertension. Approximately two-thirds of the vascular bed must be obliterated before the resting pulmonary artery pressure rises; or, stated another way, only one-third of the vascular cross-sectional area is needed for the conduction of the resting cardiac output at normal pressures. On the other hand, if two-thirds of the vascular bed is unavailable, any increase in cardiac output will be dependent on a rise in the driving pressure. This in turn will require increased work of the right ventricle. Studies have been made of the pressure increments imposed by this reduction in cross-sectional area. Figure 5-4 (p. 112) shows the relationship between flow rate and pressure in normal individuals and in those who have undergone pulmonary resection. If the pulmonary vascular bed is obstructed or obliterated by any other process, presumably the same relationships would hold true.

There are a number of diseases which lead to destruction of the pulmonary vascular bed. The most obvious of these are chronic infectious processes like bronchiectasis, tuberculosis, etc., which destroy the alveolo-capillary network. If a region of lung to be resected has been destroyed by an infection, its removal will not significantly alter the cross-sectional area of the vascular bed. Most chronic infectious processes which require pulmonary resection destroy the pulmonary vascular bed in the area. However, if normal lung must be included in the resection of diseased lung, the functional cross-sectional area of the vascular bed obviously will be further decreased.

Degenerative Lung Disease.   Aging of itself leads to some diminution in the size of the pulmonary vascular bed, due both to obliteration and to obstruction of small vessels. This normal aging process is not associated with any elevation of pulmonary artery pressure, even with moderate exercise. As the aging process proceeds, the peaks of possible physical activity diminish, and so the demand for high flow rates also falls. Therefore the loss of vascular bed in the normal aging process in the lung is rarely a limit to an individual's exercise tolerance. The degenerative diseases such as obstructive emphysema or diffuse fibrosis obliterate large portions of the vascular bed. These diseases disrupt both the ventilatory and circulatory mechanics of the lung.

In obliterative disease, particularly that associated with emphysema, vasoconstriction plays an important role in aggravating the pulmonary hypertension. An acute respiratory illness which increases difficulty with ventilation leads to hypoxemia and acidemia, which in turn add vasoconstrictive obstruction to the anatomical obstruction of the pulmonary vascular bed. The rise in resistance due to this vasoconstriction raises pulmonary artery pressure more and further burdens the already overworked myocardium. Cardiac output falls below the need of the tissues for perfusion, so the patient is less able to do the added work of ventilation. Unless this downward spiral is interrupted by assisting ventilation, oxygen therapy, and the administration of digitalis, death is inevitable.

Pulmonary Embolic Disease.   In acute pulmonary embolism the effect of the obstructing clot or clots is compounded by a severe vasospastic reaction which may be more important than the embolic obstruction. Unless vasospasm is present, obstruction of less than two-thirds of the pulmonary vascular bed does not lead to vascular collapse. Much of the acute vascular collapse which patients have following a nonfatal embolus may be due to vasoconstriction. Peripheral emboli appear to produce more vasoconstriction than do emboli large enough to be caught in a main pulmonary artery. For example, when one of the main pulmonary arteries is obstructed with a balloon, there is little evidence of vasoconstriction; in fact, there is apparently vasodilation. During this acute obstruction the total cardiac output is accommodated by the intact pulmonary artery without significant rise of pulmonary artery pressure.

Since recent work using either isotope scanning technique or angiography shows most pulmonary emboli are lysed and circulation restored, emboli which do not obstruct more than one-half the pulmonary circulation do not require operative intervention. Repeated small emboli, particularly septic emboli can, however, slowly and permanently obstruct major portions of the pulmonary arterial tree. Idiopathic or primary pulmonary hypertension is best explained in this manner, though thrombosis rather than emboli may be the underlying pathological process. In any case, repeated small pulmonary emboli can lead to severe pulmonary hypertension and cor pulmonale. Their prevention, by isolating the source before extensive damage is done, is the only clinically and physiologically sound basis of controlling this disease. When pulmonary hypertension exists, there is no presently feasible therapy.

Obstruction of the vascular bed by multiple thrombosis or pulmonary emboli has the same effect on the capillary bed as obliteration due to infection, fibrosis, or emphysema. But since such obstruction may not have as much deleterious effect on pulmonary mechanics as fibrosis or emphysema, it may be better tolerated.

Elevated Filling Pressure of the Left Heart.   If increased pressure is required to fill the left ventricle, a chain of events can be initiated which leads to serious pulmonary hypertension. The most common causes of pulmonary venous hypertension are mitral valve disease and left heart failure. A rise in pulmonary artery pressure associated with a rise in pulmonary venous pressure is required to maintain the same driving pressure. Arterial pressure does not need to rise as much as venous pressure to maintain the flow rate, because vascular resistance decreases as vessels are distended as a result of the high intraluminal pressure. At this stage of disease, correction of the cause of obstruction to venous outflow will restore pulmonary arterial pressure to normal.

More commonly, the pulmonary arterial pressure is elevated to a degree which cannot be accounted for by the rise in venous pressure. Correction of the element causing increased pulmonary venous pressure in these instances may not restore the pulmonary artery pressure to normal. This complex type of pulmonary hypertension is associated in its earlier stages with constriction of the precapillary bed, followed later by obliteration due to sclerosis and obstruction by thrombosis of the small precapillary vessels.

Whether vasoconstriction in pulmonary hypertension initiated by a high pulmonary venous pressure is protective or not is controversial. It does increase the work of the right ventricle further. However, by increasing the tension required to increase the right ventricular output, the vasoconstriction can damp elevation in capillary pressure due to the surges in right ventricular output and, therefore, pulmonary artery flow and pressure. The constriction also would damp the transmission of the pressure pulse to the capillaries. In this manner, vasoconstriction, though it further burdens the right ventricle, decreases the likelihood of acute rise in intracapillary pressure and resultant pulmonary edema.

Often patients with mitral stenosis or insufficiency are reported to have a very high pulmonary vascular resistance. Despite this apparent high resistance, surprising degrees of pulmonary hypertension disappear following operative repair or replacement of the valve. Most patients in whom the hypertension persists have associated degenerative disease of the lungs or are near-terminal functional Class IV patients at the time of operative repair. Often the reported increase in resistance is spurious and results from failure to subtract the mean left atrial pressure from the mean pulmonary artery pressure in calculating the resistance. The decrease in pulmonary vascular resistance after operative repair of the mitral valve is usually due both to vasodilatation and to reversal of vessel wall thickening.

In patients with high-flow ventricular septal defect or patent ductus arteriosus, there may be significant elevation of left atrial and pulmonary venous pressure due to a required increase in the left ventricular filling pressure. Dogs in which a large systemic pulmonary shunt is acutely created die of pulmonary edema due to left ventricular failure before significant pulmonary hypertension develops. If by some means the ventricle is conditioned to the increased cardiac output prior to creation of the shunt, flow great enough to cause pulmonary hypertension can be maintained without left ventricular failure.

Pulmonary Hypertension in Patients with Congenital Heart Disease. Patients with ventricular septal defect or patent ductus arteriosus who have high pulmonary blood flow may have pulmonary hypertension. In ventricular septal defect or patent ductus arteriosus there are two major resistances in series that impede the flow of blood from the systemic circulation through the pulmonary circulation. These are the impedance to flow offered by the defect and that offered by the pulmonary vasculature. The flow to the systemic circuit must overcome only the systemic vascular resistance. In patent ductus arteriosus or ventricular septal defect, the distribution of the left ventricular output between systemic and pulmonary circuits will depend on the relative values of the sum of the series resistances to flow through the defect and through the pulmonary vascular tree versus the resistance in the systemic vascular circuit.

A hypothetical example can be worked out for a patient with a patent ductus arteriosus. If the resistances in the systemic and pulmonary vascular beds are the normal amounts of 0.9 and 0.1 mm. Hg per cubic centimeter per second, respectively, and their two resistances are in parallel, then with no intervening resistance the arterial pressures in the two circuits would be the same. If we disregard venous pressure for the moment, the flow to the pulmonary bed would be nine times that to the systemic bed.

$$Q_P = \frac{P}{R_P} \qquad\qquad Q_S = \frac{P}{R_S}$$
$$= \frac{90}{0.1} \qquad\qquad\quad = \frac{90}{0.9}$$
$$= 900 \text{ cc./sec.} \qquad = 100 \text{ cc./sec.}$$

Where Q_P = pulmonary artery flow
$\quad\quad\quad\ Q_S$ = systemic flow
$\quad\quad\quad\ \ P$ = systemic pressure
$\quad\quad\quad\ R_P$ = pulmonary vascular resistance
$\quad\quad\quad\ R_S$ = systemic vascular resistance

If the ductus creates some resistance, then the flow to the pulmonary artery will decrease in an amount proportional to this added resistance.

$$Q_P = \frac{P}{R_D + R_P} \qquad R_D = 0.23, R_P = 0.1$$
$$= \frac{90}{0.23 + 0.1}$$
$$= 270 \text{ cc./sec.}$$

Where R_D = resistance across the ductus

In this example the ductus raises the resistance, so that only three times as much flow goes through the pulmonary circuit as goes through the systemic circuit. In fact, the pressure in the pulmonary artery would be lower than that in the aorta, so the calculations are more complicated than is indicated. Using 34 mm. Hg as the pulmonary artery pressure, 0.1 mm. Hg per cubic centimeter as the pulmonary resistance, 90 mm.

Hg as the systemic pressure, and 0.23 mm. Hg per liter per second as
the resistance, the calculations would be:

$$Q_P = \frac{P_P}{R_P}$$
$$= \frac{34}{0.1}$$
$$= 340 \text{ cc./sec.}$$

and

$$Q_{SH} = \frac{P_S - P_P}{R_D}$$
$$= \frac{90 - 34}{0.23}$$
$$= 240 \text{ cc./sec.}$$

Where Q_P = pulmonary flow
P_P = pulmonary artery pressure
R_P = pulmonary resistance
Q_{SH} = shunt flow
R_{SH} = shunt resistance
P_S = systemic pressure
R_D = resistance across ductus $(= R_{SH})$

It is apparent that the flow and pressure in the pulmonary circuit are
controlled by the pulmonary, systemic, and shunt resistance. An increase
in pulmonary vascular resistance can likewise affect the distribution of
flow by raising the pulmonary resistance toward that in the systemic bed.
For example, if P_P is 55 mm. Hg, R_P is 0.2 mm. Hg per cubic centimeter, P_S is 90 mm. Hg, and R_{SH} (shunt resistance) is 0.2 mm. Hg per
cubic centimeter,

$$Q_P = \frac{P_P}{R_P}$$
$$= \frac{55}{.2}$$
$$= 280 \text{ cc./sec.}$$

and

$$Q_{SH} = \frac{P_S - P_P}{R_{SH}}$$
$$= \frac{90 - 55}{0.2}$$
$$= 180 \text{ cc./sec.}$$

In the study of patients with patent ductus arteriosus and ventricular septal defect it has been found that if the communicating defect exceeds 1 sq. cm. per square meter of body surface area, there will be little resistance to flow across it (Fig. 5-10). A defect this large or larger offers so little resistance to flow that pressures in the ventricles are equalized, and flow to the pulmonary bed is entirely controlled by the pulmonary vascular resistance.

If pulmonary blood flow and total pulmonary resistance are compared with the systolic gradient across the defect, patients with a high gradient across the defect have normal pulmonary resistance and near-normal pulmonary blood flow. The defect is in this case contributing a significant effective resistance to flow. As the systolic gradient between ventricles decreases, the pulmonary vascular resistance increases a small amount and flow increases markedly. As the gradient across the defect approaches zero, the pulmonary vascular resistance increases so much that the pulmonary flow is usually lower than in defects with some gradient across them. Thus, nonobstructive communications between the two ventricles or between the aorta and pulmonary artery result in high resistance in the pulmonary circuit.

The increased resistance to pulmonary blood flow in patients with high-pressure left-to-right shunts is due to a number of causes. There is good evidence that the resistance vessels are constricted. In addition, in many cases there is definite evidence of structural changes. The microscopic anatomy of the pulmonary arteries and arterioles is very similar to that seen in patients raised at high altitudes. There is also individual variation in the degree of preservation of the fetal pattern which suggests a difference in sensitivity to increased flow and driving pressure, just as there is a difference in sensitivity to chronic hypoxia. In patients with severe pulmonary hypertension, the anatomical changes often have progressed to complete sclerosis and multiple thrombosis of significant portions of the vascular bed.

When this pattern of structural change progresses to endarteritis and obliteration and obstruction of vessels, it prohibits successful surgical

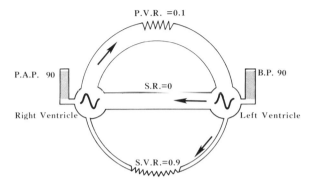

A Defect is greater than $1cm.^2 / M.^2$ body surface, with normal P.V.R.

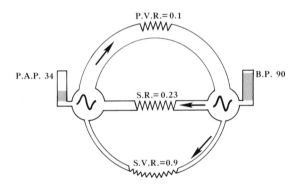

B Smaller defect with normal P.V.R.

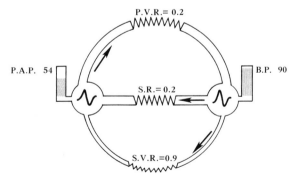

C Same size defect as in **B**, but with P.V.R. doubled

repair of the communication between the two circulations. Elevation of the pulmonary systolic pressure at rest to above 70% of the systemic systolic pressure has been found to be a warning signal that patients may have reached this stage and will not tolerate operative closure of defects.

By determining both pulmonary artery pressure and pulmonary artery flow, a better index of the state of the pulmonary vascular bed can be made. If the pressures are high and the pulmonary flow low, so that the pulmonary resistance is above 70% of the systemic vascular resistance, this high resistance signifies the presence of advanced vascular disease with obliteration and obstruction of the vessels. If the pulmonary flow is high, the resistance is lower, and the hypertension is due to the large shunt flow; in these cases the results of closure are more favorable. Those who have no fall in pulmonary artery pressure and who survive operation may be little improved. Those who do not survive die due to progressive pulmonary obliterative vascular disease. An even better method of differentiating the good- from bad-risk patients may lie in more complete analysis of all the factors impeding flow. These are discussed in the final section of this chapter.

In patients with atrial septal defects there is also high flow through the pulmonary vasculature, so the circulation is hyperkinetic. This condition is different than in the high-pressure defects, because the right ventricle is interposed between the defect and the pulmonary vascular bed. The distribution of blood to the two ventricles therefore depends

---

Fig. 5-10. The effects of change in diameter of ventricular septal defect and relative resistances of the pulmonary and systemic vascular beds on shunt flow and pulmonary artery pressure (P.A.P.). *S.R.*, shunt resistance; *P.V.R.*, pulmonary vascular resistance; and *S.V.R.*, systemic vascular resistance. The width of the lines joining the right and left ventricles are proportional to the flow rate through each. The size of the symbols for resistance is inversely proportional to the resistance in the circuit. In all examples resistance in the systemic bed is 0.9 mm. Hg per cubic centimeter per second, and flow is 100 cc. per second (6 liters per minute), and mean aortic pressure (B.P.) is 90 mm. Hg.

(A) The ventricular defect exceeds 1 sq. cm. per square meter body surface area, so it does not have effective resistance. Pulmonary artery pressure is equal to systemic pressure, and pulmonary resistance is normal, 0.1 mm. Hg per cubic centimeter per second. Flow through the pulmonary artery is 9 times that through the aorta, and flow across the shunt is 8 times that through the aorta.

(B) The defect is smaller and has a resistance of 0.23 mm. Hg per cubic centimeter per second. This results in decreased flow across the shunt; and, with the same pulmonary vascular resistance, the pulmonary artery pressure decreases to 34 mm. Hg, the pulmonary flow to 3.4 times the systemic flow, and the shunt flow to 2.4 times the systemic flow.

(C) Here the pulmonary resistance has risen to 0.2 mm. Hg per cubic centimeter per second and pulmonary artery pressure to 54 mm. Hg, reducing the pressure across the shunt and the resultant flow across the shunt to 1.8 times the systemic flow and the pulmonary flow to 2.8 times the systemic flow.

on the resistance across the defect and the resistance to filling of the two ventricles.

The right ventricle is thinner and requires less filling pressure than the left ventricle. Since pulmonary vascular resistance usually remains low in patients with atrial septal defects, very large shunts may exist without significant elevation of the pulmonary vascular pressure. In fact, alterations in pulmonary vascular resistance would have no direct effect on shunt flow; only increased resistance to filling of the right ventricle will alter this. The increased work load of the ventricle leads to ventricular hypertrophy, and this in time can alter shunt flow by increasing resistance to right ventricular filling. If the high flow results in pulmonary vascular disease, which increases pulmonary vascular resistance, pulmonary hypertension will develop. The pulmonary hypertension in turn will further increase the load on the right ventricle. This increased load may result in right ventricular failure, which elevates filling pressure of the right ventricle above that of the left and reverses the shunt from left-to-right to right-to-left.

Patients with atrial septal defects develop pulmonary hypertension and obliterative vascular disease later in life than patients with high-pressure defects, due to the interposition of the right ventricle; it protects the pulmonary vessels from the high pressure in the left ventricle. The factors operating in control of flow in atrial septal defects are very similar to those present during exercise. Increased right heart filling leads to increased output and pulmonary vasodilatation. Only when the ventricle fails or when the vasculature is damaged by the continued high flow does pulmonary hypertension result.

NEWER CONCEPTS IN THE STUDY OF BLOOD FLOW AND PRESSURE RELATIONSHIPS

In the preceding discussions the assumption was often implicit that pulmonary blood flow obeys Poiseuille's law. However, all the conditions for Poiseuille's law are not met by the pulmonary circulation. The vessels are not long, straight, smooth, narrow, and round; the viscosity does not remain unchanged at different rates of flow; and tube geometry is affected by pressure. It is likely that further understanding of pulmonary circulatory dynamics will be impossible unless the true conditions are analyzed. At present too many people despair of understanding the true conditions. The knowledge and methods for better understanding are being worked out, however, and in this section a brief discussion of some of the new approaches are presented.

TURBULENT FLOW

Poiseuille's law deals only with orderly laminar flow. In fact, the pulmonary flow is not all orderly. When turbulent flow is present, it has been found empirically that forward flow is proportionate to the square root of the pressure rather than linearly related to pressure. The amount of turbulence that will occur depends in part on the Reynold's number (see Appendix, p. 333). Since blood as it enters the pulmonary artery is not flowing in an orderly pattern but is rather sloppy, even at low flow rates, turbulence does exist. Turbulent mixing is apparent from the lack of the usual cone of streamlined flow in the pulmonary artery. The cone is replaced by a flat front, which shows that there is disorder in the flow pattern.

Turbulent flow is a problem only in the larger vessels, since the Reynold's number falls as the radius and velocity of the flowing blood decrease. The cross-sectional area of the vascular bed increases as it branches, and so, from the continuity equation, velocity of blood must decrease as blood moves along from arteriole to capillary. The radius of the individual vessels also decreases as the vascular tree branches. It is, therefore, very unlikely that in the small vessels the Reynold's number at which turbulence occurs will be exceeded.

CHANGES IN KINETIC ENERGY

Another effect of the change in cross-sectional area and thus the slowing of the velocity of blood flow is seen in the conversion of kinetic to potential energy. In Poiseuille's equation, both the driving pressure and the kinetic energy (energy of motion, or velocity) are assumed to be constant. The slowing of the velocity of the blood as it moves along from the arteries to the capillaries requires energy transfer, i.e., the conversion of some of the kinetic energy of motion to potential energy of hydrostatic pressure. This gained potential energy is not all reconverted to kinetic energy in the veins as the cross-sectional area decreases and velocity increases. In the veins blood flow is no longer pulsatile, and this smooth-flowing blood has only approximately one-fifth as much kinetic energy as is present in pulsatile blood flow in the arteries. In the pulmonary vascular tree, the actual situation is such that the slowing of the blood converts kinetic to potential energy; which may be equivalent to an addition of as much as 3 mm. Hg to the driving pressure.

DISTENSIBILITY OF VESSELS

In addition to the special conditions created by turbulence and by the conversion between potential and kinetic energy as blood progresses down the vascular tree, there are special conditions due to the fact that the vessels have elastic walls. The distensible bed will be stretched to different degrees relative not only to the mean pressure but also to the pulse pressure. To determine only pulmonary vascular resistance from mean pressure divided by mean flow is an incomplete description of the factors controlling impedance of flow in the pulmonary vascular bed.

The vascular elements of the lung consist of series of parallel vessels which have elastic properties. The pulsatile flow requires acceleration and deceleration of blood in each segment of the vascular tree, a process which is superimposed on the overall slowing of blood velocity from arteries through the capillaries. Pulsatile flow continues into the pulmonary capillary bed, and when the bed is widely opened in the hyperkinetic states, this pulse is of considerable magnitude. It is apparently damped out by the time blood reaches the veins but may still be present in the venules. To fully describe the forces impeding flow or the energy cost of pushing blood through the vascular network requires a determination of the relation of flow and pressure from moment to moment during each pulse cycle. There is a difference in calculated dissipation of power using mean and pulsatile terms because the mean terms do not consider inertial and compliant reactance. To describe this complex system, impedance, not resistance, must be measured.

Reactance is dependent on frequency and so will be altered by changes in pulse rate. If the pulse wave were a pure sine wave, the impedance could be calculated by knowing the amplitude and frequency of the flow and pressure waves. The pulse wave is not a pure sine wave; it is a complex wave which can be conceived of as a wave made up of the sum of a number of waves of different amplitude and frequency. By using a Fourier analysis, these waves can be broken into their component sine waves and the impedance for each harmonic calculated. This then will permit approximate calculations of physical characteristics of the system.

POWER DISSIPATION

A useful way of analyzing the effect of pulse in the vascular bed is to calculate the actual power dissipated as blood traverses the bed compared to that calculated using mean pressures and cardiac output. By multiplying instantaneous flow times instantaneous pressure and summing or integrating the products during a given period, the actual power dissipated can be calculated. If a simultaneous calculation is made of mean pressure times mean flow, the difference is the power dissipation resulting from the pulsatile nature of flow. In normal subjects approximately 30% of the power dissipated is due to the pulsatile character of

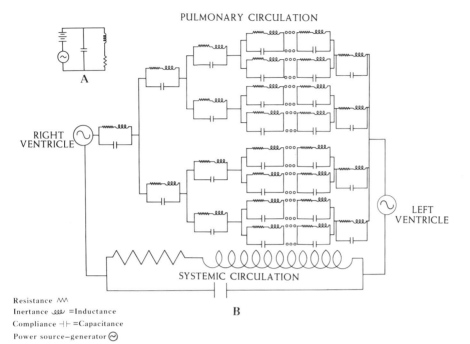

PULMONARY CIRCULATION

RIGHT
VENTRICLE

LEFT
VENTRICLE

SYSTEMIC CIRCULATION

Resistance ⋀⋀⋀
Inertance ⠶⠶ =Inductance
Compliance ╢╟ =Capacitance
Power source–generator ⊘

B

Fig. 5-11. Electrical analogs of the pulmonary vascular bed. (A) Representation of the vascular bed as a simple circuit. The generator is the right ventricle; the battery depicts the fact that the valve does not allow pulmonary flow to be bi-directional, i.e., flow is a pulsed D.C. flow in which the pressure and flow oscillate around the mean values. The inertia and resistance of the system are represented by the resistance and inductance in series. Since the direction of stretch of the elastic vessel walls is at right angles to the direction of flow, the capacitor representing this is in parallel to the series resistor and inductance. As pressure and flow rise during systole, some of the blood volume is stored in the increased volume of the vessels resulting from their increased diameter due to the stretch of the walls. During diastole, the pressure falls and vessels contract, discharging volume and maintaining flow. Since current cannot flow through a capacitor, if a capacitor was in series with the resistance and inductance, blood could not flow through the pulmonary vessels. The charge stored during systole in the parallel circuit shown flows out of the capacitor through the coil and resistor during diastole in the same direction as flow takes during systole.

(B) A more complete electrical analog of the pulmonary vascular bed. It is made up of a number of circuits as shown in (A) minus the power source (battery and generator). Each segment of the pulmonary artery between branchings is in essence an element as shown in (A). As the arteries branch, there is an ever-increasing number of these elements in parallel, reaching the hundreds of millions in the capillaries. The generations of branchings beyond the fourth are represented by OOO. On the venous side the number of subcircuits decreases each generation to reach four at the main pulmonary veins. The systemic circulation is similar, having a larger resistance, capacitance, and inertance because of its larger volume and longer course. Treating the pulmonary circuit by summing these elements as shown in (A) is a reasonable and simple analogy.

the flow. However, under some hyperdynamic situations in which phase angle between flow and pressure exceeds 90 degrees, the power dissipated with pulsatile flow may be less than the calculated power dissipated using mean terms.

PULMONARY VASCULAR IMPEDANCE

Increases in cardiac output are achieved usually by increases in both pulse rate and stroke volume (Fig. 5-11). The increase in stroke volume would lead to an increase in pulse pressure amplitude if the impedance remained the same. In the normal subject the changes in pressure amplitude are small when stroke volume increases. Stated differently, there is a small but measurable rise in systolic pressure with increased stroke volume. If the pressure remains constant and the flow increases, the impedance must fall. This could be due principally to fall in resistance and little change in compliance, or to increase in compliance and a lesser fall in resistance.

Increase in resistance will ordinarily lead to increase in power dissipated due to the pulse. Likewise, decrease in compliance of the vessels will bring the phase of pulse and pressure closer together. It is probable that as pulmonary vascular disease progresses, the resistance increases and the compliance falls. These simultaneous occurrences tend to increase the power dissipation per unit of flow. On the other hand, in the hyperdynamic state of the pulmonary circulation, resistance is usually low and compliance is normal or increased and together they minimize the power dissipation per unit of flow. Hyperdynamic and low-flow hypertension represent the extremes: an intact versus a severely damaged pulmonary vascular bed. The problem for the surgeon is to define the middle ground more precisely, so that he may predict the type of vascular bed which will revert toward normal after surgical correction of the initiating cause of pulmonary hypertension.

6. DIFFUSION

IN the early part of this century there were two major explanations of the transfer of gases across the alveolo-capillary membrane. Haldane contended that there was an active transport mechanism which could transfer gases against pressure gradients, while Krogh and Barcroft presented evidence that the gas exchange was dependent entirely on pressure gradients. At present, evidence supports the contention of Krogh and Barcroft, and so it is necessary to understand clearly the effects of pressure gradients on the transfer of gases.

DIFFUSION OF GASES

All molecules of gas are in constant random motion. If two gases of different composition are placed in the same container, this random motion should result in mixing of the two gases until the concentration throughout the mixture is uniform. In 1829, before molecular theory was developed, the English chemist Graham set down the fundamental law of diffusion, that the diffusion rate of gases is inversely proportional to the square root of their density. The density of a gas is directly proportional to its molecular weight, and the speed of motion of the molecules is inversely proportional to the molecular weight of the gas. Graham's law stated in modern terminology is that the diffusion of gases is inversely proportional to the square root of their molecular weight, or directly proportional to the kinetic energy of the molecules of the gas.

Fick's law defines the other factors controlling diffusion of molecules in a gas from an area of high to one of low concentration.

$$\frac{Q}{t} = K \times S \times \frac{c_1 - c_2}{d}$$

The equation states that Q, the amount of gas that diffuses in t, a given time, is equal to K, the diffusion coefficient, times S, the area across which it diffuses, times $c_1 - c_2$, the concentration gradient, divided by d, the distance. Concentration gradient can be expressed as difference in grams per cubic centimeter, or, in the terms used for measuring gases in physiological studies, as difference in partial pressure of the gas between two points. It is apparent that for any two gases in an alveolus, the only two variables in Fick's equation will be difference in partial pressure, or concentration gradient, and diffusion coefficient. From Graham's law we know that the diffusion coefficient (DC) is proportional to the square root of the molecular weight; therefore, the relative rates of diffusion of carbon dioxide, molecular weight 44, and oxygen, molecular weight 32, are:

$$\frac{DC \text{ for } CO_2}{DC \text{ for } O_2} = \frac{\sqrt{\text{mol wt } O_2}}{\sqrt{\text{mol wt } CO_2}} = \frac{\sqrt{32}}{\sqrt{44}} = \frac{5.6}{6.6}$$

This means that in the gaseous phase carbon dioxide diffuses only 0.85 times as fast as oxygen.

If diffusion is to be an effective means of transport and mixing of gases in the lung, it must be complete in the time available during a respiratory cycle. Solution of Fick's equation for carbon dioxide and oxygen shows that, because of the time limitations of the respiratory cycle, diffusion is an effective means of gas transport only over very limited distances. In a lobule or alveolus with a diameter of 0.5 mm., mixing by diffusion is 80% complete in .002 second; while a fourteenfold increase in the diameter of the alveolus to 7 mm. results in increasing the time for complete mixing by diffusion to 0.38 second, a one hundred and ninetyfold increase. Diffusion in units larger than the primary lobule is too slow for respiratory gas exchange. However, in a normal alveolus of 100 μ, mixing by diffusion is almost instantaneous; and within a lobule of normal size, diffusion is fast enough that the partial pressures of gas in the lobule are essentially uniform. If the alveolus or lobule is enlarged for any reason, mixing by diffusion may not be complete (Fig. 6-1).

To reach the blood, alveolar gas must pass from the gas phase in the alveolus into the liquid phase in the body fluids. Exner in 1875 showed the rate of diffusion of gas from one phase to another was directly proportional to the solubility of the gas in the liquid and inversely proportional to the square root of the molecular weight. This relationship shown by Exner is described by a combination of Henry's and Graham's laws. Henry's law states that the amount of gas dissolved in a liquid is equal to the solubility coefficient of the gas times the partial pressure. If the gas has a high solubility coefficient, there will be a higher concentration of gas at the surface, i.e., a higher number of molecules of dissolved gas per molecule of solute. If there are more molecules of dissolved gas, the concentration gradient between gas molecules at the surface layer of the liquid and the deeper layers will be greater than if the gas has a low solubility coefficient. If the concentration gradient in the liquid surface is greater, the rate of diffusion will be faster. For example, carbon dioxide diffuses 0.85 times as fast as oxygen but is 24.3 times more soluble than oxygen. As a result, carbon dioxide moves from the gas to the liquid phase 20.7 (0.85×24.3) times as fast as oxygen.

The above facts can be summarized in the following equation which

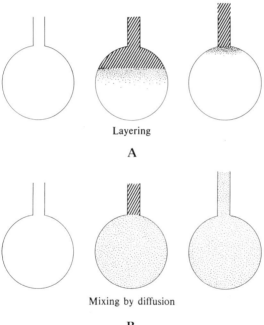

Layering

A

Mixing by diffusion

B

Fig. 6-1. The role of diffusion in mixing of gases in the alveoli. (A) If diffusion did not take place, the inspired gas would layer at the top of the alveolus, as shown in the center diagram, and the recently inspired gas would then be expelled without mixing during expiration (right-hand diagram). (B) Newly inspired gas (center) almost instantaneously diffuses to mix with air already in the alveolus (middle diagram) resulting in a uniform alveolar gas concentration on expiration (right side). There is no boundary between gas of different concentrations. If the alveolus is large, so that diffusion is not complete, the situation shown in (A) will occur.

describes the factors controlling the rate of diffusion of a gas into or out of a liquid.

$$\text{Diffusion/min.} \sim \frac{PG \times CA \times S}{D \times \sqrt{M.W.}}$$

A larger amount of gas will diffuse with (1) increase in pressure gradient, PG; (2) increase in cross-sectional area, CA; or (3) increase in solubility of the gas, S. A smaller amount of gas will diffuse with an increase in distance for diffusion, D; and increasing molecular weight, M.W. The amount of a gas that diffuses across the alveolo-capillary membrane will thus depend on the pressure gradient across the membrane, the area of the alveolo-capillary surface, and the distance across the alveolo-capillary membrane.

THE ANATOMY AND PHYSIOLOGY OF DIFFUSION

The anatomical factors affecting diffusion of gas from gas to blood are the length of the path between gas and the interior of the red cell and the surface area of contact between blood and alveolar air. To travel from an alveolus to a hemoglobin molecule, a molecule of oxygen must pass through: (1) the film of fluid containing surfactant that lines the alveolus; (2) the alveolar epithelium; (3) the basement membrane; (4) the capillary endothelial lining; (5) plasma in the capillary; (6) the red cell membrane; and (7) the intracellular fluid in the cell. At the thinnest point this distance is 0.2 μ and oxygen can diffuse across very rapidly with minimal pressure gradient. However, in substantial areas the path across the alveolo-capillary membrane is as much as three to four times longer than the minimum path. Some of these areas are at the sites of alveolar cells, at turns in capillaries, and in the collecting tubules.

Disease can lengthen any of the layers of this complex pathway between hemoglobin molecule and alveolar air. The film of fluid lining the alveolus can be increased due to lack of surfactant or due to exudation of fluid into the alveolus. The alveolar lining may be thickened by increased thickness of alveolar cells or fibrosis. Edema fluid can accumulate between the epithelium of the alveolar lining and the capillary endothelium due to inflammation, decreased lymphatic function, or increased hydrostatic pressure in the capillary. Dilation of the capillaries by increased venous pressure or distortion of the geometry can increase the intracapillary diffusion distance. Abnormal erythrocytes may lengthen the path within the red cell. All diseases in which there is an increase in the distance between the alveolus and the red cell offer a physical block to gas diffusion. Diseases in which an alveolo-capillary block is the primary defect are the only true disorders of diffusion.

The surface area of the alveolo-capillary membrane is affected not only by the structural anatomy of the lung but also by the functional anatomy. The surface area of the alveoli which is covered by the fine network of capillaries (described in the section on morphometrics in Chapter 1, "Functional Anatomy") is the surface area of the alveoli available for diffusion. This area is usually 50 to 70 square meters and can be increased to 90 square meters when the lungs are fully inflated. Any process which alters the number of pulmonary capillaries perfused with blood will change the capillary surface area. With exercise or change from upright to supine posture, more capillaries are opened and the diffusion surface is increased. Occlusion of a pulmonary artery or surgical shock decreases the surface area because portions of the bed are unperfused.

If the number of alveoli being ventilated is increased or decreased, the surface area for diffusion will be changed. Following a yawn the slow erosion of the surface area is restored as unventilated alveoli are opened up and restored to normal ventilation. Exercise or voluntary hyperventilation increases the number of alveoli ventilated and thus the surface area available for diffusion. If the alveolar walls are destroyed by coalescence, as in emphysema, both the alveolar and capillary surface areas are diminished.

The amount of gas that diffuses across the membrane is also dependent on the difference in mean partial pressure of gas in the alveoli and in the capillaries. The mean partial pressure of a gas in a capillary is not equal to the partial pressure of the venous blood, or the partial pressure of the arterial blood, or the average of the two. It depends on a complex set of factors. These are whether the blood makes chemical combination with the gas, the speed of transit along the capillary, and the concentration of the gas in the venous blood. It is particularly difficult to get a reasonable value for mean capillary pO_2, because the amount of oxygen in the mixed venous blood and the rate of transfer across the membrane is altered by the constantly changing partial pressure difference as the addition of oxygen to the blood decreases the gradient from alveolus to capillary.

The mean alveolar concentration of a gas is also dependent on a number of factors. These are the partial pressure of the gas in the inspired mixture, the ventilation of the alveoli, and the rate at which the gas is removed by the blood.

In summary, the factors determining the amount of a gas that is transported from the gas phase into the liquid phase in the lung are: (1) the mean distance from the alveolar surface to the inside of the red cell, (2) the effective area of the membrane, which is dependent on the number of capillaries perfused and alveoli ventilated, (3) the mean alveolar gas partial pressure, which is dependent on the inspired air partial pressure and the amount and distribution of ventilation, and (4) the mean capillary blood-gas partial pressure, which is dependent on mixed venous gas content or saturation, the rate of blood flow, and whether chemical combination occurs in the blood. If the amount of a gas transported per minute is diminished, it could be the result of any or all of these factors. To delineate the factors involved, physiologists have developed methods of measuring the diffusion capacity.

PULMONARY DIFFUSING CAPACITY

The purpose in measuring the diffusing capacity, D_L, is to determine the resistance to, or force required for, transportation of a unit of gas volume across the alveolo-capillary membrane. By convention, physiologists have used a term that expresses this quantity in terms of the ability of the membrane to conduct gas across it, the conductance. To determine this conductance the rate of gas flow across the membrane is divided by the forcing pressure.

$$D_L = \frac{\text{milliliters of gas transported per minute}}{\text{mean alveolar partial pressure} - \text{mean capillary partial pressure}}$$

The diffusing capacity is presumably a function of the area and thickness of the alveolo-capillary membrane and is independent of the alveolar and capillary partial pressures. The level of ventilation can affect the diffusing capacity only by changing the number of alveoli ventilated and thus the number of alveoli taking part in gas exchange. Blood flow alters diffusing capacity only by changing the number of perfused capillaries and thus the number of capillaries taking part in gas exchange.

To determine diffusing capacity, it is necessary to measure the amount of gas that moves between alveolar air and capillary in a given time and the mean partial pressure between alveolar air and capillary blood. As pointed out earlier (p. 149), it is difficult to determine the mean partial pressure of oxygen in capillary blood. Carbon dioxide cannot be used because the fast diffusion rate results in a pressure gradient so small as to be impossible to determine. If a breath of the soluble foreign gas nitrous oxide is inhaled, the nitrous oxide diffuses across the alveolar membrane very promptly because of its high diffusion coefficient and quickly reaches equilibrium in all the tissues. In other words, it is like carbon dioxide in its speed of diffusion. After the first short period, when the lung tissues are saturated with nitrous oxide, any continued exchange from alveolar gas to blood is dependent on the flow of blood through the capillaries to transport the nitrous oxide away from the lungs. Thus the rate of removal of nitrous oxide from an alveolus is a function of blood flow, not membrane thickness or area.

To measure diffusing capacity, D_L, requires a gas with a significant alveolo-capillary partial pressure difference that permits accurate determination of uptake and measurement of mean capillary and mean alveolar partial pressures. Carbon monoxide has been found to be useful for this purpose. In nonsmokers there is no carbon monoxide in venous blood. Hemoglobin combines with carbon monoxide 100 times more than with oxygen, so carbon monoxide that diffuses into the capillary blood will be promptly bound to hemoglobin whether blood is flowing or not. Only when all the hemoglobin is saturated with carbon monoxide at that partial pressure, will transfer cease. Thus carbon monoxide diffusion is not dependent on the rate of blood flow in the capillaries but rather on the area and thickness of the membrane. The same is true of oxygen; however, carbon monoxide has the advantage that the great affinity of hemoglobin for carbon monoxide and the absence of carbon monoxide in venous blood make it valid to assume that the pCO of capillary blood is zero when the concentrations of carbon monoxide breathed are low enough to prevent saturation of hemoglobin.

To measure diffusing capacity for carbon monoxide (D_{LCO}), gas with 0.3% carbon monoxide is taken in a single breath or breathed for 2 to 3 minutes and the volume of carbon monoxide transferred is measured by determining the functional residual capacity and the percent of carbon monoxide in alveolar gas at the beginning and end of the period of measurement. The mean alveolar pCO is calculated in the breath-holding method and is assumed to be constant in the breathing method. If the diffusing capacity for carbon monoxide is known, theoretically the diffusing capacity for oxygen can be calculated by multiplying D_{LCO} by a factor to correct for the difference in solubility and diffusion coefficient between carbon monoxide and oxygen. In normal individuals D_{LCO} is most closely related to lung volume and therefore is related to body size and to increases with increase in body size. The diffusing capacity for oxygen is 1.23 times the diffusing capacity for carbon monoxide. In a normal male D_{LCO} is 25 cc. per minute per millimeter of mercury, and this gives a D_{LO_2} of 31 ml. per minute per millimeter of mercury.

Since exercise, hyperventilation, and change from erect to supine posture increase the resting diffusing capacity, the term *capacity* is a misnomer. As used to define oxygen capacity of the blood, the term oxygen *capacity* is the maximum or full ability of blood to combine with oxygen; the diffusing capacity is not the maximum capacity of the lung to transport carbon monoxide or oxygen but rather the measured ability under a particular set of circumstances. This misnomer has led to difficulty in interpreting the results of different investigators, because the conditions of measurement are often not recorded carefully enough or are not considered in the interpretation of the results.

FACTORS ALTERING DIFFUSING CAPACITY

In normal individuals diffusing capacity is larger during exercise than at rest, presumably due to perfusion of greater areas of the pulmonary capillary bed (Fig. 6-2). Even in well-trained athletes, during exhausting exercise, when all the capillaries are perfused at a maximum, diffusion can be a limiting factor to oxygen transport. During exhausting exercise both the arteriovenous oxygen difference and the speed of flow through the capillaries increase markedly. As a result, a greater amount of oxygen must diffuse from alveolus to red cell in a shorter period of time. In exhausting exercise the time each aliquot of blood spends in the alveolar capillary is inadequate for enough oxygen to be transported to saturate the hemoglobin, so moderate arterial oxygen unsaturation occurs. Studies have shown that the degree of oxygen unsaturation during exhausting exercise in well-conditioned athletes is greater than in untrained individuals. In well-trained individuals the greater arterial oxygen unsaturation may be due to faster blood flow, greater tolerance to low arterial oxygen, or faster oxygen extraction in muscles causing large arteriovenous oxygen differences.

In patients with congenital heart disease and left-to-right shunts, pulmonary blood flow is increased and resting diffusing capacity approaches levels seen in exercising normal subjects. Presumably the increased pulmonary blood flow perfuses larger areas of the capillary bed than in a normal subject. In pregnant women, who have an elevated cardiac output, the diffusing capacity is not increased as it is in patients with left-to-right shunts. Since blood flow increases with anemia and falls in polycythemia, one might expect diffusing capacity to rise in a patient with anemia and fall in a patient with polycythemia. However, the opposite is true; diffusing capacity falls with anemia and rises with polycythemia. Diffusing capacity in these diseases may depend on the rate of transfer across the red cell membrane rather than on pul-

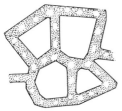

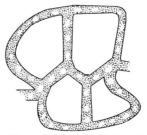

INCREASE

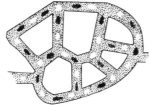

NORMAL

Dilatation of capillary bed

Hyperventilation of alveoli

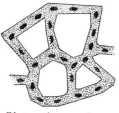

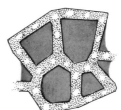

Obstruction or closure
of capillary bed

Failure to ventilate

DECREASE

Destruction of alveolar septa
and capillaries

Increased length of
diffusion path

Fig. 6-2. Factors altering diffusion capacity. At the center is the normal condition, in which one-half the capillaries are open. Above the normal are factors increasing diffusion capacity. The upper left diagram illustrates the case during exercise or in patients with a left-to-right shunt: The entire capillary bed is opened, resulting in an increase in surface area. The upper right diagram shows hyperventilation opening all the alveoli. The factors that decrease diffusing capacity are emboli; obstruction or closure by vasoconstriction of a regional vascular bed; failure to ventilate some alveoli; destruction of alveolar septa and capillaries, which decreases surface area; and lengthening of the diffusion path by edema (see Fig. 5-9, p. 123).

monary bood flow. In surgical shock pulmonary blood flow is decreased and many areas of the capillary bed are unperfused. In shock the decrease in the number of capillaries perfused decreases the diffusing capacity. Increased pulmonary venous pressure opens more of the capillary bed, so heart disease leading to elevation in left atrial pressure also might be expected to increase diffusing capacity. However, when diffusing capacity is measured in patients with mitral stenosis, it is decreased, not increased. This presumably is due to occlusion of areas of the capillary bed by fine vessel disease or to spasm associated with perivascular edema or, perhaps, to dilation of capillaries and increase in diffusion path.

Following surgical procedures in which lung is not resected, diffusing capacity falls and does not return to normal for 7 to 14 days. The reduction is as much as 25% if the thorax is opened and is slightly greater following cardiac bypass. This reduction in diffusing capacity is due to change in the volume of lung being ventilated as well as to change in total lung volume. It may be largely the result of microscopic areas of atelectasis. When lung is resected, the acute changes in diffusing capacity seen with other types of operation are exaggerated. The late decreases in diffusing capacity following pulmonary resection are less than would be expected from the portion of lung volume removed, presumably because there is increased blood flow through the remaining lung.

Pneumothorax reduces diffusing capacity if the lung is significantly collapsed; the increase in flow to and ventilation of the intact lung partially compensates by increasing the diffusing capacity of the intact lung. Acute pulmonary embolism likewise decreases diffusing capacity, though a few weeks afterward diffusing capacity is back to near-normal levels. Inflammation of lungs, such as occurs in pneumonia, also reduces diffusing capacity in approximate proportion to the reduction in lung volume. In patients with emphysema, diffusing capacity is decreased by destruction of capillary and alveolar surfaces consequent to the disruption of alveolar septa. The uneven distribution of ventilation aggravates this reduction, since uneven distribution of ventilation and perfusion decreases total diffusing capacity even if the diffusing capacity of individual alveoli is normal.

In acute pulmonary edema resting diffusing capacity is not markedly reduced until significant numbers of alveoli are filled with fluid and thus not ventilated. Presumably diffusing capacity would be reduced before this if the pulmonary membrane were diffusely thickened. Some thickening does occur but is not great enough to affect diffusing capacity until areas of lung are unventilated due to fluid accumulation within the alveoli. The fall in diffusing capacity in patients with chronic pulmonary congestion, as seen in mitral stenosis or chronic left heart failure, is due to chronic interstitial edema of the lungs which probably leads to fibrosis later and permanent reduction in diffusing capacity.

Arterial thickening or distortions of alveolar membrane are not common. They are seen principally in the chronic nonspecific inflammatory lung diseases which result in chronic fibrosis. Reductions in diffusing capacity or arterial oxygen saturation are far more commonly the result of alterations in ventilation or perfusion, or in the coordination of ventilation and perfusion.

7. COORDINATION OF VENTILATION AND PERFUSION

NEITHER ventilation of areas of the lung that are inadequately perfused with blood returning from the systemic venous system nor perfusion of areas of the lung lacking adequate ventilation provide efficient exchange of oxygen and carbon dioxide between blood and the volume of air breathed in and out. Even in the normal individual there is some incoordination between ventilation and perfusion which is diminished during exercise and aggravated by disease. The control of distribution of pulmonary blood flow and ventilation is dependent upon the mechanical properties of the lung and upon physical forces acting on the various areas of the lung.

MIXING OF GAS AND BLOOD

The concentration of oxygen and carbon dioxide in the blood is different in each of the three vessels entering the right atrium—the superior vena cava, inferior vena cava, and coronary sinus. In the right ventricle and main pulmonary artery the blood from these three vessels is completely mixed so that the concentration of carbon dioxide and oxygen is uniform in the blood entering the various alveolar capillaries. Since blood is pumped unidirectionally through the lungs with separate passages for ingress and egress, blood that has not yet perfused the capillaries is not mixed with blood that has exchanged gas with alveolar air. Gases entering and leaving the alveoli, however, must use the same set of conducting airways for ingress and egress. The volume of air in the alveoli is augmented with air rich in oxygen and low in carbon dioxide during inspiration. If this inspired air is to dilute the alveolar air effectively, it must be uniformly mixed with the air already present in the alveoli. In the airways proximal to the primary lobule this mixing occurs as a result of turbulence in the airways, but the mixing by turbulence in the major airways accounts for only 10 to 15% of the total mixing that occurs in the lungs. The major portion of the mixing of inspired air with air already in the lung takes place after the air reaches the primary lobule. The primary lobule is small enough so that the time available is adequate for complete mixing of the air within it by simple diffusion. Since air in the airway proximal to the primary lobule is mixed only by mass movement and turbulence, the boundary between dead space gas and alveolar gas is at the level of the alveolar ducts (see Fig. 6-1, p. 147).

In patients with diseases such as emphysema, in which the alveolar air spaces are enlarged, diffusion in the lobule may be incomplete in the time available for mixing during each respiratory cycle. Although 85 to 90% of the mixing that occurs in the lungs occurs in the lobules, the gas concentrations in them will not be uniform if the gas reaching the various lobules varies in amount and composition. Likewise, variation in the amount of perfusion of the alveolar lobules will alter alveolar gas concentration, even though the blood going to the alveolar capillaries has uniform gas concentration. Uneven distribution of ventilation and perfusion will thus lead to nonuniformity of the expired gas concentrations coming from various lobules.

FACTORS LEADING TO NONUNIFORM VENTILATION AND PERFUSION

As shown in Chapter 5, "Pulmonary Circulation," p. 114, in the upright posture, perfusion of the apices of the lung is least and the amount of perfusion increases down the lung until a maximum amount occurs at the bases. This is due to the hydrostatic effect of the column of blood. In the lateral decubitus position the dependent lung is perfused more than the superior lung. In the supine posture the apices and bases are perfused equally. No studies have been made to prove it, but it is likely that in the supine position the posterior portions of the lung are better perfused than the anterior portions.

NITROGEN WASHOUT TESTS

Much of the common use of the stethoscope has been to listen to various parts of the chest to determine the difference in breath sounds or ventilation to various areas of the lung. Physiologists have confirmed the presence of uneven ventilation even in normal individuals by studying the washout of nitrogen from the lungs. In a normal subject after seven minutes of 100% oxygen breathing, the concentration of nitrogen in the expired air should drop to 2.5% or less. In such a test nitrogen concentration in expired air is measured on a final deep expiration. If some alveoli were hypoventilated, the nitrogen concentration in the expired alveolar air would remain above 2.5% at the end of seven minutes. During the oxygen breathing the hypoventilated alveoli would be more slowly washed out than normal alveoli and at the end of the period would have a higher nitrogen concentration than the well-ventilated alveoli. Since the underventilated alveoli empty on the final deep breath, the air from these alveoli adds excess nitrogen to the expired air at the time the measurement is made and so increases the final measured nitrogen concentration.

If a patient hyperventilates during the period of nitrogen washout and thus speeds up nitrogen elimination from all alveoli, the concentration of nitrogen in the underventilated alveoli may be at normal levels and a false-negative test may result. This error can be avoided by using the single-breath nitrogen washout test, which is a more accurate and useful method of determining the distribution of ventilation since it is unaffected by hyperventilation. It is performed by having the subject take a single breath of 100% oxygen and recording simultaneously the concentration of expired nitrogen and volume throughout the period of exhalation. Recordings can be made with varying breathing patterns, including normal breathing, deep breathing, varying periods of breath-holding, panting, etc. If the distribution of gas to the many primary lobules comprising the lung were uniform, the concentration of nitrogen in the expired mixture should be the same throughout the expiration after washout of the 100% oxygen from the dead space. If individual lobules contribute expired gas of different concentrations (due to variation in perfusion) but empty simultaneously, the expired air should be a mixture of these gases and should have a uniform nitrogen concentration. When a single-breath nitrogen washout test is done, however, the concentration of nitrogen is not uniform but rises slowly during expiration. This means that the various areas of the lung must have different alveolar gas concentrations, ratios of ventilation to perfusion, and that some lobules must empty faster than others.

PARALLEL VENTILATION THEORY

To explain the differences in the amount of ventilation of various lobules of the lung, the parallel ventilation theory of gas distribution has been developed. This theory assumes that the flow of air in and out of each area of the lung depends on the relative values of the airflow resistance in the bronchus leading to each area and upon the compliance of each

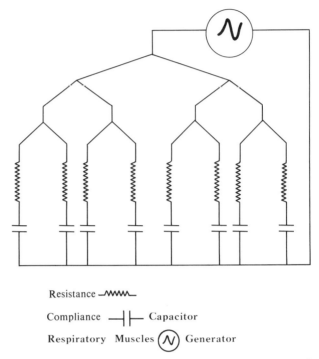

Resistance ─/\/\/\/\─

Compliance ─┤├─ Capacitor

Respiratory Muscles Ⓝ Generator

Fig. 7-1. Parallel ventilation theory. A simplified analog of the respiratory tree can be likened to an electronic circuit, as shown in this picture. (For a more complete analog see Fig. 4-3A, p. 60). The trachea branches into two main bronchi, which in turn branch into lobar bronchi, etc. Each subdivision of the lung consists of resistance and compliance units connected in series, and these compliance-resistance combinations are connected in parallel with one another; this is the origin of the term *parallel ventilation theory*. The respiratory muscles, or generators, develop the same pressure across each subsegment. The amount of air going to each depends on the relative values of the compliance and resistance of each subdivision (see Fig. 7-2).

area of lung. The resistance and compliance of each area is considered to be in series, and each of these series circuits is connected together in parallel (Fig. 7-1). Each series circuit has a time constant determined by its resistance and compliance. If a forcing pressure is applied across a resistance and compliance connected in series, 66% of the complete response will occur in a time period equal to the product of the resistance and compliance. If two such resistance-compliance units are connected in parallel, as are the subdivisions of the lungs, the ventilation going to each will be controlled by the relative values of the compliances and resistances of each.

It is apparent that the resistance in the airways leading to all the lung lobules is not the same and likewise that the compliance of these lobules is not the same. While the resistance and compliance of various areas of the lung differ, it is thought that in each part of the normal lung the product of the resistance and compliance, which is the time constant, is the same as that in another. The distribution of gases is determined by all three factors, the resistance, compliance, and the time constant.

The types of gas distribution that are predicted by the parallel ventilation theory can best be shown by some examples of the effects on distribution of varying values of compliance and resistance and their product.

Resistance Change.   First consider that the compliance of two areas is the same but the resistance is different (Fig. 7-2); both areas end up with the same volume if the time available for inspiration or expiration is at least three times the time constant (the time necessary for a 95% response), because the limiting factor is not flow through the resistance but the amount the translobular pressure can stretch the lobule. However, if the time of the half-cycle is less than three times the time constant of the high-resistance lobule, the alveolus with the higher resistance receives less air because its greater resistance and thus longer time constant will not allow complete response in the time available. The obvious explanation for this fact is that it takes longer for air to flow past the resistance and fill the alveolus. A clinical example of a disease state in which different areas of the lung have different resistances is seen when one pulmonary artery is occluded. The resultant alveolar hypocapnia causes ipsilateral bronchoconstriction which increases airway resistance and decreases ventilation to the lung with the occluded pulmonary artery.

Compliance Change.   Next consider a case in which the resistance is uniform and relatively low throughout the lung (thought by some to be the case in normal individuals), while the compliance of one area is greater than another. The more compliant area has the longer time constant. If the time available during a normal breathing cycle exceeds three times the time constant of the most compliant area, a given forcing pressure stretches the lung to a larger volume than if the compliances were uniform and equal to that of the least compliant area. The more compliant area receives more ventilation because the applied pressure stretches it to a larger volume than the less compliant area. If the time available is less than three times the time constant of the more compliant area, the more compliant area still receives the greater amount of ventilation. The absolute amount of air added to the more compliant unit is less, however, than if a longer time were available to permit a

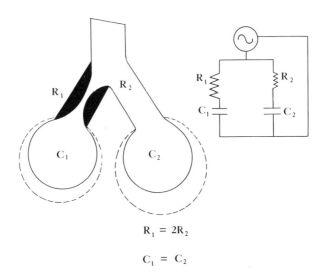

$$R_1 = 2R_2$$

$$C_1 = C_2$$

A

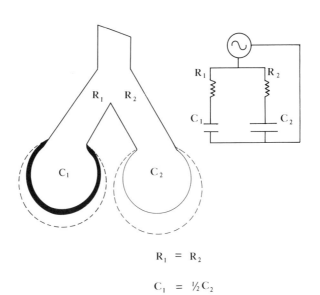

$$R_1 = R_2$$

$$C_1 = \tfrac{1}{2}C_2$$

B

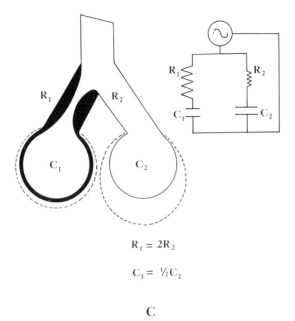

$$R_1 = 2R_2$$

$$C_1 = \tfrac{1}{2}C_2$$

C

Fig. 7-2. Distribution of ventilation. Each figure consists of an electrical analog and a mechanical representation. On the mechanical analog the solid lines represent the original volume and the dotted lines volume at the end of the inspiratory cycle.

(A) The compliances are the same, C_1 and C_2, but the resistance to the subsegment on the left, R_1, is twice that of the one on the right, R_2. More air enters the segment on the right. If time was unlimited, the one on the left would reach a volume equal to the one on the right.

(B) R_1 and R_2 are equal, but C_1 is one-half of C_2, so that C_2 expands to a greater volume. No matter how long the cycle, C_2 will contain more air than C_1.

(C) R_1 is twice R_2, and C_1 is one-half C_2. The difference in volume of the two subsegments is further exaggerated by the combination of low compliance and high resistance to the subsegment on the right. If the time of the cycle were prolonged, the effect of increased resistance would disappear and the subsegment on the right would reach a volume equal to that shown in (B).

full response. The more compliant area receives more ventilation despite its longer time constant because the low-compliance area requires a greater pressure to stretch it to a given volume and thus less pressure is left to overcome airflow resistance in the low-compliance area than in the high-compliance area. The smaller pressure difference across the resistance in the low-compliance area results in a lower flow rate, so there is slower filling.

The effects of differences in compliance of two lungs on ventilation are seen when ventilation to each lung is measured in an individual lying in the lateral decubitus position. The weight of the mediastinal structures shifts them toward the dependent hemithorax. This dead weight stretches the superior and compresses the inferior lung but maintains the pleural pressures equal. The result is that the inferior lung is more compliant than the superior lung, and so when a forcing pressure is applied by contraction of the muscles of inspiration, more air flows into the dependent than into the superior lung.

Change in Resistance and Compliance. An area of lung with high compliance and low resistance will receive more ventilation than an area with low compliance and high resistance. In this case the time constant for both areas may be the same, but in the area with the low resistance and high compliance a smaller pressure drop will be required to overcome the resistance for any given flow rate and to stretch the more compliant area to any given volume. Low resistance and high compliance will have additive effects to increasing volume in this area, and the effect of rise in compliance in increasing time constant is offset by fall in resistance, so that for any given period of time the percent of total response is the same as that of the area with high resistance and low compliance.

The parallel theory of ventilation postulates that the distribution of gases to the various areas of the lung is determined by the resistance, compliance, time constant, and duration of each breath or frequency of the breathing cycle. If there are regional increases in resistance such as occur in postoperative patients with retained secretions, the time constant to these areas will be increased; a fast ventilatory rate will tend to increase the unevenness of ventilation, and a slow rate will decrease it.

VENTILATION-PERFUSION RATIOS

Study of ventilation-perfusion ratios can be very useful in an understanding of the effectiveness of ventilation. The ventilation-perfusion ratio (V_A/Q) is defined as the ratio of ideal alveolar ventilation to perfusion. A normal individual has a V_A/Q at rest of approximately 0.8; this means that the volume of blood perfusing the lungs is 1.2 times greater than the volume of air ventilating the alveoli. With exercise the V_A/Q rises because ventilation increases at a faster rate than perfusion. Efficient gas exchange is maintained because the blood-gas arteriovenous difference widens so each aliquot of blood can transport more oxygen and carbon dioxide. The V_A/Q concept can be introduced by studying two extreme situations: no ventilation and normal blood flow (right-to-left shunt); and no blood flow with normal ventilation.

RIGHT-TO-LEFT BLOOD SHUNT

When there is a right-to-left shunt of blood, ventilation is zero and so the V_A/Q is zero. The principles discussed apply whether the mixed venous blood gets to the systemic arterial blood through an atelectatic lung, an intracardiac right-to-left shunt, or a pulmonary arteriovenous fistula. For purposes of illustration consider the case when one lung is completely atelectatic (Fig. 7-3). Assume that 50% of the right-heart blood output goes to each lung and that the blood has an oxygen capacity of 20 volumes percent. Blood coming from the atelectatic lung will have the same oxygen saturation as venous blood, 65%. With normal hemoglobin concentration (oxygen capacity 20 volumes percent), this will be equivalent to an oxygen content of 13 cc. per 100 cc. Blood coming from the ventilated lung cannot be more than 97.5% saturated, which will be equivalent to an oxygen content of 19.8 cc. per 100 cc. The systemic arterial blood will be a mixture of equal parts of blood with 13 and 19.8 cc. of oxygen per 100 cc., which will give it an oxygen content of 16.5 volumes percent or an oxygen saturation of 82%.

An oxygen saturation of 82% represents severe hypoxemia, and the patient might be expected to hyperventilate to increase his arterial oxygen saturation. Such hyperventilation will in fact accomplish little. Marked hyperventilation can raise the alveolar pO_2 from 100 to only 125. Because the upper part of the oxygen dissociation curve is flat, the oxygen saturation content of the arterial blood will be raised to only 98.5%. The dissolved oxygen will be increased even less (.075 cc. per 100 cc.). Breathing 100% oxygen would be little more effective; the oxygen saturation would rise to 100% and dissolved oxygen to 2.5 cc. per 100 cc., giving an oxygen content of 22.5 cc. per 100 cc. in blood coming from the ventilated lung. This blood, when mixed with venous blood containing 13 cc. per 100 cc., would raise the oxygen content of arterial blood to 17.7 cc., giving an arterial oxygen saturation of 88%. When a shunt permits venous blood to reach the systemic arteries without passing through ventilated alveoli, arterial unsaturation will persist despite administration of 100% oxygen.

While a patient with atelectasis or right-to-left shunt of any kind has a low pO_2, the arterial pCO_2 is usually normal. The depressed pO_2 causes some hyperventilation, and if pCO_2 were elevated, more hyperventilation would result. Hyperventilation of the intact areas of lung lowers the carbon dioxide content of blood returning from the normally perfused lung. The pCO_2 of the blood will be lowered in direct proportion to the increase in ventilation because the carbon dioxide dissociation curve is a straight line and has no flat portion, as does the oxygen dissociation

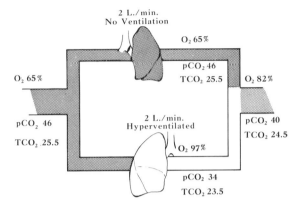

A Equal blood flow in both lungs.

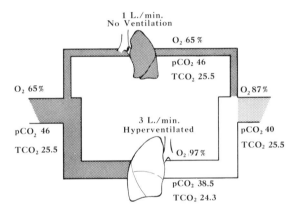

B Blood flow to left lung ⅓ flow to right.

Fig. 7-3. Blood shunt. The left lung is atelectatic and unventilated, so blood going through it is unchanged. (A) Flow to the left lung equals flow to the right lung, but the right lung is hyperventilated, lowering the pCO_2 to 34 mm. Hg and total CO_2 (TCO_2), to 23.5 mEq but raising the oxygen saturation to only 97%. The mixture of blood from these two sources, the hyperventilated and unventilated lung, has an oxygen saturation of 82% and normal pCO_2 and TCO_2.

(B) Flow to the atelectatic lung is one-third that to the ventilated lung. The ventilated lung is hyperventilated to the same degree as in (A). The pCO_2 of blood leaving the lungs falls to 38.5 mm. Hg and TCO_2 to 24.3 mEq; oxygen saturation is 97%. When mixed with blood from the unventilated lung, pCO_2 and TCO_2 are again normal, but oxygen saturation is 5% higher, or 87%. Arterial pCO_2 is largely determined by the total amount of ventilation and is little affected by shunts. Oxygen saturation is more dependent on the size of the shunt and is little affected by ventilation.

curve. Thus when the blood of low carbon dioxide content from the hyperventilated lung is mixed with venous blood of high carbon dioxide content from the shunt, a mixture with a near-normal carbon dioxide content will result. The blood from only the hyperventilated lung has normal oxygen content, however, and when it is mixed with blood of low oxygen content, the mixture remains desaturated (see Fig. 2-9, p. 38).

If the right-to-left shunt is small, the measurement of systemic arterial oxygen saturation may not indicate the presence of the shunt because the arterial blood is diluted with only a small amount of venous blood; the fall in arterial oxygen saturation will be slight because the decrease lies on the flat part of the oxygen dissociation curve. If the pO_2 rather than oxygen saturation were measured, a small shunt would become evident because admixture of only a small amount of venous blood would significantly lower the systemic arterial pO_2.

If the systemic arterial oxygen content, mixed venous oxygen content, and oxygen content of the blood draining the ventilated lung are known, the amount of blood perfusing the unventilated lung (the amount of blood shunted) can be calculated. The oxygen saturation of blood draining the ventilated lung may be assumed to be 98%, or, if the patient is breathing pure oxygen, 100% (with 2.5 cc. of dissolved oxygen), and only mixed venous and arterial blood samples are required. The absolute amount of shunt can be calculated if the oxygen consumption is known; without this information the relative amount of shunt can be determined.

$$\frac{O_2 \text{ consumption (cc./min.)}}{\text{Arterial } O_2 \text{ cont.} - \text{mixed venous } O_2 \text{ cont.}} = \frac{\text{cardiac output}}{\text{or total flow}} \quad (1)$$

$$\frac{O_2 \text{ consumption (cc./min.)}}{\text{pul. venous } O_2 \text{ cont.} - \text{mixed venous } O_2 \text{ cont.}} = \frac{\text{flow through}}{\text{ventilated lung}} \quad (2)$$

Equation 1 — Equation 2 = shunt flow

If oxygen consumption is unknown, 100 can be substituted for the oxygen consumption figure. The answer obtained will give the relative shunt fraction.

VENTILATORY SHUNT

If a pulmonary artery to one lung is acutely occluded, as by an embolus or a balloon catheter, the total cardiac output must fall in half or all the blood must go through the intact lung (Fig. 7-4). To maintain adequate

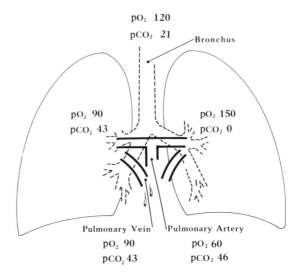

A   Both lungs equally ventilated without hyperventilation.
Left lung unperfused.

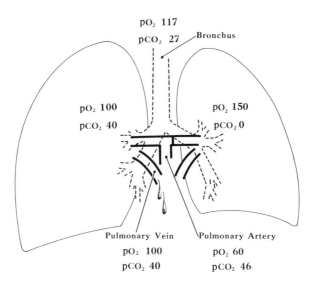

B   Right lung ventilated twice as much as left lung.
Left lung unperfused.

cardiac output, the flow to the intact lung will be doubled. If the ventilation to the perfused lung does not increase in proportion to its increase in perfusion, the ventilation will be inadequate to maintain normal alveolar and arterial pCO_2 and pO_2. The alveolar pCO_2 will rise and the alveolar pO_2 will fall, with a resultant rise in arterial pCO_2 (and total carbon dioxide) and fall in arterial pO_2 (and oxygen content). These changes in systemic arterial blood gas concentrations stimulate the respiratory center and lead to increased ventilation to restore the blood gases to near-normal values. If there is reasonable coordination of ventilation and perfusion in the lung with intact blood supply, the pO_2 and pCO_2 of its alveolar gas will be nearly the same as that in the arterial blood. In the unperfused lung the alveolar gas will have a higher pO_2 and lower pCO_2 than the arterial blood, since no oxygen is removed or carbon dioxide added to this alveolar gas.

The ventilation of unperfused areas of lung provides no exchange of gas with the blood, just as the ventilation of the anatomical dead space in the airways provides no gas exchange. Ventilated unperfused areas of lung have been given the name of *alveolar dead space*. Alveolar dead space cannot be directly measured. Physiological dead space, which is the anatomical dead space plus the alveolar dead space, can be determined using the Bohr equation, which is:

$$V_D = \frac{\left(Pa_{CO_2} - P_{E_{CO_2}}\right) V_E}{Pa_{CO_2}}$$

where V_D = volume of physiological dead space
Pa_{CO_2} = arterial pCO_2
$P_{E_{CO_2}}$ = expired air
V_E = expired volume

Fig. 7-4.   Ventilatory shunt. The left lung is unperfused but ventilated. (A) Ventilation to the two lungs is equal and total ventilation normal. Twice as much blood goes to the right lung, so the ventilation is inadequate; the pO_2 falls and pCO_2 rises in the arterial blood and alveolar air of the right lung. The alveolar air of the left lung has the same pO_2 and pCO_2 as room air. The mixed end-tidal or alveolar air from both lungs has a high pO_2 of 120 mm. Hg and a low pCO_2 of 21 mm. Hg, an A–a pO_2 gradient of 30 mm. Hg, and a pCO_2 gradient of 22 mm. Hg.

(B) The right lung is hyperventilated to produce a normal arterial pO_2 and pCO_2. The low pCO_2 in the left lung causes bronchoconstriction, so ventilation to the left lung is one-half that to the right. The mixed alveolar pO_2 is 117 and pCO_2 is 27 mm. Hg, giving an A–a pO_2 gradient of 17 mm. Hg and a CO_2 gradient of 13 mm. Hg.

This equation is based on the assumption that gas coming from normally perfused alveoli has the same pCO_2 as arterial blood. For example, if a patient had an expired volume of 600 cc., a pCO_2 in expired air of 16 mm. of Hg, and an arterial pCO_2 of 40 mm. Hg, the physiological dead space could be calculated, using the formula, as

$$V_D = \frac{(40 - 16)\ 600}{40}$$
$$= 360\ cc.$$

The anatomical dead space in adult males is about 150 cc., leaving an alveolar dead space, or ventilatory shunt, of 210 cc. per breath; the ventilation of perfused alveoli is $600 - 360$, or 240 cc. per breath. When the statement is made that the physiological dead space has increased, it is an indirect and perhaps obtuse way of describing incoordination of ventilation and perfusion characterized by ventilation of poorly perfused or unperfused alveoli.

ALVEOLAR–ARTERIAL OXYGEN DIFFERENCES

Ventilatory and blood shunts can be relative rather than absolute. One way of measuring such shunts is to determine the difference in gas partial pressure between alveolar air (A) and arterial blood (a), or the A–a difference.

In a normal person breathing air, the systemic arterial oxygen tension is 5 to 10 mm. lower than the oxygen tension in the alveolar gas, an A–a oxygen difference of 5 to 10 mm. This difference is due to the systemic venous admixture, a small shunt of about 2%, and to variation in V_A/Q in different parts of the lung. The A–a oxygen difference can also be increased when there is a diffusion block at the alveolo-capillary membrane or when, as in exercise, the flow rate of unsaturated blood through the alveolar capillaries exceeds the capacity for transfer of oxygen between alveolar air and capillary blood, a functional diffusion block. Since differences in A–a oxygen can be due to any combination of these four factors, other studies are necessary to determine whether there is a shunt, an abnormal ventilation-perfusion ratio, or a diffusion block.

One of these tests is to have the patient breathe 100% oxygen for a period of five minutes. The rise in alveolar pO_2 due to 100% oxygen breathing will increase alveolo-capillary pO_2 gradient so that any alveolo-capillary diffusion block will be overcome. Also, if there are some alveoli that are underventilated (but do have some ventilation), 100% oxygen breathing will increase the oxygen concentration in these poorly ventilated alveoli enough to provide adequate oxygen to saturate the hemoglobin despite the relative hypoventilation. Persistent arterial oxygen unsaturation or depression of arterial pO_2 below 300 mm. Hg after five minutes of breathing 100% oxygen must be due to perfusion of an unventilated portion of the lung or to an anatomical right-to-left shunt of some other sort. It is not due to a diffusion block or to alveolar hypoventilation.

In normal individuals there is no significant A–a carbon dioxide difference. Because of the linear nature of the carbon dioxide dissociation curve and the small arteriovenous pCO_2 difference, an absolute shunt as large as 10% would produce a barely measurable A–a carbon dioxide difference of only 0.5 mm. Carbon dioxide diffuses so fast across the alveolar membrane that the limits of diffusion are not reached. The differences found in A–a carbon dioxide are almost exclusively due to ventilation-perfusion incoordination. The alveolar pCO_2 is lower than the arterial pCO_2 in all types of ventilation-perfusion incoordination, whether it is overventilation and underperfusion or overperfusion and underventilation. The corollary is that an alveolar pCO_2 lower than the arterial pCO_2 indicates ventilation-perfusion incoordination. The mechanism of production of the A–a carbon dioxide differences in various types of ventilation-perfusion incoordination involves the interplay of the difference in concentrations of carbon dioxide in the alveolar gas and in arterial blood from the various regions of the lung and the proportion of the expired alveolar air or blood leaving the lung that is contributed by each region of lung (Fig. 7-5).

In situations in which some areas of lung are overventilated (or underperfused), the alveolar air and blood leaving the overventilated areas will have a lower pCO_2 than that from the normally ventilated areas. From the hyperventilated areas blood and alveolar gas with low pCO_2 will mix with blood and alveolar gas with normal pCO_2 from the normally ventilated areas. Since the blood and alveolar gas coming from the hyperventilated areas have the same pCO_2 on mixing, the degree to which they depress the pCO_2 of blood and gas from normally ventilated areas will depend on the volume of blood or gas from the hyperventilated areas added to that from the normal areas. If the area is hyperventilated and underperfused, there will be relatively more gas with low pCO_2 than blood with low pCO_2 coming from the hyperventilated areas. As a result, the alveolar pCO_2 will be depressed more than the arterial pCO_2.

A lower alveolar than arterial pCO_2 can also result from overperfusion (or underventilation) of areas of lung. Under these conditions blood and gas coming from the overperfused area will have a higher

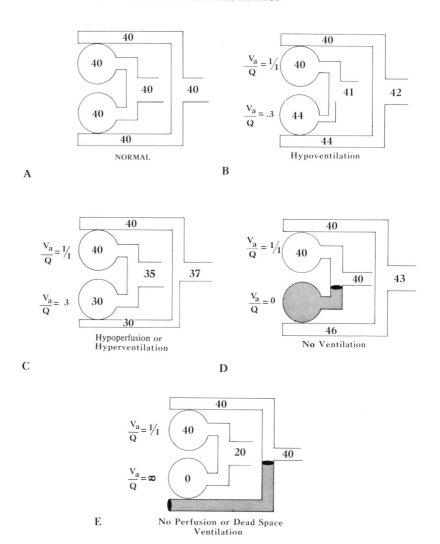

Fig. 7-5. Effect of changes in V_A/Q on A–a carbon dioxide difference. In the normal condition (A) there is no A–a carbon dioxide difference. (For simplicity's sake, the normal V_A/Q in these diagrams has been considered to be 1 rather than the actual value of 8.)

(B) The lower lung has its ventilation cut to one-third, $V_A/Q = 0.3$, so the alveolar and the pulmonary venous pCO_2 rise to 44 mm. Hg. The ventilation remains unchanged in the unaffected (upper) lung. The blood is made up one-half of blood with pCO_2 of 40 and one-half of blood with pCO_2 of 44 to give an arterial pCO_2 of 42 mm. Hg. There is three times as much alveolar air coming from the upper lung as from the lower lung, so the mixed alveolar carbon dioxide rises to only 41, an A–a carbon dioxide difference of 1 mm. Hg.

pCO_2 than blood and gas from normally perfused areas. Overperfused areas of lung have greater blood flow than ventilation, so that the volume of blood with high pCO_2 is relatively large. When mixed with that from other areas with normal V_A/Q, arterial pCO_2 will be increased more than will the alveolar pCO_2 when the small volume of gas with high pCO_2 is added to that from alveoli with normal V_A/Q. Since the amount of gas with high carbon dioxide is less than the amount of blood with high pCO_2, the alveolar pCO_2 will not be raised as much as the arterial pCO_2.

The A–a carbon dioxide differences are small when alveoli are over-perfused (or underventilated) because the difference between arterial and venous pCO_2 is so small—6 mm. of Hg. Therefore, blood from an overperfused alveolus cannot have a pCO_2 more than 6 mm. higher than that from a normally perfused alveolus. Air in a hyperventilated (or underperfused) alveolus may have a pCO_2 of zero (40 mm. less than normal). Hyperventilation can thus cause larger differences in A–a carbon dioxide gradient than can hyperperfusion (or underventilation). Measurement of A–a carbon dioxide difference is not useful in determining the presence of small V_A/Q imbalances present in healthy individuals, because alveolar pCO_2 varies throughout expiration and the size of the shunt would depend on the time chosen as representative of mixed alveolar air. Measurable differences in A–a carbon dioxide gradient are usually due to ventilatory shunts, so-called physiological dead-space ventilation. Measurement of A–a nitrogen differences more

(C) The ventilation to the two lungs is equal, but perfusion to the lower lung $V_A/Q = 3$ is cut to one-third that of the upper. The lower lung can be considered to be either hypoperfused or hyperventilated. The alveolar and arterial pCO_2 of the upper lung is 40. When alveolar air from the upper lung is mixed with an equal amount of alveolar air of pCO_2 30 from the lower lung, the mixed alveolar pCO_2 is 35 mm. Hg. Since only one-third as much blood of pCO_2 30 from the lower lung is available to mix with blood from the upper lung, the arterial pCO_2 only falls to 37, an A–a carbon dioxide difference of 2, twice the difference in (B). Thus both hypoventilation and hyperventilation result in a lower alveolar than arterial pCO_2.

(D) and (E) illustrate why the difference is exaggerated by hyperventilation or hypoperfusion more than by hypoventilation. In (D) there is no ventilation to the lower lung; in (E), no perfusion. Because in (D) venous pCO_2 is only 46, the pCO_2 of blood draining the unventilated lung can only rise to 46 and the arterial pCO_2 goes up only to 43 while alveolar pCO_2 remains 40, an A–a carbon dioxide difference of 3 mm. Hg. In (E), where there is no perfusion to the lower lung, the alveolar pCO_2 is zero, while that from the perfused area is 40; the mixture of equal parts of gas from each lung has a pCO_2 of 20 mm. Hg. Blood comes only from the upper lung, and so arterial blood has a pCO_2 of 40, resulting in an A–a carbon dioxide difference of 20 mm. Hg. Ventilation of unperfused alveoli is like ventilation of dead space, and large A–a carbon dioxide differences indicate ventilation of unperfused areas of lung.

accurately quantitates mean V_A/Q imbalances than A–a oxygen or A–a carbon dioxide differences, but the methodology is difficult and not widely used. Part of the reason such methods are not used more often is that measurements of A–a differences signify only whether ventilation-perfusion incoordination is present. They cannot localize the site of incoordination.

MEASUREMENT OF REGIONAL VENTILATION-PERFUSION RATIO DIFFERENCES

Differential bronchospirometry is the first method used for measuring differences in ventilation and oxygen uptake of the two lungs. The ratio of ventilation to oxygen uptake in each lung gives a rough measure of V_A/Q if the oxygen uptake is used as an indication of perfusion. Bronchospirometry is a cumbersome method and useful only to separate one entire lung from another. Another method using direct sampling of expired gas concentrations is to pass a small radiopaque catheter into various areas of the lung under fluoroscopic control and to withdraw air samples to determine differences in oxygen and carbon dioxide partial pressures in the sample. Any differences in gas partial pressure from two sampling sites indicate uneven distribution of ventilation and perfusion. This method has shown that alveolar pCO_2 is lower in the upper lobes of the lungs than in other regions.

Other methods of study produce further information. Pulmonary angiography can demonstrate gross changes in the distribution of blood flow and can precisely identify sites of anatomical block in major pulmonary arteries and, with special techniques, in medium-size vessels. It cannot show changes in small vessel circulation. Scanning over the entire chest after the intravenous injection of microaggregated radioactive human serum albumin can identify gross areas of decreased perfusion.

More elegant techniques involve the breathing of carbon dioxide made with oxygen 15. Perfusion can be determined by measuring the rate of removal of the radioactive carbon dioxide with scintillation counters placed over various regions of the chest. Xenon 133 can be used in a similar manner. Perfusion is measured by determining the maximum number of counts in various areas of the lung after the intravenous injection of Xe^{133} dissolved in saline. Ventilation is determined by measuring the rate of decay of radioactivity as the xenon is removed from the alveoli by ventilation. Xenon also can be placed in the inhaled gas mixture and its distribution monitored to measure the relative ventilation of various areas of the lung.

These new techniques of measuring ventilation and perfusion have demonstrated that at rest, when the subject is in the upright posture, the V_A/Q in the lungs varies from 3.3 at the apices to 0.63 at the bases. Ventilation is fairly uniform, but perfusion of the apices is less than perfusion of the bases. In the upright posture, gravity increases the hydrostatic pressure of the column of blood in the pulmonary vessels at the bases and decreases it at the apices, thus lessening resistance to blood flow to the bases as compared to the apices. In the supine posture, the difference in perfusion between the apices and bases disappears. Since local alveolar hypocapnia from the relative hyperventilation of the apices causes reflex bronchoconstriction, ventilation of the lung apices is less than that of the bases but is not decreased nearly as much as perfusion. In the lateral decubitus posture, blood flow is greater to the dependent than to the superior lung. As pointed out earlier, ventilation of the dependent lung is also greater because the dependent lung is more compliant. There is, therefore, less imbalance of ventilation and perfusion between the two lungs in the lateral decubitus posture than there is between apices and bases in the upright posture.

When, as with exercise, the gas exchange apparatus is called on to do more work, the degree of uneven perfusion diminishes, as blood flow to the apices increases more than does blood flow to the bases. With the increase in blood flow during exercise, pulmonary vascular resistance decreases and the relative effect of gravity on the various regions of the lung is lessened. As exercise becomes more strenuous, the ratio of ventilation to perfusion may increase as much as four times throughout the lungs. By increasing the arteriovenous oxygen difference, each cubic centimeter of blood flowing through the lungs can acquire more oxygen and, when it goes through the systemic circulation, give up more oxygen. To fully saturate the hemoglobin, the alveolar pO_2 must be kept at the same level regardless of rate of oxygen exhalation; as a result, ventilatory volume increases more than cardiac output.

The incoordination of ventilation and perfusion resulting from the uneven perfusion of the lungs must lower the efficiency of the system. In normal individuals the actual decrease in efficiency is small, less than 5%. Since the discrepancy between ventilation and perfusion diminishes with exercise, even this small loss of efficiency decreases when the greatest demand is placed on the exchange system. In disease, however, incoordination of ventilation and perfusion can seriously compromise the efficiency of the gas exchange system.

DISEASE AND THE VENTILATION-PERFUSION RATIO

The changes in V_A/Q with disease may be due primarily to circulatory or to ventilatory disturbances or a combination of both. Hypovolemic shock decreases the perfusion pressure and slows pulmonary circulation. This results in the closure of vessels to many areas of the lung. In patients in shock this decrease in perfusion associated with increase in ventilation induced by acidosis causes a great increase in the physiological dead space or ventilation of virtually unperfused lung, which is a wasted effort the shocked patient can ill afford.

Pulmonary hypertension diminishes the uneven distribution of blood flow. As the pulmonary artery pressure rises, the relative importance of the hydrostatic pressure diminishes and blood flow to the lung apices is nearly the same as blood flow to the bases. Left-to-right shunts without marked pulmonary hypertension decrease the unevenness of perfusion in the same manner as does exercise. The lowered vascular resistance and increased flow tend to decrease but not wipe out the uneven flow pattern.

When pulmonary venous pressure is raised as a result of mitral stenosis or left heart failure, flow to the lung apices is greater than that normally found in the upright posture. In advanced stages of heart disease, when pulmonary congestion is present, flow may be greater to the apices than to the bases. The rise in venous pressure dilates the vessels, decreasing resistance. Since venous pressure exceeds alveolar pressure throughout the lungs, all the capillaries are open and the Starling resistors are not functioning. If the rise in venous pressure is enough to cause interstitial edema in the dependent portions of the lung, the pulmonary vascular resistance in these areas will rise markedly, shunting blood to the less edematous apices. Lowering of pulmonary venous pressure reverses the process and increases flow to the dependent portions of the lung. Friedman and Braunwald have shown that measurement of regional perfusion is an indication of the degree of mitral stenosis. The reversal of flow pattern in upright patients with mitral stenosis is directly related to the degree of valvular stenosis.

Patients undergoing major thoracic and upper abdominal surgical procedures have a persistently depressed systemic arterial pO_2 and, usually, a normal pCO_2. Since administration of 100% oxygen to these patients does not raise the pO_2 to the expected levels, there must be areas of the lung that are being perfused and not ventilated. These areas are presumably regions of microatelectasis caused by a cough inadequate to effectively clear the airways and by failure to take deep breaths. The initiating cause of the microatelectasis is pain associated with the operative incision, which inhibits normal motion of the chest. The depression of pO_2 is greatest after thoracic operations, but after laparotomy, particularly in the upper abdomen, arterial pO_2 is commonly depressed for two to five days.

When the chest is opened or the chest wall disrupted by multiple rib fractures, in addition to the microatelectasis resulting from failure to cough or take deep breaths, large areas of lung can be poorly ventilated due to the disturbance in the mechanical integrity of the chest wall, which alters the forces applied to the lung and thus the distribution of the inspired air.

Obese patients frequently have serious respiratory problems and may have serious hypoxemia and hypercapnia postoperatively. This is partly the result of decreased alveolar ventilation, but, in addition, there are significant ventilation-perfusion abnormalities in the very obese individual. While perfusion is maximal in the lower zones of the lung in obese patients, as it is in nonobese patients, ventilation of the lower zones of the lungs is much reduced. The ventilation-perfusion incoordination and alveolar hypoventilation can cause reduced arterial oxygen tension in the obese patient at rest. If even a moderately obese patient undergoes laparotomy, pain and muscle spasm together with obesity reduce further the ventilation of the lower lung regions, aggravating the preexisting ventilation-perfusion incoordination.

Both atelectasis and pneumonia produce depressed arterial pO_2 levels due to perfusion of unventilated areas of the lung. Fortunately, the perfusion of areas of collapsed or consolidated lung is markedly diminished due to a local increase in pulmonary vascular resistance, and so the arterial unsaturation is not as great as if perfusion was maintained at normal levels.

The distribution of ventilation becomes progressively less uniform with age. This change is probably related to long-term inhalation of noxious agents. In heavy cigarette smokers disturbances in V_A/Q may occur at an earlier age than in nonsmokers. In patients with so-called obstructive emphysema, one of the principal difficulties may be uneven distribution of inspired volume. The compliance and resistance increase more in the most affected parts, and this leads to alterations in distribution of inspired air (see p. 164). In some areas the increase in compliance and airway resistance results in extreme trapping of air, causing further disruption of the normal distribution of ventilation. Because of ventilation-perfusion incoordination and large physiological dead space, most patients with emphysema must increase their minute ventilation to maintain a normal arterial pCO_2 and pO_2. They often have decreased pO_2 despite a normal pCO_2, indicating that some of the perfused areas of the lung are underventilated. Usually the administration of 100% oxygen to patients with emphysema brings the pO_2 to expected levels, which means that the absolute shunts are small. The principal problem is underventilation of some areas of the lung and overventilation of others. In addition, the disruption of alveolar septa may result in some peripheral air sacs being so large that mixing by diffusion is incomplete in the time available during respiration. This incomplete mixing in the primary lobule has the same effect as uneven distribution of ventilation to the lobule.

The incoordination of ventilation and perfusion that occurs in aged or obese patients or in those with emphysema will be aggravated by injury or surgical procedures. Respiratory insufficiency can result.

With the development of improved techniques of studying ventilation-perfusion ratios, it is becoming increasingly apparent that incoordination of ventilation and perfusion is the principal cause of oxygen desaturation in disease and that only infrequently are diffusion defects important causes of systemic arterial oxygen unsaturation. With the growth of knowledge concerning mechanical factors leading to ventilation-perfusion incoordination, better therapeutic measures inevitably will be developed to correct these disturbances.

8. CHEMICAL AND REFLEX REGULATION OF RESPIRATION

THE regulation of respiration involves a highly complex, integrated set of sensing devices for input to the control centers. The sensory inputs consist of chemoreceptors, which respond to changes in pO_2, pCO_2, and hydrogen ion concentration, and proprioceptors of various sorts, which respond to stretch of bronchial smooth muscle and/or relaxation of respiratory and perhaps other muscles of the body. The response devices controlled by the centers are equally complex and involve activation and inhibition of somatic muscles of respiration and smooth muscle of the airway system, cardiac muscle, and the vasculature of the entire body. The respiratory centers are in effect a complex network of computing centers for the integration of the inputs from the various neural pathways and the generation of signals to the appropriate end organs. In surgical patients the control system is usually not deranged except during anesthesia or as the result of direct cranial injury. However, alterations in the circulation, in pulmonary, chest wall, and upper airway mechanics, and in the concentrations of gases in inspired air all change the stimuli to the sensory inputs and thus the information fed to the respiratory center. Any abnormal information causes the center to direct the end organs to change markedly the pattern of ventilation.

The automatic regulation of respiration at rest is not altered significantly by removal of cerebrum and cerebellum, though clearly they are able to affect the respiratory pattern. What their integrative function is in the response to exercise is not known. The medulla and upper spinal cord possess the necessary neural hardware to maintain respiratory automaticity at rest at least. These centers do not contain any sensory elements. All the sensing elements are in remote chemoreceptors and proprioreceptors.

THE PERIPHERAL CHEMORECEPTORS

The peripheral chemoreceptors provide the major input for alterations in pO_2 and the fast response system for alterations in pH and pCO_2. These peripheral chemoreceptors are in two anatomical sites—the aortic bodies, which lie between the arch of the aorta and the pulmonary artery, and in the carotid bodies. The afferent fibers to the aortic bodies run up the vagus nerves with the left recurrent laryngeal nerve, and their blood supply comes from a branch of the coronary system or from a vessel arising directly from the aortic arch. The afferent impulses from the carotid bodies travel to the brain by the ninth cranial nerves and by the vagus nerves; their blood supply is from the occipital artery, which is a branch of the external carotid artery. Stimulation of the peripheral chemoreceptors causes increased tidal volume and respiratory rate, constriction of the vessels of the extremities, bradycardia (carotid bodies) or tachycardia (aortic bodies), increased systemic arterial pressure, and increased bronchomotor tone. Increase in arterial pressure, which stimulates the aortic and carotid baroreceptors, decreases ventilation; and a decrease in arterial pressure increases ventilation. The antagonistic effect of the responses of these peripheral receptors is an index of the problems involved in analysis of the effects of a particular stimulus.

The peripheral receptors are the principal mediators for changes in pO_2. There may be some sensory input from central receptors when extreme falls in pO_2 occur, but this is of minor importance in the general regulation of respiration. The peripheral chemoreceptors are sensitive both to the level of pO_2 in the systemic arterial blood and to the amount of blood flowing to them. They have a very rich blood supply, and efferent blood has nearly the same pO_2 as afferent blood. If the perfusion falls, so that the efferent pO_2 is depressed, respiratory stimulation occurs. The effect of decrease in the afferent blood pO_2 is variable from individual to individual and depends on the inherent sensitivity of the individual's receptors. In most subjects a drop in pO_2 from 100 to 80 mm. Hg has no effect; only a very small effect is seen until the pO_2 drops to 40 mm. Hg. This is the point of sharp break in the oxyhemoglobin dissociation curve (see Fig. 8-2). A drop in both blood flow and pO_2 has greater respiratory stimulus effect than the sum of the change of each stimulus acting alone. In patients with anemia and carbon monoxide poisoning, the arterial pO_2 is not depressed, and unless enough of the oxygen-carrying capacity of hemoglobin is lost so that inadequate oxygen is provided for the metabolism of the aortic or carotid chemoreceptor cells, thereby leading to low efferent pO_2, ventilatory level is normal.

The peripheral chemoreceptors are also sensitive to changes in arterial hydrogen ion concentration resulting from changes in bicarbonate ion concentration and changes in arterial pCO_2. The peripheral chemoreceptors respond to changes in acid-base balance, apparently as the result of change in intracellular hydrogen ion concentration. Since carbon dioxide can diffuse across the cell membrane very rapidly, a change in arterial pCO_2 results in a rapid change in intracellular hydrogen ion concentration and an acute rise or fall in ventilation. Diffusion of bicarbonate ions across the cell membrane is slower than the diffusion of carbon dioxide, so that changes in extracellular hydrogen ion concentration due to fall in bicarbonate ion concentration have more delayed effect on intracellular hydrogen ion concentration of the peripheral receptors. The response of the peripheral chemoreceptors to changes in arterial blood pCO_2 and pO_2 is very prompt, occurring within one minute. Due to the slow diffusion of bicarbonate ions across the cell membrane, the peripheral chemoreceptors have a slow response to changes in arterial blood hydrogen ion concentration resulting from metabolic acidosis or alkalosis.

Just as when low blood flow and low pO_2 occur together, when the chemoreceptor cells are stimulated simultaneously by both a fall in pO_2 and rise in pCO_2, the response to the combined stimulus will be greater than the response induced by the sum of the individual stimuli if they were acting alone. In other words, a cell stimulated by a low pO_2 is more sensitive to a given rise in pCO_2 than a cell which is bathed by blood with a normal pO_2 (Fig. 8-1).

THE CENTRAL CHEMORECEPTORS

The discovery of peripheral chemoreceptors explained some of the ventilatory responses to alterations in acid-base and blood-gas concentrations of blood. However, other responses to alterations in blood acid-

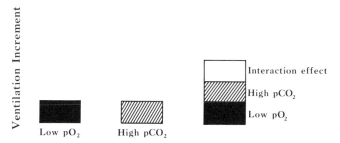

Fig. 8-1. The increment in ventilation with single and combined stimuli. In addition to the stimulus of low pO_2 and high pCO_2 alone, there is an interaction stimulus when both are altered.

base balance indicated that the respiratory centers had to act in a unique manner, as both sensing and coordinating regions of the brain which were somehow insulated by a protective membrane from acute alterations in perfusing blood. This was a puzzling concept, since it would be unique for this one region and control system of the brain. More recent studies have proved that the central receptor system is not in the substance of the brain. On the ventrolateral surface of the upper medulla, near the roots of the ninth and tenth cranial nerves, there are some special receptors which are uniquely sensitive to changes in environmental hydrogen ion concentration. These receptors are in contact with the cerebrospinal fluid and are influenced by the hydrogen ion concentration of the spinal fluid rather than by changes in arterial blood hydrogen ion concentration. These central receptors are insensitive to changes in pO_2. Because of their surface location, they are affected by hypothermia and by high intracranial pressure. Their superficial location also makes them vulnerable to low concentrations of local anesthetic agents. If the output of medullary sensors is completely blocked in a sedated patient, apnea may result, thus explaining the occurrence of complete apnea with high spinal anesthetics. Stimulation or inhibition of these receptors has no direct effect on the cardiovascular system.

The sensitivity of the central chemoreceptors to changes in cerebrospinal fluid hydrogen ion concentration explains many of the paradoxes found between alterations in blood-gas and acid-base concentrations and level of ventilation. The cerebrospinal fluid is not a simple ultrafiltrate of plasma. The processes determining the composition of cerebrospinal fluid are passive diffusion through the barrier between blood and cerebrospinal fluid, secretion by the choroid plexus, and active transport. Cerebrospinal fluid has a higher concentration of sodium and hydrogen ions and lower concentration of bicarbonate and potassium ions than plasma. These differences in concentration can be maintained only by an active transport mechanism. This mechanism is capable of restoring cerebrospinal fluid hydrogen ion concentration to normal against a concentration gradient in the plasma which deviates from normal.

The hydrogen ion concentration of cerebrospinal fluid is maintained by two mechanisms. The first mechanism is familiar: the regulation of the pCO_2 of the blood. Just as carbon dioxide can diffuse with ease across the cell membrane to reach equilibrium between intracellular and extracellular pCO_2 concentrations, it also can diffuse freely across the blood–brain barrier, resulting in fairly prompt equilibrium between blood and cerebrospinal fluid pCO_2 levels. The second mechanism is the slower regulation of cerebrospinal fluid hydrogen ion concentration with regard to blood by the active transport mechanism. Acute changes in blood

pCO_2 may induce a prompt ventilatory response due to the change in cerebrospinal fluid hydrogen ion concentration resulting from the diffusion of carbon dioxide into the spinal fluid; this response will then be altered as the hydrogen ion concentration of cerebrospinal fluid is restored to a more normal level by the active transport system increasing the bicarbonate ion concentration of spinal fluid. There are still some gaps in the theory, which places the central regulation of ventilation under the influence of central chemoreceptors sensitive to a cerebrospinal fluid hydrogen ion concentration which is regulated by active transport. However, such a theory fits best the known facts of chemoreceptor sensitivity and central nervous system response.

THE CHEMICAL REGULATION OF RESPIRATION

If the direct neural regulation of the level of respiration is ignored for the moment, the level of breathing resulting from stimuli originating from the central hydrogen ion concentration receptors and the aortic and carotid bodies can be given as a unified concept in conditions such as low oxygen atmospheres, metabolic acid-base disturbances, and following chronic elevation or depression of arterial pCO_2 (Fig. 8-2). When the inspired oxygen partial pressure is low, as when one ascends to high altitude, the low arterial pO_2 stimulates the aortic and carotid chemoreceptors, which results in increased ventilation. The increased ventilation in turn lowers the pCO_2, which tends to suppress in part the aortic and carotid chemoreceptors. The cerebrospinal fluid hydrogen ion concentration also falls, since pCO_2 is able to diffuse out of the cerebrospinal fluid quite rapidly, just as it can cross the cell membrane with ease. This results in a further depression of the stimulating effect of a low arterial pO_2. Over the course of a few days the active transport mechanism in the cerebrospinal fluid restores cerebrospinal fluid hydrogen ion concentration to normal by lowering the bicarbonate ion concentration in the cerebrospinal fluid and removing the inhibiting effect of a low cerebrospinal fluid hydrogen ion concentration on the ventilatory response to low pO_2. This theory explains the late increase in hyperventilation that occurs with chronic exposure to low oxygen tensions without invoking the concepts of "adaption" or any change in "sensitivity" of the chemoreceptors or of the central response to chemoreceptor discharge. When the individual returns to sea level and the stimulus due to low pO_2 is removed, ventilation decreases, causing a rise in cerebrospinal fluid pCO_2 and a rise in cerebrospinal fluid hydrogen ion concentration. The rise in cerebrospinal fluid hydrogen ion concentration causes continued hyperventilation until active transport

A   Ascent to Altitude

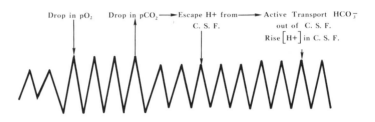

B   Descent from Altitude

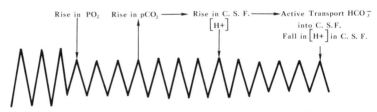

Fig. 8-2. In these illustrations the height of the spirometer tracing is proportionate to ventilatory response. An arrow going from a label toward a spirometer tracing signifies that the described alteration caused a change in ventilation. An arrow going from a tracing to a label indicates the change in minute ventilation caused by the change noted. Arrows between labels signify that the described change resulted in the subsequent alteration.

(A) With ascent to altitude, inspired air pO_2 falls, which increases minute ventilation. The increased ventilation lowers pCO_2, and hydrogen ions escape from the cerebrospinal fluid. This lowers the stimulus to breathing, and minute ventilation decreases. Bicarbonate ions are then removed from the cerebrospinal fluid by active transport, returning the cerebrospinal fluid hydrogen ion concentration to normal and resulting in a stimulus to ventilation.

(B) Descent from altitude. The rise in inspired air pO_2 lowers ventilatory stimulus, which in turn causes a rise in pCO_2, which raises cerebrospinal fluid hydrogen ion concentration, which in turn increases ventilation. Active transport of bicarbonate ions into the cerebrospinal fluid restores cerebrospinal fluid hydrogen ion concentration slowly to normal, and ventilation returns to normal levels.

(C) The effect of metabolic acidosis on ventilatory volume. The rise in hydrogen ion concentration at the peripheral receptors increases ventilation. This in turn lowers pCO_2, which causes cerebrospinal fluid hydrogen ion concentration to fall and decrease ventilation. Active transport of bicarbonate ions restores cerebrospinal fluid hydrogen ion concentration to normal, and ventilation increases.

(D) Correction of metabolic acidosis. Rise in blood bicarbonate ion concentration causes hydrogen ion concentration to rise in peripheral receptors, which decreases ventilation. The decrease in ventilation raises pCO_2, which increases cerebrospinal fluid hydrogen ion concentration and stimulates respiration. Active transport of bicarbonate ions into the cerebrospinal fluid slowly lowers cerebrospinal fluid hydrogen ion concentration to normal, and ventilation returns to normal levels.

C   Metabolic Acidosis

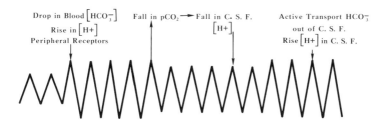

D   Correction Metabolic Acidosis

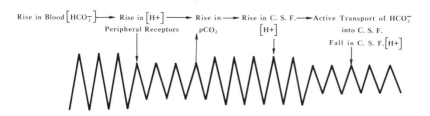

E   Prolonged Mechanical Hyperventilation

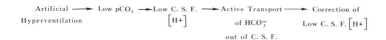

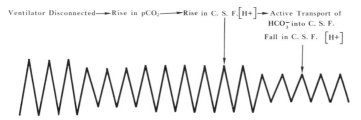

(E) Prolonged mechanical hyperventilation. Artificial hyperventilation lowers pCO_2, which lowers cerebrospinal fluid hydrogen ion concentration and initiates active transport of bicarbonate ions out of the cerebrospinal fluid to restore low cerebrospinal fluid hydrogen ion concentration to normal levels. When the ventilator is disconnected, pCO_2 rises, which raises cerebrospinal fluid hydrogen ion concentration and stimulates the subject to hyperventilate. Active transport starts to slowly restore cerebrospinal fluid bicarbonate ion concentration to normal, and hyperventilation ceases. It is best to decrease the minute ventilation to allow this correction prior to discontinuing the respirator. (Note similarity to B.)

F   Chronic Respiratory Insufficiency

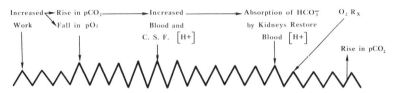

Fig. 8-2 (cont.).   (F) Chronic respiratory insufficiency. Increased mechanical work lowers effective ventilation and causes a fall in pO_2 which directly stimulates ventilation. The decreased effective ventilation also raises the blood and cerebrospinal fluid pCO_2 and hydrogen ion concentration, and these changes in turn further increase ventilation. Reabsorption of bicarbonate ions by the kidney and active transport of bicarbonate ions into the cerebrospinal fluid restores blood and cerebrospinal fluid hydrogen ion concentration to nearly normal and lowers the stimulus to respiration. Administration of oxygen to correct the low pO_2 lowers the stimulus further, and, in consequence, pCO_2 may rise to anesthetic levels.

restores cerebrospinal fluid bicarbonate ion concentration to normal concentrations.

In acute metabolic acidosis, carotid and aortic hydrogen ion concentration receptors are stimulated, resulting in hyperventilation and a fall in arterial pCO_2. The fall in arterial pCO_2 lowers cerebrospinal fluid pCO_2 and hydrogen ion concentration. The fall in cerebrospinal fluid hydrogen ion concentration inhibits ventilation and partially dampens the stimulating effect of the high arterial hydrogen ion concentration on the peripheral receptors. Over the course of twenty-four hours the cerebrospinal fluid hydrogen ion concentration is restored to normal, and its inhibiting effect is removed, and ventilation increases. If chronic metabolic acidosis is acutely corrected, the stimulatory effect of low hydrogen ion concentration on the peripheral receptors will be removed and ventilation will decrease, resulting in rise of arterial pCO_2 toward normal. The rise in arterial pCO_2 will elevate the cerebrospinal fluid pCO_2 and hydrogen ion concentration and stimulate the central hydrogen ion receptors. This explains the continued hyperventilation which occurs following the acute correction of chronic blood acid-base disturbances.

If a patient has been mechanically hyperventilated long enough, the depressed arterial and cerebrospinal fluid pCO_2 activate the transport mechanism to remove bicarbonate ions from the cerebrospinal fluid to restore hydrogen ion concentration toward normal. If the patient has a normal alveolar ventilatory volume, when mechanical hyperventilation is discontinued, his arterial pCO_2 will rise, resulting in a rise in cerebrospinal fluid pCO_2 and hydrogen ion concentration. The increase in cerebrospinal fluid hydrogen ion concentration will stimulate the medullary receptors, making the patient try to hyperventilate. As the slow active transport mechanisms restore cerebrospinal fluid bicarbonate ion concentration to normal the stimulus to hyperventilation is removed. A patient removed from a mechanical ventilator may be capable of maintaining a normal level of ventilation but not the hyperventilation required from his temporarily deranged control mechanism. In such patients it is often necessary to slowly correct the hypocapnia by decreasing the amount of ventilation gradually to allow the restoration of cerebrospinal fluid bicarbonate ion concentration to normal prior to completely discontinuing respiratory support.

In large part the alterations in ventilatory response in chronic hypercapnia can be explained by the same type of reasoning. However, a more complete theoretical explanation is possible if some of the other neural inputs which the respiratory center coordinates are considered first.

REFLEX REGULATION OF RESPIRATION

There are many reflexes which arise from proprioceptors in the lungs and chest wall. While some of these were among the first control mechanisms described, their description and integration into a coordinated theory of respiratory control is much less complete than the blood-gas control theory. Least understood is the relation between the neural proprioceptive reflexes and the chemoreceptor control system.

The Hering-Breuer reflex, or inflation and deflation reflexes, were described in 1868, but their roles in human respiratory control are still controversial. The proprioceptors for the Hering-Breuer reflexes are in the walls of the small bronchioles. If the lung is hyperinflated or the airway is blocked in the inspiratory position, inspiration is inhibited and the duration of expiratory effort is prolonged. If the lung is deflated or the airway is blocked in the expiratory position, expiration is inhibited and inspiratory effort is prolonged. This is well illustrated in human beings by the fact that a breath can be held longer following full inflation of the lungs than following deflation of the lungs. During breath-holding the pCO_2 steadily rises and the pO_2 falls, but with lungs inflated at the breaking point, the arterial pCO_2 is much higher and pO_2 lower than if the lungs were deflated. Apparently full inflation inhibits the respiratory center, while deflation stimulates it. Thus in the inflated position the inflation reflex and the blood-gas changes are antagonistic, and in the deflated position they are additive. The deflation reflex, which causes increased frequency and force of breathing, may play a role in increasing the rate of breathing in patients with pneumothorax, postoperative atelectasis, or chest wall splinting due to pain.

The most important effect of the Hering-Breuer reflex may be in the regulation of the work of breathing. The most economical control system for ventilation would be one that not only provided adequate alveolar ventilation but also achieved it with the minimum effort. In animals the respiratory frequency and volume is regulated to provide the optimal alveolar ventilation with the minimum energy expenditure. The most efficient combination of frequency and tidal volume for any alveolar ventilation will depend on the dead space, the compliance of the chest walls and lungs, and the resistance in the airways and in the tissues of the lung and chest wall. The work necessary to overcome the elastic recoil of lungs and chest wall is determined by their compliance and the tidal volume. The flow rate determines the work dissipated in flow resistance and tissue resistance. If the tidal volume is increased and the rate slowed, the elastic work per minute will increase; if the rate is speeded up and tidal volume is decreased, the resistive work per minute and the dead space ventilation increases. In man the normal tidal volume of 400 to 500 cc. and respiration rate of 15 to 18 is the ventilatory pattern requiring the least work. In a child the decreased dead space and increased stiffness of the lungs and chest wall shift the balance toward a higher rate, despite the increased resistance due to smaller airways.

When the lungs become stiff, as occurs in interstitial fibrosis, pneumonia, or edema, the shallow, rapid breathing pattern that results lowers the elastic work and thereby keeps total work at a minimum. In patients with airway obstruction due to asthma or other causes, breathing is deep and slow to minimize flow rates and, thus, the work required to get air past the resistance.

The inflation reflex may play a decisive role in setting the most efficient tidal volume and rate. When the lung is stiff, a great transpulmonary pressure could lead to greater stretch of the bronchi, resulting in inhibition of inhalation and rapid, shallow respiration. Bronchoconstriction, on the other hand, would make the airways stiffer and diminish the stretch on them, thus diminishing the firing of the bronchial proprioceptors and prolonging inspiration.

Another interesting and little understood reflex is the paradoxical reflex found by Hood in 1889. He found that if the vagus nerve was cooled, the inflation reflex was inhibited, but as the nerve was partially rewarmed, inflation led to further inflation. This reflex results in a positive feedback rather than negative feedback, the more common regulatory reflex. The importance of this reflex is unknown, though it might be the mechanism which causes the deep sigh or yawn to preserve the compliance at normal levels.

The reflex regulation of respiration is not confined to pulmonary proprioceptors and the proprioceptors and chemoreceptors of the aortic and carotid bodies. Also important are the control mechanisms which regulate muscular contraction. Little is known of their mechanism of action or how muscle contraction is augmented or new muscle groups recruited when more effort is required. To coordinate the muscular effort, the regulatory centers must receive at least as much information from sensors in the chest wall and its musculature as from the lungs and chemoreceptors.

VENTILATORY RESPONSE TO EXERCISE, COLD, AND PAIN

As the mechanisms of operation of control systems in regulation of respiration have been presented in this chapter, the progression has been from the chemocontrol system, of which there is moderately good comprehension, progressively through areas of increasing paucity of knowledge. The discussion of responses to exercise, pain, and cold can be only descriptive. The specific stimuli which increase ventilation are passive movement of limbs, even with only nerve and blood vessels intact, cold water sprayed on the body surface, and painful cutaneous stimuli. The increase in ventilation elicited by these stimuli is more powerful and faster than that elicited by any other mechanisms, but the means by which the increase comes about is not known.

Equally elusive is a satisfactory explanation of the hyperventilation with exercise which occurs prior to any change in arterial blood gases and which is precisely related to the degree of exercise. In fact, this hyperventilation seems in part to anticipate the needed level of added ventilation with exercise. The ventilation increases acutely with onset of exercise and then has a further, later increase presumably related to the alteration in intracellular hydrogen ion concentration due to accumulation of acid metabolites. Cessation of exercise causes a prompt drop in ventilation, but some hyperventilation persists until the excess of acid metabolites is aerobically burned. The increased ventilation resulting from increased metabolic demands not usually classified as exercise, such as fever, obesity, or hyperthyroidism, likewise can occur without significant changes in blood gases. The identification of the factors which allow these adjustments is completely lacking at this time.

SLEEP, ANESTHESIA, AND DRUGS

The better understood chemoregulatory system has appeared to be more important at rest than have the less well-comprehended reflex regulators. However, recent studies of respiration during sleep have shown there are still questions about chemical regulation even at rest. In deep sleep alveolar pCO_2 may rise from 40 to 46 mm. Hg. Thus sleep must decrease the sensitivity of the respiratory center to chemical stimuli. However, if the individual's airway is obstructed, he awakens immediately and struggles violently to free himself. This is clearly an instance of proprioceptive input overriding chemical control.

Anesthesia and narcotic drugs have important effects in altering the

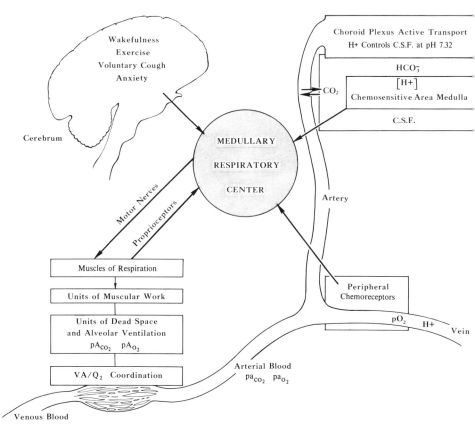

Fig. 8-3. The complex interplay of stimuli and feedback in control of respiration. The medullary center stimulates the motor nerves to the muscles of respiration. The proprioceptors of these muscles in turn send information back to the center. The muscles put out units of work. This work ventilates the dead space and alveoli, altering alveolar carbon dioxide and oxygen concentrations. The ventilation-perfusion ratio coordination and the venous blood concentration determines the effect of this ventilation on arterial pO_2 and pCO_2. These concentrations plus cardiac output in turn determine the stimuli to the respiratory center from the peripheral receptors. Likewise, acid-base composition of blood affects the central chemoreceptor stimulus. Overriding all these responses is the stimulus level from the cerebrum.

responses to various stimuli. In the awake man hyperventilation lowering pCO_2 to as low as 16 does not result in apnea. However, under anesthesia hyperventilation to a much smaller degree consistently leads to apnea. Apparently the degree of wakefulness sets the response level of the regulating mechanism. Breathing does not require a normal pCO_2 level in the awake man, but does in the anesthetized or sleeping man.

In patients in whom it is desirable to use controlled artificial ventilation, it is important to administer some sedation to depress the response level of the regulatory system. Anesthetic agents such as pentothal, cyclopropane, and fluothane can depress and even abolish the medullary center response to evaluation of arterial pCO_2, leaving only the peripheral oxygen receptors, which are not depressed as early as the other receptors. If a high inspired oxygen concentration is used, the oxygen drive may be absent and severe respiratory acidosis can result. Natural sleep and such drugs as morphine produce additive depression of the respiratory center. Knowledge of this provides the logical basis for the simplest treatment of patients with overdosage of narcotic agents, stimulation and awakening.

It would appear at this time that the role of the level of carbon dioxide and oxygen in blood is subsidiary to the neural control of ventilation, both at rest and during exercise (Fig. 8-3).

WORK OF BREATHING AND VENTILATORY RESPONSE

The respiratory center regulates the amount and pattern of ventilation to minimize work. The increment in minute ventilation in response to a given increase in concentrations of carbon dioxide in inspired air is smaller with than without an artificial resistance in the airway. Further testing suggests that a given respiratory stimulus results in a certain amount of muscular work. If the work per unit of ventilation is increased, the resulting ventilation will be less than if respiratory mechanics are normal (Fig. 8-4).

In a patient with deranged respiratory mechanics, such as is seen in emphysema, a given change in arterial pCO_2 will result in a smaller increase in ventilation than in a normal individual. Likewise, the oxygen cost of such an increase in ventilation will be greater. Because the output of the respiratory center is programmed in units of effort rather than units of ventilation, the system is further attuned to produce the most efficient level of ventilation.

This theory can best be illustrated by reviewing the response mechanisms of a patient with respiratory insufficiency and chronic elevation of arterial pCO_2 and depression of pO_2. As will be pointed out in Chapter

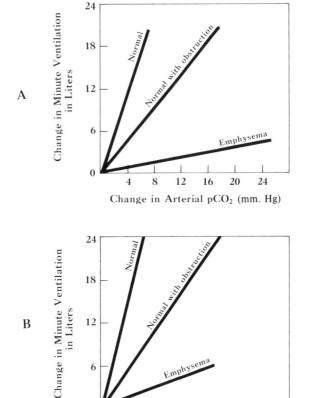

Fig. 8-4. (A) Relation of ventilatory response to arterial pCO_2. The ventilatory response to an increment in arterial pCO_2 is reduced if obstruction is introduced in the airway of a normal individual or in patients with emphysema. (B) The relation between energy or oxygen cost of breathing and change in minute ventilation. It is apparent that the decrease in ventilatory response to carbon dioxide is related to oxygen cost of a liter of ventilation. The greater the oxygen cost, the smaller the increment in ventilation.

9, elevation of pCO_2 and depression of pO_2 will increase the absolute quantity of oxygen acquired and carbon dioxide excreted per unit of ventilation. Elevation in arterial pCO_2 and hydrogen ion concentration and depression of arterial pO_2 will stimulate the peripheral chemoreceptors. The secretion of hydrogen ions by the kidneys to restore plasma hydrogen ion concentration to normal will increase blood bicarbonate toward normal and lower the hydrogen ion concentration in the periphcral receptors and so lower their stimulus to increased ventilation. The increased pCO_2 will have diminished stimulatory effect on the central receptors, because active transport in the cerebrospinal fluid system will raise cerebrospinal fluid bicarbonate ion concentration to return the cerebrospinal fluid hydrogen ion concentration toward normal. The damping of the stimulus of increased pCO_2 by the restoration of pH of plasma and cerebrospinal fluid will result in a lower minute ventilation. The decrease in ventilation will result in some rise in pCO_2, and an equilibrium between these various factors will be slowly reached. If oxygen is administered to the patient, not only is the stimulatory effect of low pO_2 removed, but the additive effect of low pO_2 and high pCO_2 is also not present. A striking decrease in ventilation can result in marked elevation of pCO_2. If the concentration of oxygen in the inspired air is kept low enough to keep arterial pO_2 below 90, the depressant effect of oxygen therapy will be small unless arterial pO_2 was markedly lowered prior to oxygen administration.

To restore ventilatory response with artificial ventilation, pCO_2 must be lowered to normal levels and maintained there long enough to permit renal excretion of the excess bicarbonate ions in the blood and active transport of excess bicarbonate out of the cerebrospinal fluid to return its acid-base distribution to normal. If, in conjunction with this, respiratory mechanics are improved (by treatment of intercurrent infection, use of bronchodilators, etc.), then a more normal pCO_2 may be maintained by the combination of mechanical improvements and compensatory acid-base adjustments. This will restore the usual stimulatory effect of changes in pCO_2 and decrease work, and so the ventilatory output for a given stimulus will return toward normal.

Much is still unknown about the hardware and software in the central computer that operates the respiratory system. However, the pieces are slowly being fitted together. Looking at any part of the system alone may be misleading, since any other stimulus may condition the response of the stimulus of immediate interest.

9. THE ENERGY COST (WORK) OF BREATHING

THIS chapter can best be introduced by quoting a statement of Comroe:*

> Gas exchange requires expenditure of energy: by the respiratory muscles to affect alveolar ventilation: by the right ventricle to pump mixed venous blood through the pulmonary capillaries; and, to a much lesser degree, by the arteriolar and bronchiolar smooth muscle to cause proper distribution of blood and gas within the lungs. Physiologists also believe that there are mechanisms which regulate frequency and total volume of breathing so that proper alveolar ventilation may be achieved with a minimal expenditure of energy.

The factors which influence the amount of energy output by the respiratory muscles and heart are (1) the mechanical properties of the lung, which include the distensibility of the lung, which in turn depends on the elasticity of the tissues and the surface forces in the alveoli and the resistance of the airways and lung tissue; (2) the mechanical properties of the chest wall and its musculature, the chest tissue resistance, and compliance; (3) the efficiency of the respiratory muscles, the condition of these muscles, and the shape and integrity of the chest wall; (4) respiratory dead space; (5) ventilation-perfusion coordination; (6) transfer of gases across alveolar membranes by diffusion; (7) the efficiency of the chemical processes in the blood; and (8) the rate and volume of respiration. (This list is nearly a complete index to this book.) A discussion of the energy cost of breathing thus is, in essence, a bringing

---

*Julius H. Comroe, Jr., "Pulmonary Gas Exchange." In D. J. C. Cunningham and B. B. Lloyd (Eds.), *The Regulation of Human Respiration*. Philadelphia: Davis, 1963. P. 45. Used by permission.

195

together of the knowledge about the respiratory system so as to quanti-
tate the effects of changes in the system in terms of the burden they place
on the individual. Even in the healthy individual the effort necessary to
get a given amount of gas exchange varies with the rate of gas exchange
required. When disease deranges the system, the energy required for
any level of gas exchange is increased. Dyspnea develops when the
energy expenditure exceeds a comfortable level. If the system is inefficient, dyspnea occurs at a low minute ventilation; if the individual is
well conditioned, it develops only at a high level of ventilation.

OXYGEN COST OF BREATHING

If an individual's oxygen consumption is measured at rest and then at
various levels of induced voluntary hyperventilation, it may be assumed
that the change in oxygen consumption is the result of the increased
ventilation. If oxygen consumption is plotted against ventilation, then
the oxygen consumed per liter of ventilation at various levels of ventilation can be determined. Such studies show that, as ventilation increases,
the oxygen consumption per liter of ventilation increases. Stated another
way, the system gets less efficient as ventilatory exchange increases.

Unfortunately the accuracy of these determinations leaves much to
be desired, as is apparent from the discrepancy of the data from different
investigators. Some of the values found show that at a resting minute
ventilation of about 4 liters per minute, the oxygen uptake per liter of
ventilation is 0.5 to 1 cc. per liter, or 2 to 4 cc. per minute, while total
oxygen consumption is 200 cc. per minute. Less than 1 to 2% of oxygen consumption is used for ventilation. As the minute ventilatory volume rises to 20 liters per minute, the oxygen uptake for each liter of
ventilation rises to 4 cc. per liter, or four to eight times as much oxygen
per liter as at resting ventilatory levels. Theoretically, if the ventilatory
volume was progressively increased, a point would be reached at which
more oxygen was being consumed by the muscles of respiration and the
heart than could be acquired by increased ventilation. In other words,
the cost of hyperventilation would exceed the returns. In normal individuals such a situation is never approached, but it can occur in patients
with altered respiratory mechanics.

Presumably, measures of the oxygen cost of breathing include the
oxygen consumption of the heart as well as the respiratory muscles,
and so the energy required to operate the whole cardiorespiratory system is measured. Thus a change in the oxygen cost of breathing can be
the result of a change in minute ventilation or in the functional integrity
of the system. A more specific measure of energy required to ventilate

the lungs can be made by measuring the mechanical work done on the lungs or the lungs and chest wall.

MECHANICAL WORK

Work equals a force moved through a distance. As pointed out in Chapter 4, "Mechanical Properties of the Respiratory System," the equation for the force in a pressure-volume machine is:

$$P_{app} = \frac{1}{C} V + R\dot{V} + L\ddot{V}$$

where P_{app} = force applied to the system
   C = compliance
   V = volume
   R = resistance
   $\dot{V}$ = flow rate
   L = inertance or mass
   $\ddot{V}$ = rate of change of flow

When considering the total respiratory system, there is an additional force involved, that of the dead weight of the chest wall and abdominal contents. The factor of dead weight can be accounted for in the term C, representing compliance. The last term in the equation, $L\ddot{V}$, the inertance term, can be neglected because inertia of the lungs and chest wall is so small. One might hope, then, to be able to calculate work done on the respiratory system if flow, volume, compliance, and resistance were known. This is not a practical way of calculating work, however, since neither compliance, nor resistance, nor flow is constant throughout a breath.

An alternative would be to determine the relationship between the force applied to the system and the rate of volume change of the system. The reasoning behind this approach is:

$$\text{Work (W)} = \text{force} \times \text{distance}$$
$$W = \text{gm.} \times \text{cm.}$$
$$\text{Pressure (P)} = \text{force per unit of area, gm./cm.}^2$$
$$\text{Volume (V)} = \text{cm.}^3$$
$$\text{Work} = \text{volume} \times \text{pressure} = \text{gm./cm.}^2 \times \text{cm.}^3 = \text{gm.} \times \text{cm.}$$

or, work done in ventilating the lungs equals pressure applied times volume change of the chest cavity:

$$\text{Work} = P_{app} \times \Delta V$$

Although measuring the change in volume of the system is simple, measuring the force on the lungs and chest wall during spontaneous breathing is impossible, because to do so it would be necessary to measure the forces applied by all the various muscles of respiration. Since muscular force cannot be directly measured, any consideration of the actual mechanical work done on the whole system is of necessity theo-

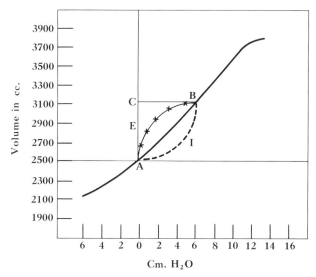

Fig. 9-1. Plot of forcing pressure to stretch the lungs and chest wall to a given volume. In all of the pressure-volume plots, the vertical axis represents change in intrathoracic gas volume in cubic centimeters and the horizontal axis represents forcing pressure. The functional residual capacity is 2,500 cc. (horizontal line); at this point the force across the system is zero and to inflate the system requires forcing pressure. In this pressure-volume plot of elastic and resistive forcing pressure versus volume, the dashed line (*I*) represents the pressure-volume change during inspiration. The cross-hatched line (*E*) represents volume-pressure change during expiration. The triangle *ABCA* represents work to stretch the lung. The area between the dashed portion of the loop and the line *AB* is the work done during inspiration to overcome resistance to air flow and tissue motion. The area between line *AB* and the cross-hatched portion of the loop represents resistive work of expiration. The distance from the loop to the line *AB* at any point represents the forcing pressure required to overcome resistance at that point. To change air flow direction during expiration, the forcing pressure must be the opposite of that during inspiration, so the difference between line *AB* and loop *E* is opposite in sign to that between line *AB* and loop *I*. The actual force for expiration comes from potential elastic energy stored during inspiration, when work was done to stretch the lungs. Some of this stored elastic energy, the area of triangle *ABCA* not filled by the loop, is dissipated as heat by the inspiratory muscles, which continue to contract during expiration.

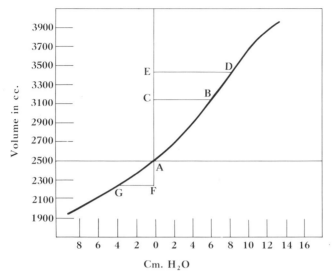

Fig. 9-2. Effect of change of tidal volume on elastic work. Over the straight-line portion of this plot a 1 cm. H_2O forcing pressure increases the volume 100 cc. To increase volume from A to B, an amount of 600 cc., the forcing pressure must change from 0 to 6 cm. Work equals force times distance, so the work is equal to the forcing pressure times the volume change. Since during the first 100 cc. of change forcing pressure is rising from 0 to 1 cm. H_2O, and during the last 100 cc. forcing pressure is rising from 5 to 6, the forcing pressure is steadily changing. The actual work is equivalent to the triangular area *ABCA,* or half the product of volume change times total pressure change. To increase volume to 900 cc. instead of 600, added work *BCEDB* must be done. As much work is done for the last 300 cc. as for this first 600 cc.

retical, but it is still useful since the bases of the theoretical analysis are sound. To make a theoretical analysis of work done on the lungs and chest wall, assume for the moment that we can measure in pressure units the force which moves the tidal volume into and out of the lungs.

SPONTANEOUS BREATHING

If the value of forcing pressure across the lungs and chest is plotted against the volume change during a single breath, a loop is described, as shown in Figure 9-1. Analysis of this loop allows one to calculate the total work of one breath, which can be broken down into the elastic work (which includes in this analysis dead-weight work) and resistive work. We shall first consider the elastic component of the total work.

If the compliance of the lungs and chest wall is 100 cc. per centimeter H_2O, then to stretch the system to contain another 600 cc. of volume will require the forcing pressure to rise from 0 to 6 cm. H_2O. Figure 9-2 is a plot of the changes in forcing pressure versus the change in volume for a system in which compliance is 100 cc. per centimeter H_2O and in which there is no resistance. The starting volume is 2,500 cc., the point at which all muscles are relaxed and the forcing pressure is zero. As stated earlier, work is equal to pressure change times volume change. However, in this case it is not 6 gm. per square centimeter $\times$ 600 cc., or 3,600 gm.-cm. Reference to Figure 9-2 shows that for the first 100 cc. increment in volume, the forcing pressure rises from 0 to 1 gm. per square centimeter, and, for the second 100 cc., from 1 to 2 gm. per square centimeter. The forcing pressure is constantly changing, so the rate of doing elastic work is constantly changing. The elastic work is equivalent to the area of triangle *ABCA,* or one-half the product of the maximum volume change times the maximum pressure change, in this case, 1,800 gm.-cm. If a breath of 900 cc. instead of 600 cc. is taken, then the total work is equivalent to the area *ABDECA*, or

$$\frac{8 \text{ gm./cm.} \times 900 \text{ cc.}}{2} = 3,600 \text{ gm.-cm.}$$

The additional 300 cc. requires as much work as the original 600 cc. This is because as the lung and chest wall are stretched to a large volume, the pressure across them must be greater, so the forcing pressure per 100 cc. increase in volume must also steadily increase. Actually, the elastic work of breathing goes up as the square of the increase in tidal volume. If air is expelled 300 cc. beyond the resting volume, the mechanical work required to compress the system is equal to *AGFA,* the same 900 gm.-cm. as are required to inhale 300 cc.

These calculations suggest that if tidal volume must be increased, the elastic work would be least if half of the increase was from the expiratory reserve and half from the inspiratory reserve. Since one can measure neither the actual force required from the expiratory muscles to compress the chest versus that required to expand it nor the effect of compression on resistive work, this apparently logical conclusion rests on incomplete evidence. In fact, only with maximum respiratory effort is the reserve volume used for ventilation.

If compliance is abnormal, elastic work will be altered. In Figure 9-3 line *AD* represents a compliance one-half of normal. For a 600 cc. breath elastic work will be twice that required with normal compliance, or equal to the area *ADCA*. If the compliance is doubled, line *AE,* the work will be half the amount required with normal compliance, or area *AECA.*

During inspiration the force applied to expand the volume of air in the lungs stretches the elements of the lung and chest wall. If the forcing

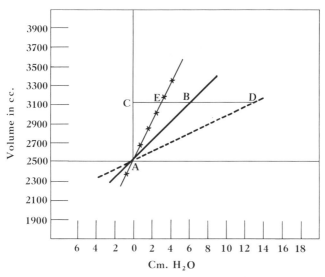

Fig. 9-3. Effect of change in compliance on elastic work. Line *AB* represents normal compliance of 100 cc. per centimeter H_2O. Line *AD* represents a compliance of 50 cc. per centimeter H_2O. This fall in compliance doubles the work of stretching the lungs; area *ABCA* is one-half the area *ADCA*. Line *AE* represents a compliance of 200 cc. per centimeter H_2O; here the elastic work is cut in half and area *ABCA* is twice area *AECA*.

pressure is released, the system will contract back to the original volume. Speaking in energy terms, during inspiration potential elastic energy is stored in the chest wall and lungs in an amount equal to the elastic work done on the chest wall and lungs. This potential elastic energy is then available to do work during expiration.

The dashed line in Figure 9-1 is a true record of pressure-volume changes during inspiration. The triangle *ABCA* in Figure 9-1, as in Figure 9-2, represents the elastic work done during inspiration for a 600 cc. breath. During inspiration, in addition to the work required to stretch the lungs and chest wall, work must be done to overcome resistance. In Figure 9-1 the forcing pressures required to overcome inspiratory resistance are equal to the distance from the dashed loop to line *AB*; the inspiratory resistive work is represented by one-half the elipse, the area *AIBA*. During expiration the flow reverses, so the forcing pressure must also reverse its direction. In algebraic terms, the signs of both flow and pressure reverse. The cross-hatched portion of the loop starting at *B* and going to *A* is a plot of the forcing pressure and volume during expiration. The expiratory flow resistive pressures are equal to the distance from line *BA* to the cross-hatched loop. The area of half of the elipse to the left of line *BA* represents the resistive work of expiration. In this case it lies entirely within the triangle *ABCA,* which represents elastic potential energy stored during inspiration and which, in this case, provides all the force necessary to overcome resistance during expiration.

The area of the triangle *ABCA* not filled by the expiratory loop represents potential elastic energy which is dissipated as heat by the inspiratory muscles, which continue to contract during the early part of expiration. If the resistance in the system increases, the pressure necessary to overcome resistance will increase unless flow decreases. The loop will become fatter, as in Figure 9-4. In this case, during part of the expiration the loop lies outside the triangle *ABCA.* The potential energy stored during inspiration is insufficient to push air out, and active work is required of the expiratory muscles.

Increase in the number of breaths per minute, even without change in tidal volume, increases the resistive work per breath. The faster flow rate necessary to move the tidal volume in and out in a shorter period

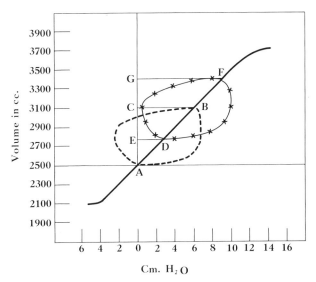

Fig. 9-4. Effect of increased resistance on pressure-volume relations. The increased resistance requires increased forcing pressure, so the loop becomes fatter. During expiration the dashed loop falls outside the triangle *ABCA,* and muscle force is required to create a pressure to push air out of the lungs. This force collapses the bronchi and so fattens the expiratory loop more than the inspiratory loop. If this muscle force cannot be provided, all of the inspired air will not be expelled during the expiratory half of the cycle. The expiratory reserve volume then will increase until the stored elastic energy is adequate to force all of the air out of the thorax, area *EDFGE* (see Fig. 9-1).

of time requires an increase in forcing pressure to achieve the higher flow rate, and so work is increased. The increase in forcing pressure is further elevated if increased turbulence results from increased flow. The force necessary to overcome resistance to turbulent flow equals the resistance times the square of the flow rate, $R\dot{V}^2$, rather than $R\dot{V}$. If there is more turbulence, which can result from the higher flow rates due to the high respiratory rate, more force is required to move a given volume and so more work is done per cubic centimeter of ventilation. If the expiratory muscles are required to force air out of the lungs to achieve the higher flow rates, the contraction of these muscles raises the pleural pressure. The increased pressure compresses the small bronchi, narrowing their lumina and increasing resistance to air flow through them.

To increase minute ventilation, either tidal volume or respiratory rate must be increased; in either case, flow rate will have to rise. Thus, increased rates of gas exchange increase resistive work per breath because to move the same volume in less time requires a higher flow rate, which in turn leads to a higher proportion of turbulent flow and greater resistance to air flow due to compression of bronchi during expiration. Since increase of either tidal volume or respiratory rate increases work per liter of minute ventilation, as minute ventilation increases, the efficiency of the ventilatory system decreases.

ARTIFICIAL RESPIRATION

Since during spontaneous breathing the muscular forces driving the chest wall cannot be measured, there are no actual experimental data to calculate work done on the system. The total mechanical work done on the lungs and chest wall can be measured only when a relaxed patient is artificially ventilated with a respirator. Such measurements are not accurate reflections of the conditions during spontaneous breathing, but they are of some interest. During inspiration the pressure created by the respirator at the opening of the airway is the driving pressure which stretches the lung and chest wall and overcomes the resistance in the system. During expiration the air must be forced out of the lungs by the elastic recoil of the system. If the elastic recoil force is inadequate to expel all the air pumped in by the respirator, the end-expiratory volume will be increased and the system will be partially stretched at the start of the next breath. The pressure required at the beginning of the second breath will not be zero but rather will be equal to the end-expiratory pressure found at the new residual volume. The elastic work required to inflate the lung and chest 600 cc. on the next breath will be increased. Figure 9-4 (above) depicts this change when, at the start of the second breath, the residual volume is increased 300 cc. The inspiratory elastic work is represented by the trapezoid *DEFGD*, which is equal to the 3,600 gm.-cm. of work needed to stretch the system, as opposed to the 1,800 gm.-cm. (area *ABCA*) required in the first breath. This greater stretching force applied to inflate the chest stores more potential elastic energy during inspiration so there is adequate force to expel air during the expiratory cycle.

If the resistance to air flow is increased in a patient ventilated with a respirator, residual volume will increase until the elastic recoil of the lungs and chest wall can supply the force necessary to expel the tidal volume. While total mechanical work done on lungs and chest wall can be measured only during artificial ventilation, work on the lung can be measured in spontaneously breathing subjects.

In most chest diseases treated without surgery the principal disorder is in the lungs, not the chest wall, so measurements of work done on the lung alone accurately reflect the major changes in work. However, in surgical patients the mechanical derangements may involve the chest wall as much as the lungs, and measurements of work on the lung may not accurately reflect the energy cost of breathing in postoperative and postinjury patients.

WORK ON THE LUNG

Work done on the lungs can be measured during spontaneous breathing because the expansion and contraction of the lungs is not dependent on muscles within the lung. The lungs passively respond to changes in the pressure across them, which is the difference between pressure at the opening of the airway and pressure in the pleura. This transpulmonary pressure can be measured with a differential manometer, one side of the manometer being connected to a balloon catheter in the esophagus and the other to the inlet of the airway. Figure 9-5 is a diagram like Figure 9-2 but showing the elastic work done on the lungs in addition to the previously depicted triangle *ABCA* for total work done on the system. The solid line *ABF* is the compliance line of the whole system. The dashed line *EBG* is steeper and represents the greater compliance of the lung alone. It is displaced to the right because at end-expiration the interpleural pressure is not zero. The cross-hatched line *DCH* is the compliance line of the chest wall and is displaced to the left a distance equal to the displacement to the right of the lung compliance line. These compliances are assumed to be linear over the 1,200 cc. of volume change shown.

As in Figures 9-1 and 9-2, the total work done to stretch the system by the muscles for a 600 cc. breath is *ABCA*. At the start of inspiration the intrapleural pressure is −3 cm. H_2O. The lungs are not at resting

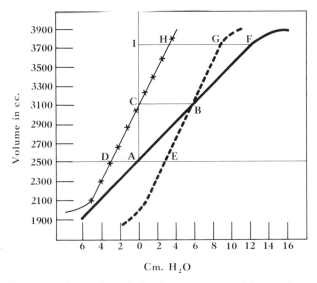

Fig. 9-5. Pressure-volume plot of elastic component of lungs alone and chest wall alone. The solid line is the elastic pressure-volume of lungs and chest wall, as shown in Figure 9-1. Line *EBG* is that for the lungs. The compliance of the lungs alone is twice that of the lungs and chest wall, and at zero pressure the volume falls 600 cc.; i.e., at functional residual volume the lung is stretched by a force of 3 cm. H_2O. The chest wall likewise has a compliance twice that of the lungs and chest wall, and at zero pressure its volume increases 600 cc. At functional residual capacity the lungs are pulled out by the chest wall and the chest wall is pulled in by the lung with a force of 3 cm. H_2O. During inspiration part of the work done to expand the lung, the area *AEBA*, is provided by the stored potential energy in the compressed chest wall, area *ACDA*. When a large breath of 1,200 cc. is taken, for the last 600 cc. the chest wall as well as the lungs must be stretched, the area bounded by *AFIA*. The elastic work on the whole system exceeds that on the lung during the last half of the breath. This is represented by the area *BFGB*, which is equal to the area *CHIC*, the work needed to stretch the chest wall the last 600 cc.

volume but are partially stretched; therefore, the work to stretch the lungs is equal to the area of trapezoid *AEBCA*. More work is done to stretch the lungs alone than to stretch the entire system. The negative intrapleural pressure at the start of inspiration means that at the starting point the lung is partially stretched and the chest wall is partially compressed. Part of the force to stretch the lung during inspiration is provided by the potential elastic energy of recoil in the compressed chest wall area *ADCA*. During expiration, the chest wall is pulled in by the lung and the potential elastic energy transferred by the chest wall to the lungs during inspiration is returned to the chest wall during expiration. In Figure 9-5 this is shown by the fact that the area of the triangle *AEBA*, which represents the amount of work done on the lung in excess of the total work done on the system, equals the area of the triangle *ADCA,* which represents the stored potential energy that was present in the compressed chest wall at the start of inspiration.

If a larger breath, 1,200 cc., is taken, the chest wall as well as the lungs must be stretched during the last 600 cc. of the breath. In this case total elastic work for the last part of the breath exceeds elastic work done on the lungs alone by an amount equal to the force needed to stretch the chest wall. Total elastic work is equivalent to triangle *AFIA;* elastic work on the lung equals *AEGIA*. During the last 600 cc., the excess of total elastic work over that done on the lung is equal to *BFGB* and this, in turn, is equal to the elastic work done on the chest wall, *CIHC*.

It is impossible to determine either the amount of energy transferred by the chest wall to the lungs during inspiration or the energy transferred back to the chest wall from the lungs during expiration, because during spontaneous breathing the forces acting on the chest wall cannot be measured. When work on the lung is measured by determining pleural pressure, some indeterminate portion of the measured elastic work does not require muscular effort.

The resistive work done on the lungs alone is calculated exactly as it is for the lungs and chest wall. In quiet breathing and when resistance is normal (Fig. 9-6), the expiratory portion of the loop lies within trapezoid *AEBCA,* which represents elastic energy stored in the lungs or lungs and chest wall during inspiration. If the apparent resistance is increased by disease or by fast flow rates, the elastic potential energy is inadequate and positive muscular effort is required to expel air. As shown in Figure 9-6 part of the dashed loop is to the left of the zero line, representing the fact that pleural pressure has swung to a positive value during the latter part of inspiration. Just as was shown for the total system (Fig. 9-4), the force needed for expiration could be supplied by increasing the end-tidal volume 300 cc. rather than by expiratory muscular effort. In Figure 9-6 this is depicted by the cross-hatched loop. The inspiratory elastic work increases from 2,700 gm.-cm., area *AEBCA,* to 3,100 gm.-cm., area *HDFGH,* and there is adequate stored potential energy to expel the inspired volume on the second breath.

A DIRECT METHOD OF CALCULATING MECHANICAL WORK

The method of graphic plotting of the pressure-volume loop on an x-y axis and measuring the areas identified in the discussion above is very time-consuming. The process is simplified by recording volume change and pressure change with an x-y recorder so the loop is directly plotted.

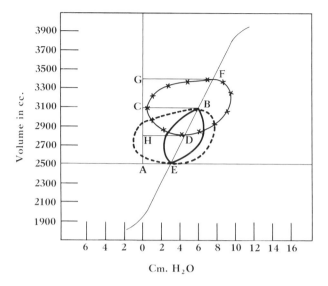

Cm. H$_2$O

Analog recordings of above loops

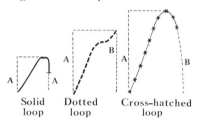

| Solid | Dotted | Cross-hatched |
| loop | loop | loop |

Fig. 9-6. Resistive work done on lungs. Line *EF* is the compliance line of the lungs. Area *AEBCA* represents the elastic energy (2,700 gm.-cm.) stored in the lungs during inspiration. The expiratory portion of the solid-line loop lies within this area, and stored elastic potential energy provides all the force necessary to expel the inspired air. The dashed loop represents the situation if resistance is increased. The force to do the work represented by the area to the left of line *ACG* will have to be done by the expiratory muscles. If functional residual capacity is increased 300 cc., the energy stored during inspiration, *HDFGH* is increased to 3,100 gm.-cm. and the cross-hatched loop lies within the trapezoid *HDFGH*. Stored potential energy is adequate to push air out of the lungs.

The bottom half of this figure shows analog computer recordings of the integrated product of pressure times flow during a cycle. The first recording represents normal. Work is stored during inspiration, the peak of the tracing, and some is regained during expiration, the fall. The distance from the end of the tracing to the zero line is equivalent to resistive work. The dashed tracing rises until the end inspiration, break in curve, and then rises further during expiration as more work is done to expel air. In the last curve elastic work has been increased during inspiration; the peak of curve is higher, so adequate energy is stored to expel air during expiration.

Even with this aid, measurement of the various areas requires 15 to 20 minutes per breath. To gather significant amounts of data requires a simpler method.

Power is the rate of change of work and has the dimensions gm.-cm./sec. The dimensions of pressure are gm./cm.,^{2} and of flow, cm.^{3}/sec. The product of pressure times flow is:

$$\text{Pressure} \times \text{flow} = \frac{\text{gm.}}{\text{cm.}^2} \times \frac{\text{cm.}^3}{\text{sec.}} = \frac{\text{gm.} \times \text{cm.}}{\text{sec.}}$$

So the product of flow times pressure is power. If a certain amount of power is expended in a system each second, and if the units of power for the period of interest, for example, the period of one breath, are added one to the other, the sum is equal to the work done on the system during that period. In calculus this sum is the integral of the quantity for that period of time. If measured transpulmonary pressure is multiplied by the flow rate continuously and the product integrated over the course of a breath, the result is equal to work done on the system.

$$\text{Work} = \int_S^E P \times \dot{V} dt$$

where   S = time at start of breath
          E = time at end of breath
          P = transpulmonary pressure
          $\dot{V}$ = airflow
          dt = derivative of time

With an analog or an analog-to-digital computer this can be simply done.

Since flow rate reverses during expiration, changing the algebraic sign, unless the algebraic sign of pressure also reverses (when resistance is high), the value of the integral decreases during expiration. The maximum value of the integral will occur at the end of inspiration. The total work, the value of the integral at the end of expiration, equals the energy not regained from the elastic potential energy stored during inspiration, and it is equal to the resistive work. If positive expiratory effort is needed to expel air from the lungs, the resistive work may exceed the total work (see Fig. 9-6). With this simplified method of calculation, values for work on the lung or total work in a patient on a ventilator can be determined as fast as the patient breathes.

Studies of mechanical work using various available methods of measurement have shown that the respiratory control system is attuned to minimize the work required for a given level of ventilation. A formula has been worked out by Otis to predict the work at a given level of ventilation. It is an imposing formula, but its solution agrees with the theory that the rate and tidal volume chosen by an individual minimizes ventilatory work.

$$W = \frac{f}{2C_{tot}} \left(\frac{\dot{V}_A}{f} + V_D \right)^2 + \frac{\pi^2 R_{tot}}{4} (\dot{V}_A + fV_D)^2$$

$$+ \frac{2\pi^2 K}{3} (\dot{V}_A + fV_D)^3$$

where W = work per minute
      C_{tot} = total compliance
      R_{tot} = total linear resistance
      f = frequency of respiration
      $\dot{V}_A$ = alveolar ventilation
      V_D = dead space ventilation
      K = constant for turbulent resistance

ENERGY COST OF BREATHING AND METABOLIC RATE

Since the metabolic demands of the individual determine the amount of ventilation necessary, the energy cost of breathing is determined both by the mechanical efficiency of the system and the metabolic rate. Lying in bed a normal man burns 1,650 calories per day; if he is eating during this period of bed rest, 1,850 calories are required; sitting in a chair requires 2,000 to 2,250 calories per day; and a laborer may use 6,000 to 7,000 calories daily. If the metabolic rate, which is the need for oxygen and carbon dioxide exchange, increases for any reason, there must be an increase in the amount of ventilation and pulmonary blood flow as well as those changes in metabolic rate associated with changing levels of activity.

Many types of injury markedly increase metabolic rate. For example, a burn patient may use 3,000 to 4,000 calories per day to provide heat of vaporization for water lost from the denuded body surface. Fever likewise increases metabolic rate, and, according to some reports, metabolic rate is up in the postoperative period.

This discussion has pointed out that the mechanical work of breathing per unit of ventilation increases when either tidal volume or respiratory rate is increased. The increase in oxygen consumption and carbon dioxide production with a rise in metabolic rate requires an increase in minute ventilation, and so an increase in metabolic rate leads to a loss of efficiency in the ventilatory system. When ventilation increases, an increasing proportion of the oxygen and carbon dioxide exchange is used by the respiratory muscles. No respiratory symptoms will result from mild increases in metabolic rate in the normal individual. If the respiratory apparatus is abnormal, however, only mild increases in metabolic rate may result in dyspnea. On the other hand, if the individual is well conditioned physically, large increases in metabolic rate may be tolerated with minimal dyspnea. As all individuals know, lack of exercise leads to dyspnea with exertion at lower levels of ventilation than when physical training is maintained. No accurate information is available to explain the effect of conditioning on the level of exercise tolerated without unpleasant dyspnea. It is thought that conditioning alters the shortening of muscles and makes them more efficient. Dyspnea is probably a symptom which is closely related to the efficiency of the respiratory apparatus; it acts to put a ceiling on the level of voluntary exercise and thus the demands made on the respiratory system.

If the efficiency of the respiratory system is markedly compromised, the energy cost of the ventilation to exchange oxygen consumed and carbon dioxide produced may be more than the patient can sustain, even at rest. If the patient cannot do the necessary work of breathing, ventilation will fall below the levels required to excrete the carbon dioxide produced by the tissues. This inadequate ventilation will cause carbon dioxide to build up in the body, and an oxygen debt will be accumulated. The carbon dioxide accumulation will increase the arterial pCO_2 and, in turn, alveolar pCO_2 and the oxygen debt will decrease the arterial and alveolar pO_2. Figure 9-7 illustrates the results of the changes in the excretion rate per 100 cc. of alveolar ventilation when arterial pCO_2 and pO_2 are altered. The fall in alveolar pO_2 and rise in alveolar pCO_2 permits exchange of more carbon dioxide and oxygen for each 100 cc. of alveolar ventilation. The patient can carry out the necessary gas exchange at a lower level of ventilation. The lower alveolar pO_2 does not result in an extreme decrease in arterial oxygen saturation, because pO_2 is still high enough to fall on the flat portion of the hemoglobin dissociation curve. An excessive rise in arterial hydrogen ion concentration is also avoided if the accumulation of carbon dioxide occurs slowly because renal reabsorption of bicarbonate ions partially compensates for the accumulation of carbon dioxide. Respiratory acidosis is thus a last-ditch method of adjustment when the efficiency of the gas exchange system is disrupted.

This general discussion of the energy cost of breathing can be of great practical as well as theoretical value. A study of the extra effort

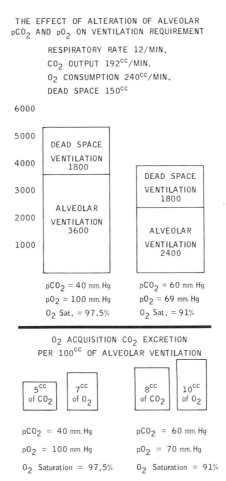

Fig. 9-7. The effect of rise in pCO_2 on the alveolar ventilation needed to exchange carbon dioxide and oxygen. Top shows the effect of decreasing alveolar ventilation from 3,600 to 2,400 cc. when carbon dioxide output is 192 cc. per minute and oxygen consumption is 240 cc. per minute: The pCO_2 rises and pO_2 falls. Despite the large fall in pO_2, the oxygen saturation fall is only modest because at this pO_2 the oxyhemoglobin dissociation curve is still flat. The bottom half shows how much more oxygen is acquired and carbon dioxide excreted per 100 cc. of alveolar ventilation when pO_2 and pCO_2 are elevated (right diagram) than when they are normal (left diagram).

or energy cost required of the patient under various conditions and in various degrees and types of illness is very helpful in understanding the mechanism of cardiorespiratory disease in designing specific therapy. The next chapters review some of the more common clinical problems from this viewpoint.

10. THE EFFECTS OF ENVIRONMENT AND THE LEVEL OF ACTIVITY

THE preceding discussions of the normal operation of the respiratory system as well as how particular functions are altered by activity level, age, trauma, or disease are the background for the next three chapters, which will discuss the cardiorespiratory system as it is affected by its environment, the level of physical activity, aging, and various clinical and disease conditions. There will be some repetition, but this is necessary to bring together and correlate the previous, more basic discussion. Two factors fundamental to all clinical conditions but often not considered by the physician are the environment the patient is in and the activity level required.

THE ENVIRONMENT

As man ventures into space, probes the depths of the oceans, and discharges wastes into the atmosphere, the effect of the environment on respiration assumes a steadily increasing importance. The primary function of respiration is to exchange oxygen and carbon dioxide; however, the other constituents of the atmosphere—nitrogen, argon, and pollutants—are also inhaled.

THE ATMOSPHERE

A brief discussion of the makeup of our atmosphere will provide useful information in understanding the effect it has on man and vice versa. The atmosphere is divided into several layers. As the altitude above the earth increases, the pressure and concentrations of the various gases decrease. The fraction of the total partial pressure or the percentage composition does not change significantly, however, until the outermost layer is reached, 360,000 feet above the earth. There is considerable mixing of gases in the atmosphere. It is estimated that 20% of the air in one atmospheric hemisphere is mixed with that in the other every six months, which means the turnover time of air in the atmosphere is 2.2 years.

The composition of the atmosphere is slowly changing. The primitive atmosphere contained hydrogen, helium, water, methane, and ammonia. Solar radiation has split the hydrogen from nitrogen, carbon, and oxygen, allowing helium and hydrogen, the fastest and lightest particles, to escape, and leaving an atmosphere of oxygen, nitrogen, and carbon dioxide, the most stable compounds.

Without life, all of the carbon would be burned up by oxygen. The plants' ability to restore free oxygen from carbon dioxide has created a kinetically steady state of concentration of nitrogen and oxygen in the atmosphere.

Carbon dioxide was probably in a steady state until one hundred years ago. The increased release of carbon dioxide into the atmosphere has been due both to increased fossil fuel combustion with the coming of the industrial revolution and to the denuding of the world's forests. The percentage of carbon dioxide in the atmosphere in 1900 was 0.0290; at present it is 0.0310, or an increase of 7% in just under 70 years. This increase in carbon dioxide leads to warming of the atmosphere and should increase the rate of photosynthesis, if vegetation is not further destroyed. It is estimated that 500 years from now the percent of carbon dioxide in the atmosphere will be between 0.085 and 0.27, depending on how much of the carbon dioxide can be absorbed by the ocean and then dissolve the calcium carbonate sediments in the ocean floor. The rates of the latter two reactions are slower than the increase in production at this time.

The final net result of the geochemical experiments of man in releasing added carbon dioxide into the atmosphere may influence his environment significantly. The increase of carbon dioxide and the slower depletion of oxygen are occurring at a very slow rate, and we have time to deal with the problem and perhaps even to find a new, suitable atmosphere in another solar system. The immediate danger is that we will poison the atmosphere with other substances, either industrial and/or atomic, and strip the earth of its essential vegetation long before the chemical depletion of the atmosphere.

AIR POLLUTANTS

The immediate danger of polluting the atmosphere with noxious gas in the form of wastes from the burning of fossil fuels is upon us. One of the most important of these pollutants is nitrogen dioxide, NO_2. This is the principal air pollutant from gasoline engine exhausts, which, for example, release 200 to 300 tons of nitrogen dioxide daily into the atmosphere in Los Angeles. Nitrogen dioxide is also produced in arc welding and from the burning of explosives and is the noxious agent in silo-filler's disease. In man, an exposure of a few minutes up to one hour to 500 parts per million (ppm) of nitrogen dioxide results in acute pulmonary edema and death; a somewhat lesser exposure causes diffuse bronchopneumonia which kills in two to ten days. Exposure to 150 to 200 ppm leads to bronchiolitis and fibrosa obliterans, which is fatal in three to five weeks. Exposure to 50 to 100 ppm causes a bronchiolitis with focal pneumonia, from which recovery takes six to eight weeks. Chronic intermittent exposure causes pulmonary fibrosis and a picture which mimics obstructive emphysema with a decrease in maximum expiratory flow rate due to increased expiratory resistance.

Cigarette smoke has 200 to 650 ppm of nitrogen dioxide. No acute toxicity results, probably because exposure is intermittent. The nitrogen dioxide in the smoke may be the etiological agent, or one of them, in the production of emphysema, since chronic exposure to nitrogen dioxide can produce a picture very similar to that seen in obstructive emphysema. In areas such as Los Angeles the residents, and particularly the children, are exposed to chronic excessive levels of nitrogen dioxide. This may in the next few decades leave us with an incidence of premature emphysema of epidemic proportions.

One solution suggested to stop the pollution of the atmosphere with nitrogen dioxide has been the electric car. This may not be a panacea unless we stop burning fossil fuels to generate electricity. Sulfur dioxide and trioxide, SO_2 and SO_3, are major pollutants from the burning of both coal and industrial-grade fuel oil. Some of the major oil companies are now constructing refineries to remove sulfur from these industrial fuels, and the increasing use of atomic power to generate electricity may prevent increasing pollution by sulfur.

Five to thirteen ppm of sulfur dioxide cause increased flow resistance in the airways, probably due to the irritant effect on the bronchial mucosa causing bronchoconstriction. Apparently, chronic exposure to sulfur dioxide in arid atmospheres has little irritant effect. In humid atmospheres such as are encountered in paper mills, there is an increased incidence of nasopharyngitis; greater frequency of cough, expectoration, and dyspnea on exertion; and increased acidity of the urine. These differences may be due to the presence of noxious agents in the humid atmosphere which are absent in the arid one, or to aerosols carrying the gas into the tracheobronchial tree.

Ozone, O_3, is the third of the major air pollutants. Ozone is produced by electrical discharge on oxygen or air by some chemical reactions such as the oxidation of phosphorus. It is formed in the upper atmosphere by ultraviolet light of less than 2,200 A, and it is decomposed by ultraviolet light of 3,000 to 2,000 A. Clean air has a higher ozone content than that in built-up areas, where smog filters out ultraviolet light and prevents the conversion of oxygen to ozone. Welders exposed to 9 ppm of ozone develop marked dyspnea, chest pain, and cough with minimal findings in the chest, though such an injury has a long morbidity requiring nine days to nine months for complete recovery.

Cough, dyspnea, and some decrease in carbon monoxide diffusion capacity and forced expired volume have been reported on exposure to only 1 ppm of ozone. Ozone also affects visual acuity. Chronically exposed animals develop tolerance to the instant effects of ozone, but they then develop chronic bronchitis and bronchiolitis, and emphysematous and fibrotic changes occur in the pulmonary parenchyma.

Carbon monoxide is another major pollutant of our atmosphere. It is produced by the incomplete burning of fossil fuels. Toxic levels of this gas have been found in the streets of our cities, where it may be a causative agent in many motor vehicle accidents. Carbon monoxide is particularly dangerous because it is an odorless, nonirritating gas which insidiously poisons an individual by impairing his consciousness. The impairment of function depends on the proportion of hemoglobin that is converted to carboxy hemoglobin, which in turn depends on the percentage of carbon monoxide in the inspired air and the duration of exposure.

A useful formula for determining impairment is the number of hours of exposure times the parts of carbon monoxide per 10,000. If the product is less than 6, then the exposure will have no effect on the subject. If the factor rises to 9, the individual may develop a frontal headache, drowsiness, and lassitude. When the product reaches 15, there is danger of loss of life. Another measure of impairment is the degree of saturation of hemoglobin with carbon monoxide. When HbCO saturation is above 15% but below 25%, the mild symptoms of headache, lassitude, and drowsiness are present. When it rises to 25% or more, the symptoms at rest are still slight, but exertion causes dyspnea, hyperpnea, disturbance of vision, and clouded mentality. When HbCO is 50%, vision becomes dim and getting up from a chair, walking, or thinking become difficult; if exposure is continued, death can result. The faster the metabolic rate, the sooner the onset of symptoms. This is why canaries are kept in mines as an index of carbon monoxide conccntration; their accelerated metabolic rate will make them succumb to carbon monoxide poisoning at levels not yet toxic to man.

The toxic effects of carbon monoxide are also exaggerated at high altitudes, where the partial pressure of oxygen is reduced. This characteristic may make low levels of carbon monoxide a significant cause of aircraft accidents, just as its presence at high concentration levels makes it a significant factor in accidents on the highway.

Carbon monoxide poisoning should be treated by removing the individual promptly from the carbon monoxide atmosphere and providing high concentrations of oxygen. It takes about 250 minutes to drop the blood level of HbCO to half its original value when an individual breathes air. Breathing pure oxygen reduces this time to 40 to 50 minutes, a five- to sixfold increase. The addition of 5 to 6% carbon dioxide to the inspired gas mixture to cause hyperventilation or placing the patient in a hyperbaric chamber can further speed the elimination of carbon monoxide.

SMOKING

All of the above-mentioned pollutants have been found in the atmosphere of our cities in excessive amounts. All of them (with perhaps the exception of ozone) are also found in excessive amounts in cigarette smoke. The pollution of the inhaled air by sucking on a cigarette does not cause dramatic results except in the nonsmoking novice, because tolerance develops with chronic exposure to pollutants. Unfortunately this tolerance does not seem to be protective and may actually represent suppression of protective mechanisms. Recent studies have shown that even in the college-age group, smokers have a definite increase in morbidity of respiratory infections and a decrease in maximum expiratory flow rate, vital capacity, and maximum breathing capacity.

A study of 400 young U.S. Air Force recruits undergoing physical conditioning showed definite differences between smokers and nonsmokers. Endurance performance was inversely related to the number of cigarettes smoked daily and the duration of habitual smoking. Those who had smoked less than six months were not significantly affected. The response to the training program was also impaired in the smokers. All of these findings point to an accumulative, deleterious effect of smoking on cardiopulmonary function. The deficits are those which might be anticipated from chronic injury by pollutants in the inhaled smoke.

The increase in morbidity and the deficit in function in these young people suggest that the changes seen in later life of obstructive emphysema may be the cumulative effect of continued injury by the noxious agents in cigarettes. The role of cigarettes in the production of cancer may prove to be insignificant compared to their effect on the structural integrity of the lungs.

Another aspect of our environment which affects the function of the cardiorespiratory system is barometric pressure. Some effects of going from near sea level to mountain altitudes have already been discussed on pages 129–131. As man increases his mobility and makes more use of the upper atmosphere and ocean floor, increasing numbers of individuals will be subject to major changes in barometric pressure.

High Altitudes. Since the amount of hemoglobin that is saturated with oxygen is determined by the partial pressure of oxygen in the alveoli, not the percentage of oxygen in the atmosphere, the saturation of hemoglobin will decrease as one ascends in the atmosphere. Table 10-1 lists the barometric pressure and partial pressures of oxygen in the inspired air at various heights above sea level. At an altitude of 10,000 feet the partial pressure of oxygen is down to a level such that a significant decrease in oxygen saturation occurs. At this level the changes in ventilation occur as described in Chapter 8 (pp. 183–186). Above 10,000 feet air must be enriched with oxygen unless the individual has been carefully acclimatized. Even a pure oxygen atmosphere has a deficit in inspired oxygen partial pressure at 40,000 feet, because water vapor added to the air in the upper airways equals 46 mm. Hg, leaving an inspired oxygen partial pressure of only 95 mm. Hg (see Appendix).

In commercial aircraft of even the most luxurious type, cabin pressure

Table 10-1. Changes in Barometric Pressure and Inspired Oxygen Pressure at Various Altitudes

Altitude (feet)	Barometric Pressure (mm. Hg)	Partial Pressure Inspired Oxygen (mm. Hg)
Sea level	760	159
5,000	635	133
10,000	523	109
15,000	429	90
20,000	349	73
25,000	282	59
30,000	226	47
35,000	179	37
40,000	141	30

is not maintained at ground level, because the requirements for cabin structural strength and superchargers would be excessive. These cabins are maintained at a pressure not less than 575 mm. Hg, equivalent to 7,500 feet altitude.

Compensation for reduced partial pressure of oxygen at high altitudes is achieved by hyperventilation, though the maximum stimulus of such hypoxia only doubles the minute ventilation. A healthy man can go to 20,000 feet breathing air with hyperventilation; without hyperventilation he can go to only 17,000 feet. Breathing oxygen he can survive at 47,000 feet with hyperpnea and 44,000 feet without. If an aircraft is at an altitude of 40,000 feet and the cabin pressure of 575 mm. Hg is suddenly dropped to the outside atmospheric pressure, 141 mm. Hg, the passengers will suffer acute decompression as well as oxygen deficiency. If the air passages are kept closed, the pressure difference between the air trapped in the chest and the atmosphere would be nearly 400 mm. Hg, and alveolar rupture leading to air emboli may occur. If the air passages are opened, air will rush out and no harm will result.

A patient with pneumothorax may develop serious difficulty breathing when the atmospheric pressure drops from 760 mm. Hg (at sea level) to the pressure of 575 mm. Hg at the simulated altitude of 7,500 feet in commercial aircraft cabins. This change would cause each 100 cc. of air in the chest cavity at ground level to occupy 130 cc. of the thoracic volume at 7,500 feet. Decompression to 140 mm. Hg at 40,000 feet would cause each 100 cc. of air to occupy 410 cc. and would be lethal if a significant pneumothorax was present. It is imperative that patients with pneumothorax be advised not to fly. If a patient has emphysematous bullae which do not empty readily, the air in the cysts expands as atmospheric pressure falls, just as does air in a closed pneumothorax space. Airline pilots with a history of spontaneous pneumothoraxes are disqualified for piloting aircraft until a corrective operative procedure has been done to prevent such occurrences.

Below Sea Level. The development of scuba diving equipment for military, industrial, and recreational use is placing growing numbers of people in environments with increased atmospheric pressures. The recent great enthusiasm for the medical use of hyperbaric oxygen-enriched atmospheres which exposed patients and staff repeatedly to increased pressures is fortunately dying.

One atmosphere is defined as a pressure of 760 mm. Hg. Since mercury is thirteen times heavier than water, one atmosphere is equal to $760 \times 13/1,000$ meters of water, which equals 9.8 meters or 32 feet of water. For every 32 feet one descends below the surface of water, the barometric pressure doubles. At 96 feet below the water surface, the pressure is three atmospheres, or 2,280 mm. Hg, and the oxygen partial pressure is 450 mm. Hg. If pure oxygen is breathed, the oxygen partial pressure will be over 2,000. High partial pressures of oxygen damage the lung, add little oxygen to the blood, and do not aid the elimination of carbon dioxide. The principal problem in hyperbaric physiology is to find how men can safely work and play in the presence of greatly increased ambient pressure; it will contribute very little to therapeutic medicine because of the toxic effects of high partial pressures of oxygen (for details see pp. 299–300 on oxygen therapy and oxygen toxicity).

It is inappropriate to consider here all of the problems created by high-pressure environments, but a few may be noted. Compression or deep diving increases the volume of nitrogen and oxygen dissolved in the blood, and the amount is dependent on the absolute atmospheric pressure and the duration of exposure. If decompression is too rapid, the gas comes out of solution in the body fluids and forms small bubbles. These bubbles may cause only the severe pain of the "bends," or they may be fatal if the bubbles occur in critical areas such as the brain or coronary circulation. Just as decompression below atmospheric pressure can cause undue expansion of gas in the lungs, so can decompression from pressures greater than atmospheric. Therefore scuba diving is dangerous for those with lung cysts or pneumothoraxes.

Oxygen is not the only gas that is toxic at high concentrations. High partial pressures of nitrogen also have a narcotic effect on the individual. In addition to the hazards facing the scuba or deep sea diver during ascent to the surface—hyperinflation of lungs and decompression sickness—nitrogen narcosis is also a threat if he stays down at greater than 100 feet for too long. The same hazards face patients or staff in hyperbaric chambers. The use of hyperbaric chambers for oxygen deficiency states is limited by the danger of oxygen toxicity and so has proved of little clinical value. Nitrogen narcosis can be prevented by using a helium atmosphere, oxygen toxicity by holding the partial pressure of oxygen below 300 mm. Hg, and the bends by slow, staged decompression. The dangers of rupture of lung bullae can also be avoided by slow decompression.

DROWNING

Drowning is a risk faced by all those who expose themselves to the possibility of having to exchange their environment of air for one of water. As exploitation of water resources and interest in water sports increase, larger numbers of individuals will take this risk. Studies in drowning are difficult, and it is hard to transfer findings in experimental drowning to human accidental drowning.

Sudden immersion of human beings in cold water causes in some an almost reflex urge to gasp or take in a deep breath, while this urge to gasp is not present on immersion in warm water. Since all drowning victims, whether rescued from fresh or salt water, have aspirated and swallowed large amounts of water, they all have acute asphyxia. In addition to asphyxia, animals drowned in fresh water develop acute electrolyte disturbances characterized by hemodilution and blood hemolysis. The acute hemodilution combined with the anoxia of asphyxiation may cause ventricular fibrillation. In salt-water drowning hemolysis does not occur, and the serum sodium and chloride are elevated. Salt-water drowning victims are less likely to develop ventricular fibrillation than are victims of fresh-water drowning. In both groups a severe acidosis develops with a fall in pO_2 due to a physiological shunt, probably the result of areas of atelectasis. Even in survivors breathing room air, pO_2 is as low as 35 to 45 mm. Hg an hour after the incident.

This depression of pO_2 is the result of pulmonary edema and patchy areas of atelectasis. The aspiration of large amounts of fluid allows regions of lung to collapse when aspirated fluid is absorbed. The first step in resuscitation is vigorous positive-pressure ventilation to reinflate the lungs. This can be done successfully only by mouth-to-mouth or bag ventilation. At this stage the composition of the gas blown into the victim's lungs is less important than that a maximum tidal volume be given to reexpand the lungs. Most victims have swallowed large amounts of water, and care should be taken to prevent further aspiration due to vomiting or regurgitation. If a pulse is not palpable, external cardiac massage must also be instituted, together with appropriate drugs such as epinephrine, calcium chloride, isoproterenol, and sodium bicarbonate.

As soon as it is available, oxygen-enriched gas should be substituted for air. Positive-pressure ventilation with a respirator should be kept up until the blood gases are restored to normal values and the patchy infiltrates that are evident on x-ray throughout the lung have cleared. Continued ventilatory support is essential if significant amounts of fluid have been aspirated. In addition to giving ventilatory support, steps should be taken to correct the metabolic acidosis. If significant hemolysis is present, diuresis should be induced with mannitol.

Surprisingly long periods of submersion may be tolerated, though the exact times are usually hard to document. However, a chilled, non-struggling child has been reported to have survived 22 minutes of submersion with only small neurological residual effects. The problem of preserving cardiopulmonary function in a drowning victim who has lost cerebral cortical function is small. Apparently, if the heart and vegetative centers survive in such cases, the neurological deficit is not great.

In summary, the drowning victim suffers asphyxia as well as fluid electrolyte abnormalities as a result of exchanges across the alveolar membrane. Victims of fresh-water drowning have a fall in serum electrolytes, hemodilution, and hemolysis and often have ventricular fibrillation. In salt-water drowning, the hyperosomolarity of the aspirated fluid results in hemoconcentration and a rise in serum electrolytes. In both groups pulmonary edema and diffuse patchy atelectasis occur, with severe acidosis and oxygen unsaturation. Emergency treatment should include immediate, vigorous hyperinflation of the lungs and closed-chest cardiac massage if indicated. The next step is to continue ventilatory support with intermittent positive-pressure ventilation using a large tidal volume. The inspired mixture should contain high oxygen concentrations. The levels of blood electrolytes and blood gases should be determined as soon as possible and appropriate steps taken to correct acidosis and restore electrolytes to normal. The oxygen concentration in the inspired air should be adjusted to keep the arterial pO_2 between 90 and 100 mm. Hg.

ACTIVITY LEVELS AND ENERGY REQUIREMENTS

EXERCISE

The normal adaptations to exercise can be used to introduce the discussion of abnormal adaptations.

If increased gas exchange is required by exercise, the tidal volume and respiratory rate must increase to increase the minute and alveolar ventilation. At low levels of exercise, most of the increase in tidal volume comes from the inspiratory reserve volume and expiration remains passive without expulsive efforts by the expiratory muscles. As exercise increases the demands for oxygen and carbon dioxide, tidal volume uses some of the expiratory reserve and the expiratory muscles raise the intrapleural pressure above atmospheric pressure in order to expel air from the lungs. Conditioning strengthens the muscles of respiration and may speed their shortening to permit faster contraction and greater ventilation.

As the exercise level increases, more areas of lung are fully ventilated and ventilation becomes more uniform. Exercise also increases cardiac output and thus pulmonary blood flow. This increase in flow, which in a well-conditioned athlete may reach 30 liters per minute, is achieved with minimal increases in pulmonary artery pressure. At the onset of exercise the cross-sectional area of the pulmonary vascular bed increases as a result of relaxation of vascular smooth muscle. This dilatation of the pulmonary vascular bed results in more uniform perfusion of the lungs, so flow to the apices is nearly as great as that to the bases of the lung. The ventilation-perfusion ratio is more uniform. Cardiac output increases less than the alveolar ventilation, because the tissues extract more oxygen from the blood decreasing the mixed venous oxygen saturation and widening the arteriovenous difference.

At maximum exercise levels the rate of blood flow through the capillaries is so great that complete saturation of blood with oxygen cannot be accomplished due to limitations in the speed of oxygen diffusion across the alveolo-capillary membrane. Thus the factor limiting oxygen acquisition in a normal individual is the diffusing capacity of the lungs. Exercise results in an oxygen debt which requires continued hyperventilation until this debt is repaid. This increased level of ventilation is evidenced by the continued dyspnea after exercise stops.

Dyspnea is the consciousness of effort to breathe and can be induced in all individuals; the exercise level at which dyspnea becomes uncomfortable varies with the efficiency of the respiratory apparatus. In all individuals, young and old, healthy or diseased, careful conditioning can increase the tolerated level of exercise and the activity level at which dyspnea becomes intolerable. If conditioning is done without regard to the functional capacity of the individual, the system can be damaged by the excessive demands and the tolerable level of exercise decreased. All coaches know that attempts to get an athlete "into shape" too fast can decrease his performance level. So can excessive demands made on an individual with cardiorespiratory disease, which, for example, can produce acute pulmonary edema. On the other hand, failure to exercise cuts down respiratory and cardiac reserve capacities; the individual with decreased pulmonary function who undertakes no conditioning program cuts down his reserve just as does the normal individual who fails to exercise.

RESPONSE TO DISEASE

Disease of itself places increased demands on the gas-exchange system. Hyperactivity due to central nervous system disease and disorientation from head injury are obvious instances of this. Fever raises the metabolic rate and increases the amount of oxygen and carbon dioxide to be exchanged. If the protective covering of skin is removed from the body, as in a surface burn or open wound, the amount of water lost by evaporation increases and more energy is required to provide heat of vaporization. Operative or accidental trauma also increases the metabolic demands on the patient. This increase varies with the severity and type of injury. In addition to increases in basal gas-exchange requirements, in disease states in most instances the energy requirements for any activity are increased, just as, for example, it is harder to limp than it is to walk naturally.

NATURAL SLEEP

At the opposite end of activity level from dyspnea-producing exercise is sleep. In natural sleep the minute ventilation decreases as a result of decreased respiratory rate and tidal volume. This causes a mean increase in arterial pCO_2 of 4 mm. Hg, but at the deepest levels of sleep the rise in pCO_2 may reach 9 mm. Hg. Ventilatory response to carbon dioxide is also depressed, but the amount of depression is hard to assess because increasing the inspired carbon dioxide concentrations awakens the subject. The excitability of the respiratory center to carbon dioxide is decreased, but the excitability due to decrease in arterial pO_2 is not altered. During natural sleep frequent sighing restores compliance, and position change prevents congestion in dependent areas of the lung.

SLEEP INDUCED BY ANESTHETIC OR SEDATIVE DRUGS

Metabolic Rate. Sleep induced by anesthetic or sedative drugs is not the same as natural sleep. The metabolic rate under surgical anesthesia decreases 15 to 30%. There are no other significant metabolic changes unless the concentration of anesthetic gases in the blood is great enough to severely depress the respiration or circulation. Under anesthesia the minute ventilation and response to carbon dioxide are decreased and in arterial pCO_2 level at which complete apnea occurs is less than that during natural sleep.

The Airways. The insertion of an endotracheal tube decreases anatomical dead space but greatly increases airway resistance. Since resistance varies as the fourth power of the airway radius, the increased resistance is relatively greater in infants and children. In all patients the increased resistance of an endotracheal tube is of more clinical importance than the decreased anatomical dead space; in fact, the decrease in the anatomical dead space is often cancelled out by the added dead space in the anesthetic apparatus.

When an endotracheal tube is not used, anatomical dead space is often increased under anesthesia since preoperative medication with atropine relaxes bronchomotor tone and increases the anatomical dead space 30 to 45%. Vagotomy, the administration of drugs such as isoproterenol and epinephrine, and hypothermia have the same effect. Whether anesthetic agents themselves cause bronchodilation or bronchoconstriction is not clear.

General Effect of Drugs. While the increase in the anatomical dead space due to bronchodilation is of little clinical consequence, the effects of drugs in producing bronchoconstriction are of great clinical importance. Among the agents that can cause bronchoconstriction are barbiturates, succinylcholine, and aspirated foreign matter. Bronchoconstriction may also occur when the tracheobronchial tree is irritated, when an endotracheal tube impinges on the carina, or when the airways are suddenly distended by an anesthetist trying to hyperinflate a patient by excessive squeezing of the anesthetic gas bag. Bronchoconstriction can be reduced or averted by the administration of atropine, although high doses are often required.

Increase in airway resistance due to bronchoconstriction is particularly difficult to deal with in patients who are being artificially ventilated, because air must be expelled from the lungs by the elastic recoil of the system. If the bronchoconstriction is severe, it may be difficult to empty the lungs, and the end-tidal volume in the lungs will increase. In patients in whom the chest is open, the elastic recoil of the chest wall does not aid expiration, and the emptying of the lungs may be severely compromised by bronchoconstriction. Increase in arterial pCO_2 causes a reflex increase in bronchomotor tone. If some bronchoconstriction prevents adequate ventilation and results in a rise in arterial pCO_2, this may aggravate the problem by further increasing the bronchomotor tone. Large doses of atropine may be the only effective means of relaxing the bronchospasm enough to permit effective ventilation. If during induction of anesthesia a serious degree of bronchoconstriction is initiated, it is advisable not to go on with the operative procedure until the bronchoconstriction is well under control. If the bronchoconstriction cannot be controlled effectively, it may even be necessary to postpone the operation to another day.

Compliance. Anesthetic agents affect the elastic as well as the resistive properties of the respiratory system. In the deeply anesthetized or paralyzed patient the total chest compliance is greater than in the awake individual. This difference occurs because the awake individual apparently cannot voluntarily completely relax the muscles of his chest wall, and the elastic forces are opposed by some force exerted by the muscles. An anesthetized patient in the prone position has a total chest compliance 30% less than in the supine position. This loss of compliance is the result of the added dead weight on the chest. If the body is supported at the hips and shoulders, the compliance can be partially restored. The Trendelenburg position also decreases total chest compliance and reduces the expiratory reserve volume, thus cutting down the inflation of the lung. If the patient is obese or has ascites, the compressing effect of this dead weight can seriously compromise respiration in any position but dangerously so in the prone or Trendelenburg position. Such patients need respiratory assistance when under anesthesia, and quite high inflation pressures may be necessary to adequately ventilate them.

Lung compliance tends to decrease during anesthesia, because the patient does not take deep breaths. The failure to breathe deeply results in collapse of some alveoli throughout the less well-ventilated parts of the lung, or microatelectasis. If the patient is breathing a high oxygen mixture, the fast rate of absorption of the oxygen from poorly ventilated alveoli can result in an acceleration of the development of atelectasis. If a major bronchus is blocked in a patient in whom the nitrogen has been washed out by 90 to 100% oxygen breathing, it is possible for the oxygen in the blocked area of lung to be reabsorbed in a few minutes, leading to complete collapse of the unventilated portion of the lung. This is the mechanism which causes acute atelectasis of one lung during anesthesia. To minimize the development of microatelectasis, the lungs should be hyperinflated every five minutes by applying a pressure of at least 30 cm. H_2O for a period of five seconds. If the patient is obese or for some other reason has decreased chest compliance, a greater pressure will be necessary.

In patients undergoing open thoracotomy, the opposing recoil forces of the chest wall and lungs are disrupted, and the end-expiratory transpulmonary pressure falls from 5 cm. H_2O to zero. This permits the lung to collapse and decreases the end-tidal volume. This decrease in end-tidal lung volume, which is equivalent to one-half or more of the expiratory reserve, aggravates the tendency toward alveolar collapse present in all anesthetized patients. Patients undergoing open thoracotomy *must* have periods of hyperinflation of the lung, or, if the surgeon can find room to work, it even is better for the anesthetist to maintain some positive pressure throughout the expiratory cycle of ventilation and thus maintain lung inflation.

Alveolar Ventilation, Ventilation-Perfusion Ratio, and Arterial Gas Concentrations. Alterations in compliance and airway resistance can cause major derangements in the coordination of ventilation and perfusion under anesthesia, and these can be reflected in serious abnormalities in arterial blood gases. Most anesthetized patients breathe gas mixtures containing high concentrations of oxygen, which makes it possible for the arterial blood to become fully saturated with oxygen, but without an adequate amount of alveolar ventilation to remove carbon dioxide from the blood. The central nervous system's response to increased concentrations of carbon dioxide is depressed by anesthetic agents, and if the hypoxic drive is removed by the administration of high oxygen concentrations, carbon dioxide can accumulate to alarming levels.

The accumulation of carbon dioxide is difficult to recognize. It may be associated with some systemic hypertension, but usually is not. If significant increases of arterial pCO_2 have been present for more than a few minutes, they can cause changes in the flux of hydrogen and potassium ions across the cell membranes. Acute correction of the hypercapnia can result in acute imbalance in the flux of these ions, leading to serious cardiac arrhythmias. If hypercapnia has been allowed to develop during anesthesia, it is safer to lower the carbon dioxide concentration slowly than to do it suddenly. In any case, one should be prepared to reverse an arrhythmia. These arrhythmias may occur as the patient awakens and the central nervous system depression decreases, causing hyperventilation in response to the increased carbon dioxide and sudden blowing off of the excessive carbon dioxide.

In anesthetized patients the alveolar–arterial carbon dioxide gradient is increased from less than 1 mm. Hg to 5 mm. Hg or more. This means that some regions of lung are being ventilated and not perfused—a ventilatory shunt. The administration of oxygen increases this gradient, as does positioning the patient in the lateral decubitus position. This ventilatory shunt is of little consequence except that it requires an increased ventilatory volume to maintain a given level of gas exchange.

If anesthesia is prolonged and periodic hyperinflation is not carefully carried out, a vascular shunt develops which can lead to serious arterial oxygen unsaturation. This shunt is caused by the collapse of perfused alveoli. Periodic hyperinflation can prevent this shunt and, if it occurs, can correct it.

SPECIFIC EFFECTS OF DRUGS AND PHYSICAL AGENTS

Narcotics.   Narcotics reduce respiratory rate, increase tidal volume, and decrease minute ventilation. They diminish the ventilatory response to carbon dioxide but only slightly affect the hypoxic drive. All the commonly used synthetic analgesic substitutes for morphine depress the respiration more at the same analgesic level than does morphine itself. Narcotics depress the respiration more in elderly patients than they do in younger ones and more in the absence of pain than in its presence. If chest wall pain is causing splinting of the chest wall, narcotics may act to increase respiratory exchange by diminishing the restriction of ventilation imposed by the pain and associated muscle spasm.

While both narcotics and anesthetic agents depress the ventilatory drive, narcotics can foster a more efficient respiratory pattern if given in association with anesthetic agents. Narcotics reduce the tachypnea of anesthetic agents, thus reducing the work of breathing and increasing efficiency by cutting down the dead space ventilation and the gas flow rate.

Barbiturates. The speed with which a barbiturate acts depends on the transfer rate across the blood-brain barrier. The fat-soluble, poorly ionized barbiturates are fast acting. Barbiturates in small doses, enough to permit the insertion of an oral airway but not at surgical anesthetic levels, do not depress respiration. Large doses definitely depress the ventilatory drive in direct proportion to the amount of drug given and thus to the level of anesthesia. The respiratory rate is not depressed as it is with narcotics, which is a good way to differentiate narcotic from barbiturate intoxication. The hypoxic drive is little affected, most of the effect being on the carbon dioxide respiratory drive. Barbiturates are safe for the induction of anesthesia, but the degree of depression of respiratory and cardiac function necessary to achieve surgical levels of anesthesia makes them unsafe as surgical anesthetics when used alone. There are no good antagonists to these drugs, and treatment depends on lowering the blood concentration; to reverse poisonings dialysis is indicated to wash the drug out of the blood.

Anesthetic Gases. The effects of ether and cyclopropane have been extensively discussed in many publications. These agents have now been abandoned almost completely for thoracic and cardiovascular surgery and so will not be discussed. Unfortunately, the studies on the newer agents are limited. Halothane decreases the tidal volume and increases the respiratory rate. It increases the respiratory rate more in children than adults. At light planes of anesthesia, alveolar ventilation is maintained; at deeper planes the carbon dioxide drive is depressed and ventilation decreases. Halothane, in contrast to cyclopropane, is a weak liberator of catacholamines. Methoxyflurane is the only agent that does not increase respiratory rate. Its other actions are similar to halothane.

Synergistic Actions of Drugs and Anesthetic Agents. Amounts of drugs or anesthetic agents which are safe alone may be dangerous when given in combination. Neomycin is a respiratory poison when given in association with anesthetic agents. The synergism of neomycin with curare-like drugs can cause respiratory paralysis due to neuromuscular blockade which may last for hours to days. This same effect has been encountered with streptomycin, kanamycin, and polymyxin B. The blockade is not reversed by neostigmine but may be helped by the administration of calcium.

Hypothermia. Hypothermia is a useful adjunct to surgery in some patients when circulation must be compromised. Hypothermia depresses the respiratory center but also the oxygen needs, so that down to a temperature of 29° to 30°C. ventilation is adequate to provide oxygen needs. At 20°C. all spontaneous respiration ceases. Hypothermia causes relaxation of bronchomotor tone, which increases the anatomical dead space. It changes the dissociation constant for blood, the pK, so that pH rises and pCO_2 decreases. Hypothermia also increases the solubility of oxygen and carbon dioxide in the blood, increasing the amount of dissolved oxygen at any given arterial pO_2. The oxygen dissociation curve shifts, so that hemoglobin is saturated at a lower arterial pO_2. Since the amount of dissolved oxygen is increased at low temperatures, quick rewarming of blood may cause formation of microbubbles as the oxygen is forced out of solution.

11. AGE, HABITUS, AND DEGENERATIVE DISEASE

PHYSICAL habitus and size affect directly the function of the lungs and also can influence the rate at which the respiratory system deteriorates. In this chapter, age, alterations in the chest cage, and degenerative disease are related to the functional integrity of the respiratory system.

THE EFFECTS OF AGING

The small size of an infant's and child's ventilatory apparatus does not provide him with the same reserve capacity as an adult has. Since resistance is inversely proportional to the fourth power of the radius, the small airways of a child under two years of age leave him little safety factor if swelling or edema of the bronchi or bronchioles occurs. This is well illustrated by the high mortality from pertussis in infants and young children as compared to older children and adults. Not only are the airways smaller in the child, but the ratio of conducting airways to alveoli is less than in the adult, which means that both the relative and absolute size of the airways is smaller. In addition to greater relative flow resistance than the adult, the child has a less compliant lung and a relatively smaller reserve volume compared to his metabolic needs. The chest bellows, on the other hand, is relatively more compliant than the adult's. All of these factors combine to make the child less able to tolerate pneumonia, pneumothorax, airway obstruction, asthma, and other problems of the lower respiratory tract.

As the child develops from infancy through adolescence, the reserve capacity steadily increases as airways enlarge, more alveoli are added, and the chest bellows becomes more effective. In the late teens and early twenties, respiratory reserve is at its maximum. At this time the system is fully developed, the ravages of noxious fumes and aging usually have not yet seriously damaged the system, and physical conditioning is at its maximum. The onset of the deterioration of lung function with aging in the apparently normal population depends on the amount of physical exercise, heredity, and the noxious gases inhaled. By the time an individual reaches his late thirties, the processes of aging begin to become apparent and by the fifties are clearly present.

With increased age the vital capacity decreases, the residual volume increases, and the ratio of residual volume to total lung capacity increases. Anatomical dead space increases, and resting tidal volume and rate increase, leading to a small rise in minute ventilation. Oxygen consumption and carbon dioxide output decrease, and evidence of uneven gas distribution develops. Maximum breathing capacity falls as a result of decrease in vital capacity and reduced muscle strength. The diffusing capacity also is decreased.

These changes with aging are the result of changes in the mechanical properties of the lung. There is little change in airway resistance, though total lung resistance may be increased. There is less elastic recoil of the lungs; consequently, at resting end-tidal volume the elastic recoil of the chest, which does not decrease, pulls the lungs out to a larger volume and increases the residual volume.

At the two extremes of life, childhood and old age, the reserve capacity of the lungs is diminished; respiratory infections, chest trauma, or compromises of airway are more likely to lead to respiratory insufficiency. (See also pp. 81–83.)

THE CONDITION OF THE CHEST WALL AND ABDOMEN

Abnormalities of the chest wall and abdomen usually limit the motion of the chest cage and diaphragms. Since it is the motion of the bellows pump which changes the volume of the lungs, chest cage abnormalities cause a reduction in static lung volumes, usually characterized as restrictive pulmonary disease. However, in some patients static lung volumes may be normal while a pattern of restriction is still present because the individual cannot maintain a level of ventilation that uses his lungs to their maximum.

PHYSICAL CONDITIONING

The most common cause of restriction in the ability to hyperventilate in the age of the automobile is poor physical conditioning. If the activity level is continually so low that hyperventilation is not necessary to provide adequate gas exchange, the respiratory muscles will be less efficient. These skeletal muscles are no different from any others; with disuse they atrophy. Precisely how graded exercise increases the work capacity, or why sudden, heavy work loads in the unconditioned person cause muscle pain and decrease in work capacity, is not known. If great demands are suddenly placed on an unconditioned set of muscles, they will be sorely taxed to produce and will have the syndrome of post-exercise soreness and decrease in efficiency. If an injurious agent makes the lungs or chest wall acutely less efficient, increased muscular effort will be necessary to maintain an adequate level of ventilation. The unconditioned subject will be poorly prepared to sustain this increased muscular effort.

All individuals, even those patients with chronic disease of the lungs, chest bellows, or heart, are more likely to survive an acute illness if they have exercised enough to stress the system so as to maintain good physical condition of the ventilatory muscles. This requires daily exercise which produces at least mild dyspnea. Such conditioning is important in the period prior to elective surgery, since surgical procedures done on the trunk compromise both chest cage and lung function. It is also important to strengthen the abdominal muscles, since they are essential to effective cough.

OBESITY

Another common cause of restrictive ventilatory dysfunction in our sedentary society is obesity. Obesity greatly increases the danger of any operative procedure, traumatic injury, or acute respiratory illness, and can, if extreme, cause respiratory insufficiency even without the presence of a complicating injury or infection. Obesity requires increased effort at every activity level; any movement requires added work to carry the added weight. Unfortunately, fat stores are so placed that they maximally compromise the function of the chest bellows. Intraabdominal fat occupies space in the abdominal cavity needed for full descent of the diaphragms, thus it limits lung expansion. In the upright posture, abdominal wall fat pulls down on the chest wall and abdomen and must be lifted by the inspiratory muscles during each inspiration. In the supine posture both the intraabdominal fat and the abdominal wall fat push up on the diaphragms and must be lifted by the chest wall and diaphragmatic muscles on each inspiration. This compression by fat decreases residual volume and can lead to collapse of portions of the lung. Most extremely obese persons cannot lie flat without intolerable dyspnea due to the great effort needed to lift the mass of fat.

Excessively obese subjects have a large decrease in chest wall compliance, from the normal of 220 cc. per centimeter of water down to 80 cc. per centimeter of water. In extreme obesity, in which respiratory insufficiency is present at rest or is produced by slight activity, total lung capacity, vital capacity, and inspiratory capacity are all reduced. Most such studies are made in the upright posture, and undoubtedly reductions would be much exaggerated in the supine posture that is usual in the acutely ill or postoperative patient. Obesity can be so extreme that even without any associated disease the ventilatory muscles cannot move the chest bellows enough to provide adequate alveolar ventilation. Such patients develop hypercapnia and hypoxia at rest. With lesser degrees of obesity, injury to the lungs or chest wall may decrease the efficiency of the system enough to cause acute respiratory insufficiency.

In such very obese patients, cardiac failure is often present along with pulmonary hypertension and systemic hypertension. Elective operative procedures should not be undertaken in excessively obese persons. If surgery is necessary, these patients should be hospitalized and starved to induce as rapid a weight reduction as possible. In addition, both pre- and postoperatively, the supine position should be maintained for as short a time as possible. The anesthesiologist must provide enough force in ventilating the patient to overcome the low chest wall compliance. Postoperatively, blood gases should be carefully monitored and respiratory assistance provided if alveolar hypoventilation develops.

ASCITES, ABDOMINAL DISTENSION, ABDOMINAL BINDERS

Ascites and abdominal distension have many of the same effects as excessive obesity. The diaphragms are pushed up, and in the supine position the weight of fluid in the abdomen must be lifted with each inspiratory effort. The normal individual can drink a liter of fluid without any effect on lung volumes. Even two liters have little effect; large amounts of fluid, probably five liters or more, are needed to compromise ventilatory capacity. Many of the effects of abdominal distension and ascites can be mimicked by a light abdominal compression and thus ventilatory derangements will be greatly aggravated by use of an abdominal binder. All the lung volumes are reduced, as is the maximum breathing capacity. If these complications of abdominal distension or ascites are superimposed on obesity, respiratory insufficiency is very likely to result. If the ascites is removed or the abdominal distension relieved, the ventilatory function promptly returns toward normal. If the decompression cannot be accomplished, respiratory support is often indicated, just as it is in the obese patient. Patients with peritonitis have disability due to abdominal distension as well as muscular spasm due to pain and increased metabolic demands of infection. This combination often leads to respiratory failure and is an indication for respirator therapy.

Gastric dilatation is a special type of abdominal distension and has effects which are perhaps in part reflex. Serious respiratory difficulty with tachypnea and tachycardia develops with an increase in intra-abdominal volume much smaller than that necessary to affect respiratory function in a patient with ascites. The lung compliance of these patients falls and airway resistance rises markedly, suggesting that there may be a reflex mechanism, probably vagal, involved. This syndrome is dramatically relieved by decompression with a nasogastric tube.

MUSCULO-SKELETAL DEFORMITIES

The Spine. Ankylosing spondylitis is perhaps the purest form of restrictive lung disease. The chest cage is completely immobilized, and all volume change must result from motion of the diaphragms. In patients with this problem, excursion of the diaphragms is increased. The vital capacity is decreased in severe cases to 40% of normal, and total lung capacity is lowered by 25%. The maximum breathing capacity may be sustained at higher levels than the vital capacity and can be increased with conditioning. These patients adapt to these conditions quite well and are reasonable operative risks, even for thoracotomy, though injury to a phrenic nerve would be totally disabling.

Kyphoscoliosis is a much more disabling skeletal deformity than is ankylosing spondylitis. The deformity can be due to muscle paralysis, trauma, absence of ribs, hemivertebras, or fibrothorax, but in the majority of cases is of unknown etiology. The most severe cases are due to neuromuscular diseases, whereas the congenital form, without obvious skeletal or muscular defects, is usually mild. There is good correlation between the degree of deformity and the severity of cardiorespiratory disability. The respiratory deficit is one of restriction, not obstruction. The lung volumes are reduced and are very like those seen following pulmonary resection, except for the residual volume, which is normal. The maximum breathing capacity is reduced more than the vital capacity, unlike the situation in other types of restrictive disease. The oxygen cost of breathing is increased, and even small increases in minute ventilation require large increments in the oxygen cost of breathing. At rest, the mechanical work done on the lung is in the normal range, but it escalates rapidly when minute ventilation is increased. Both lung and chest wall compliance are reduced to one-half or one-third normal in adults, while in children the compliances usually are near normal. Thus growth and aging cause an increase in mechanical deficiency in these patients.

In young patients and well-compensated adults with kyphoscoliosis the distribution of air is quite uniform, though studies using broncho-spirometer techniques have shown that there is little function in the lung on the side of the concavity of the deformity. Patients with severe deformities have a small tidal volume with a normal amount of ana-tomical dead space, and thus they require an increased minute ventila-tion to provide adequate alveolar ventilation. Blood gases are normal in most children and in adults without severe deformity. In those with severe deformity, ventilation-perfusion incoordination and even hyper-capnia may be present. The carbon monoxide diffusing capacity is dimin-ished, but not excessively when considered in relation to the small size of these patients.

One of the most serious complications of kyphoscoliosis is found in the pulmonary circulation. Individuals with this deformity have pul-monary hypertension with associated right ventricular hypertrophy. The changes in the pulmonary bed are probably the combined result of mechanical compression of areas of lung and thickening of the walls of pericapillary vessels, all of which are aggravated when ventilatory insufficiency is present and which leads to vasoconstriction as a result of hypoxemia and hypercapnia. Any intercurrent infection or operative procedure may cause acute cor pulmonale and require ventilatory sup-port and digitalization of the patient.

Operative procedures to correct or limit the further development of kyphoscoliosis usually do not improve pulmonary function. They may arrest further loss, but during the procedure function may diminish further and acute respiratory failure develop. This deformity limits the force of the cough, and a major problem is effective clearing of secre-tions, particularly in the postoperative period. Respiratory function is best maintained if the deformity can be limited by early spine fixation.

Congenital Deformities of Ribs and Sternum.   There is considerable controversy at this time as to whether or not congenital rib and sternal deformities limit pulmonary function. Such uncertainty is almost defi-nitely an indication of the inappropriateness of the tests of pulmonary function, not of the normality of these patients. A family history taken of a patient with a congenital chest deformity usually shows other members with a chest deformity, though not necessarily the same deformity as the patient may have. In all these congenital deformities, whether of the depression or protrusion type, the ribs are longer than necessary, an ideal situation for plastic repair. The most common of these deformities is pectus excavatum, a depression of the sternum; less common are pectus carinatum, and lateral protrusion or depression deformities of the ribs.

These deformities range from mild—of no significance other than cosmetic—to severe, with associated kyphosis. The protrusion deformities are cosmetically more objectionable to the patient because they cannot be hidden by clothes. Many adolescent boys with any type of chest deformity will not participate in activities which require removal of their shirts. Modern undress for the female makes it more difficult for them to camouflage such deformities. The cosmetic deformity is often aggravated by kyphosis and poorly developed chest wall musculature. Exercises to increase pectoral and all shoulder girdle muscles make the defect less noticeable. The most effective method we have found to satisfy the adolescent male that a mild deformity can be camouflaged is to instruct him to keep his hands in his hip pockets. This throws the shoulders back and lifts up the depression. (It is important to supply hip pockets on bathing trunks.) If the individual avoids gym or swimming because of the defect, operative repair is advisable, since it is safe and usually very effective.

While cosmetic surgery for chest wall deformities is clearly justified, the real question that arises is whether it is also justified because of deficiency in cardiopulmonary function. Certainly these deformities must limit the mechanical efficiency of the chest wall. In children there are studies which show that there is some diminution in vital capacity and maximum breathing capacity, but these limitations have not been shown in adults. There are no good studies of the mechanics of the chest wall, particularly compliance, in these deformities. Studies need to be made of the oxygen cost of breathing as well as of the ability of these patients to sustain maximal exercise.

Studies are also needed of cardiac function. Even in patients with severe deformity, all heart and great vessel pressures are normal at rest, though in some there is evidence of disturbance in right ventricular filling. Cardiac studies carried out at rest are inadequate, since deficiencies may be present only in severe exercise. Many of these patients have subjective cardiac complaints, and some have arrhythmias which usually are relieved by corrective surgery.

In summary, operative correction of chest deformities for purely cosmetic reasons is clearly indicated, and it is probably true that correction of these deformities also improves chest wall function and thus ventilatory function and hemodynamics.

DEGENERATIVE LUNG DISEASE

OBSTRUCTIVE EMPHYSEMA

Obstructive emphysema is rapidly becoming one of the major causes of disability in our modern society. It is certainly aggravated, if not caused, by smoking cigarettes and by increasing air pollution. Some of the elements of obstructive emphysema are part of the aging process, but the increase in residual volume that occurs with aging is not synonymous with obstructive emphysema. In obstructive emphysema there is a high resistance to air flow, particularly during expiration. This high resistance to air flow is due to three changes in the lung: (1) intrinsic narrowing of the peripheral airways due to chronic bronchitis, (2) the loss of radial support of the small airways by tissue elements, and (3) decrease in retractive or elastic forces of the lung.

The latter two changes are the result of disruption of the normal geometric pattern of the elastic and connective tissue elements of the lungs. If the elastic recoil of the lung is diminished, the elastic force to expel air from the lung is less, and pleural pressure must rise to provide the force. The increase in intrathoracic pressure tends to collapse the airways, and results in further narrowing of these poorly supported, intrinsically narrowed air passages.

Patients with emphysema often reach the point where compression narrows the airways until resistance rises faster than driving pressure and flow ceases despite maximum effort. To attempt to diminish these deficiencies, the patient hyperexpands his chest cage and lungs to enable the elastic recoil of the lungs to become more adequate. However, hyperexpansion of the chest makes inspiration more difficult by diminishing the mechanical efficiency of the chest wall and diaphragms, since with the increased diameter of the chest, any change in intrapleural pressure requires greater chest wall tension and therefore more muscular effort. When the diaphragms are horizontal, as in emphysema, rather than domed, as is normal, contraction of the diaphragms can no longer aid in expansion of the base of the thorax as it does normally but may actually pull in the lower thorax, thus acting against the chest wall muscles. Consequently, both during inspiration and expiration the muscular effort to ventilate the lungs is increased. In addition, the mechanical derangements make cough relatively ineffective and aggravate the bronchial obstruction.

Patients with obstructive emphysema also have severe incoordination of ventilation and perfusion. This is one of the major deficits which requires most patients with obstructive emphysema to have higher minute ventilatory volumes than normal individuals.

The rupture of alveolar septa and coalescence of alveoli result in decrease in cross-sectional area of the capillary bed. When hypoventilation results in accumulation of carbon dioxide and hypoxemia, pulmonary vasoconstriction aggravates the anatomical loss of cross-sectional area.

People with obstructive emphysema who are reasonably well compensated can develop serious respiratory insufficiency following relatively minor respiratory infections. Even operative procedures not involving resection of lung or opening of the pleural space can cause respiratory decompensation in these patients. The mechanical derangements of obstructive emphysema are seriously aggravated by the mechanical changes due to operative trauma (p. 248). Postoperatively such patients should be carefully followed with blood gas studies, and if the pCO_2 rises or pO_2 falls, respiratory assistance should be instituted. Assistance may be needed for only a short time, and in these patients, who all have serious difficulties with the tracheobronchial tree, it is safer to avoid tracheostomy if possible.

Much has been said about the danger of oxygen therapy in patients with obstructive emphysema. When hypoxemia is corrected by treatment with high concentrations of oxygen, hypoventilation increases when the hypoxic drive is eliminated. However, persistent hypoxemia is also a serious danger. The judicious use of moderately increased concentrations of oxygen will diminish hypoxemia without causing dangerous increases in pCO_2. The correction of hypoxemia decreases pulmonary hypertension, which is one of the dangerous aspects of acute respiratory failure in these patients.

It is equally important to dispel the idea that digitalis is not helpful in patients with end-stage emphysema and cor pulmonale. Its effects are not as dramatic as they are in the treatment of cardiac failure due to valvular heart disease. However, the inotropic effect may be of critical importance in providing adequate muscular strength for perfusion of these lungs, since they have diminished vascular beds that require high perfusion pressures.

Finally, it cannot be stressed enough that patients with even early evidence of obstructive emphysema should be admonished not to smoke. Certainly elective surgery should not be undertaken until the patient has ceased smoking for at least two weeks, and preferably four. During this period the patient should be trained in effective breathing and instructed to follow a regime of progressively increasing exercise (walking) to improve physical condition. If the respiratory and cardiac muscles are well conditioned, the patient will be better able to do the added ventilatory and cardiac work imposed by operative trauma. The preoperative regime is equally effective in improving the functional state of all such patients.

CYSTS AND BULLAE

Air-filled cysts and bullae may be a complication of generalized obstructive airway disease, or they may be the result of congenital or acquired anatomical abnormalities. The most dramatic and alarming of these space-occupying, hyperexpanded areas of lung is seen in newborn infants who have an abnormality in a major bronchus which permits it to collapse on expiration. On inhalation, air is pulled into the affected area of lung and trapped when the bronchus collapses during expiration. This process continues until the affected area of lung occupies so much of the available chest volume that the infant develops acute respiratory distress. On x-ray the affected area of lung is hyperlucent and the mediastinum has shifted to the nonaffected side. Aspiration of the area is ineffectve, because the hyperexpanded area is not one large cyst but is made up of many hyperexpanded alveoli. This disease demands immediate surgery to resect the affected area of lung.

Less dramatic is the slow expansion of air-filled cysts in the lungs of young, otherwise healthy individuals in the age group 15 to 25. Occurring principally in individuals with long, narrow chest cages, the cysts develop at the apices and slowly expand as air is trapped and cannot escape. These cysts then rupture, and the patient develops a spontaneous pneumothorax. These patients may have repeated episodes of spontaneous rupture of such cysts. The treatment of choice is closed-chest drainage and, if there are repeated episodes, the production of adhesions between visceral and parietal pleura by thoracotomy and abrasion of the pleura with dry sponges. More radical procedures such as pleurectomy are not only unnecessary but are contraindicated, as they immobilize the lung and make subsequent thoracotomy virtually impossible. These patients should also be advised not to smoke, since this difficulty may be evidence of a propensity to develop obstructive emphysema in later life.

A much more difficult problem is encountered in adult patients with multiple large bullae in association with varying degrees of obstructive emphysema. In these patients, it is difficult to determine the relative role of the space-occupying bullae versus that of the generalized emphysema in the reduction of respiratory reserve. The bullae act like a pneumothorax occupying space in the chest. If the space the bullae occupy is only approximately equivalent to the amount of lung destroyed by the bullous degenerative process, their removal will not be beneficial, and the restrictions of function due to thoracotomy may further reduce respiratory reserve. However, if there is evidence on x-ray examination of compression of areas of normal lung and evidence of an intrapulmonary shunt (low arterial pO_2 on 100% oxygen breathing), and if the cysts are confined to an anatomical area which would permit their ablation, the patient may be significantly improved by operative removal of the cysts. The safest and most effective method presently avail-

Surfactant /

able is to exclude the cysts by use of one of the stapling devices. Anatomical resections always result in massive leak of air from surrounding tissue and serious postoperative pleural complications.

In patients with bullous emphysema and cystic disease, the cysts often rupture and spontaneous pneumothoraxes develop. In these patients with compromised respiratory reserve, acute respiratory insufficiency often develops. Prompt release of the pneumothorax by closed-chest drainage is a lifesaving procedure. Patients with bullous cysts of the lung or pneumothorax should be cautioned not to fly (see p. 219).

CARDIAC DISEASE AND LUNG FUNCTION

A detailed pathophysiological discussion of the relation between cardiac function and the pulmonary circulation has been given in Chapter 5. In this section only a brief review of the relationship between cardiac function and cardiopulmonary failure will be given.

In the surgical treatment of heart disease, whether it be simple closure of an intraventricular shunt or a cardiac transplant, the damage previously done to the lung by chronic cardiac dysfunction may cause a brilliant technical repair of the cardiac defect to be followed by death due to pulmonary vascular degeneration. High-pressure left-to-right shunts result in relentless destruction of the pulmonary vasculature. The speed with which this destruction occurs varies, and at this time little is known about why one individual develops irreversible changes in the vessels and another does not. Likewise, little is known about which patients will have reversal in the changes after surgical repair and which will not.

The pulmonary hypertension which results from mitral stenosis or chronic left heart failure is more likely to be reversible if a good repair of the intracardiac defect restores cardiac function. In patients with acquired heart disease, irreversible changes except in extremely far-advanced disease are often the result of associated obstructive emphysema, not the direct effect of the cardiac decompensation. In patients with pulmonary hypertension due to acquired or congenital heart disease, the operative procedure, particularly cardiopulmonary bypass, further compromises pulmonary function temporarily. The pathological changes are very similar to those seen in the so-called shock lung (p. 273). These changes are exaggerated if the bypass is prolonged or if the pulmonary collateral circulation is large. In all patients, care should be taken to prevent introduction of air into the pulmonary bed, just as care is taken to keep it out of the systemic vascular bed. In those patients with an already compromised vascular bed, any further blockage by air emboli may prove fatal. Since hypoxemia and acidosis lead to vascular constriction and thus to increased pulmonary artery pressure, it is important to correct acidosis and hypoxemia with ventilatory assistance and increased inhaled concentrations of oxygen. The postoperative ventilatory changes that follow operations within the thorax also act to aggravate the preoperative and postperfusion functional deficiencies of the alveolo-capillary interface.

In patients with compromised cardiac function requiring operative correction, cardiac and pulmonary function are not restored to normal in the immediate postoperative period, but rather are further compromised. The increased work of breathing required of all postoperative patients is exaggerated by the effects of cardiac insufficiency in patients following cardiotomy. The increase in metabolic demands required to do this extra respiratory work may exceed the capacity of the heart to increase output. This results in further cardiac decompensation and pulmonary edema with the associated deterioration of respiratory mechanics, decrease in compliance, increase in resistance, and hypoxemia. The changes in lung mechanics further escalate respiratory work and cause severe dyspnea, which results in anxiety, which also increases metabolic demands.

The only effective treatment for these patients is to use all measures to increase the effectiveness of the cardiac musuclature and to decrease the work required of the individual. The latter can be accomplished by the use of a ventilator to do the work of ventilation (see Chapter 13). This therapy is accepted and used extensively by surgeons; it should be equally effective in the treatment of acute cardiac insufficiency in the nonsurgical patient, such as postcoronary patients with pulmonary edema and a low cardiac output. The use of controlled respiration permits elevation of pulmonary venous pressure to higher levels to increase left heart output, since the pulmonary mechanical derangements due to lung congestion do not require increased effort by the patient. In patients with heart disease respiratory assistance should not be withheld until evidence of respiratory insufficiency—decrease in pO_2 and increase in pCO_2—has occurred. Assistance should be instituted as soon as it is apparent that the work of breathing is excessive for the patient. The sensation of dyspnea is a good indication of excessive work demands.

PULMONARY EMBOLI

Pulmonary emboli may vary in size from small, septic emboli which lodge in peripheral small arteries, to moderate-sized emboli which occlude a major lobar artery and immediately fatal emboli which occlude the outflow of the right ventricle. Emboli of small to moderate size have a predeliction for the lower lobes and more frequently lodge in the right than the left side.

There is still a lot of controversy about the pathophysiology of pulmonary emboli. This is engendered by the difficulty of studying the process in patients and the poor experimental models represented by anesthetized animals. These difficulties are further compounded by the differences in reaction to small peripheral and large central emboli shown in experimental animals, and the problems in patients of separating the effects of preexisting disease from those due to emboli.

One of the major problems in the study of the effects of pulmonary emboli is to determine how extensive the obstruction of the pulmonary arterial tree must be before the circulation or respiration is seriously compromised. The successful removal of an entire lung dispelled the idea that ablation of half the pulmonary bed would seriously compromise either ventilation or circulation. With the advent of the balloon catheter, it has become safe and feasible to mimic intraluminal occlusion of one pulmonary artery in normal subjects. Occlusion of one pulmonary artery in normal individuals has little effect on pulmonary artery pressure, because pulmonary vascular resistance falls in the contralateral lung. If the pulmonary artery is distended, either by an obstructing element or without obstruction, the pulmonary artery pressure rises modestly, apparently due to stimulation of baroreceptors in the large arteries. In the experimental animal small peripheral emboli below 28 μ seem to cause more marked vasoconstriction. Some of this effect is considered due to release of either serotoninin and/or histamine from the lung or from the blood clot. There is an associated bronchoconstriction which may be due either to lowered alveolar pCO_2 in the area of infarct or to the action of histamine.

The clinical and laboratory manifestations of clinical pulmonary emboli add to the confusion about their pathophysiology. Patients with pulmonary emboli develop tachypnea, dyspnea, and, occasionally, apnea. These manifestations are probably reflex in origin, since they are more marked than would be expected only from changes in blood gas levels or the degree of obstruction of the pulmonary arteries. There is a fall in systemic blood pressure, which is often only transient, and a rise in pulmonary artery pressure. Often there is wheezing and other evidence of bronchoconstriction. The arterial pO_2 falls to a range of 75 to 80 mm. Hg and is not corrected by 100% oxygen breathing, so an apparent shunt develops. Because unperfused lung is ventilated, there is an increase in the alveolar–arteriolar (A–a) carbon dioxide difference. Measurement of the A–a carbon dioxide difference can give some indication of the portion of the pulmonary bed occluded. The carbon monoxide diffusing capacity is not decreased, but the oxygen diffusing capacity is. There is no clear explanation for the maintenance of a normal carbon monoxide diffusing capacity.

Immediately after a pulmonary infarct, the changes in cardiac output, systemic blood pressure, and pulmonary artery pressure are probably more marked, due to the reflex pulmonary vascular constriction, bronchoconstriction, and, perhaps, peripheral vasodilation. If the infarct is not immediately fatal, systemic blood pressure rises and pulmonary artery pressure falls. Since pulmonary embolectomy has become technically feasible, the diagnosis and measurement of the extent of embolization have become more urgent. With the development of lung scanning and precise angiography, it has been clearly shown that most nonfatal pulmonary emboli are lyzed and circulation restored to the area of lung involved. Infarction is the exception rather than the rule and may occur only in the presence of associated pulmonary disease or with infected emboli. Since most emboli lyze themselves, it is important not to operate on patients with pulmonary emboli unless life is threatened.

When a patient has a massive embolus that causes immediate collapse, vigorous cardiac massage may dislodge the embolus from the right ventricular outflow tract or main pulmonary artery by fragmenting it. Since the cross-sectional area of the bed increases as it branches, pushing the embolus distally will diminish the degree of obstruction. If there is no evidence of peripheral vascular collapse, i.e., systemic blood pressure is maintained and dyspnea is not extreme, no therapy is required other than 50% oxygen and such preventive measures as the administration of anticoagulants or interruption of the vena cava. If there is depression of systemic blood pressure, vasopressors should be given, and, if feasible, pulmonary artery or right ventricular pressure should be measured. If moderate doses of vasopressors maintain systemic blood pressure without undue elevation of pulmonary artery pressure, operative therapy is unnecessary. In other words, the indication for operation is evidence of a degree of obstruction of the pulmonary vascular bed which prevents transfer of adequate amounts of blood through the lungs without marked elevation of pulmonary artery pressure.

Following pulmonary emboli, some patients develop evidence of severe pulmonary edema in the uninfarcted areas of lung even without a marked rise in pulmonary artery pressure. There is no good explanation for this phenomenon, though it may be due to an increase in mean capillary pressure associated with high flow rate in the intact areas of the capillary bed (the same mechanism as in patients with high-altitude pulmonary edema). These patients will be helped by the use of a respirator and the administration of oxygen.

A more insidious type of pulmonary embolic disease is that which results from multiple small pulmonary emboli, often septic in nature. Patients with this problem usually have no significant physical or x-ray findings and complain only of dyspnea on mild exertion. If the alveolar–arteriolar carbon dioxide difference is determined, it is found to be large, indicative of the ventilatory shunt which results from ventilation of areas of lung with occluded vasculature. These patients usually show no evidence of obstructive disease on ventilatory function studies. All too often the disease goes unrecognized until severe pulmonary hypertension has developed, with evidence of right ventricular hypertrophy on electrocardiographic study. If the disease is recognized early, measures to prevent further embolization are mandatory. These measures should include both ligation of the vena cava and anticoagulant therapy.

12. THE EFFECT OF INJURY ON
PULMONARY FUNCTION

FUNCTION of the respiratory system can be disrupted by traumatic or operative injury to the chest cage and/or lungs or by infection or blockage of bronchi. Unfortunately, many patients suffer a combination of such insults, all of which must be treated simultaneously. This chapter relates the effect of injury on cardiopulmonary function.

EFFECTS OF TRAUMA ON PULMONARY FUNCTION

Injuries inflicted by accidental means or as planned operative therapy are similar in their effects on the patient. It is the extent, location, and nature of the injury, not the injuring agent, which determines the effects on cardiopulmonary function.

There has been surprisingly little careful measurement of the effects of trauma on the metabolic rate. It is known that with surface burns the metabolic requirements may be increased manyfold. It has also been shown that uncomplicated laparotomy is associated with very little increase in the basal metabolic rate, while after cardiac surgery the basal metabolic rate may be increased by 20%. In young, muscular subjects, there is apparently more increase in postoperative metabolic rate than in older patients; and obese, lethargic patients have little increase. Complications such as infection greatly increase the metabolic rate and require increased minute ventilation and cardiac output.

Studies are needed to determine the total metabolic demands of the postinjury patient. He cannot recover from accidental trauma if he does not increase the output of his cardiorespiratory system, and it is likely that any activities, including turning and coughing, are less efficient following trauma.

Studies of the incidence of postoperative pulmonary complications have pinpointed the importance of the site of injury. Injuries to the extremities and head and neck seldom lead to pulmonary complications, whereas injuries to the chest cage result in a high incidence of pulmonary complications. Injuries to the lower abdomen result in fewer complications than injuries to the upper abdomen. It is clear that the degree of compromise of postoperative pulmonary function is directly related to degree of compromise of motion of the rib cage and abdomen. Body habitus also influences the degree and number of complications and the degree of compromise of function. Obese individuals have far more difficulty following trauma than individuals of like body build without excessive fat. The amount of muscular development of the abdomen and trunk is also important. Women have only half as many pulmonary complications as men, and light-muscled men fewer than do men with very heavy muscular development.

POSTOPERATIVE RESPIRATORY FUNCTION

Postoperative Pattern of Ventilation and Blood Gases. In a patient with an uncomplicated postoperative course, respiratory rate increases, tidal volume decreases, and minute ventilation increases to maintain an essentially unchanged alveolar ventilation. The vital capacity is cut in half, largely due to a decrease in inspiratory reserve. The maximum breathing capacity is cut to 30% of normal, but the percent of vital capacity expelled in the first minute is unchanged. All of these changes are indicative of restriction of ventilation.

In the early postoperative period, there may be modest to slight elevation of the arterial blood pCO_2 until the depression resulting from the anesthetic agents has worn off. Persistent elevation in arterial pCO_2 beyond the period of anesthetic depression is seen only in patients with serious associated cardiopulmonary disease or dysfunction of the chest cage. Following this early rise, pCO_2 falls to normal or slightly below preoperative levels. The arterial blood pO_2 is depressed and remains so even after alveolar ventilation returns to normal or greater than normal levels. Breathing of 100% oxygen does not return the arterial pO_2 to normal, signifying the presence of an intrapulmonary shunt.

Postoperative Musculoskeletal Mechanics. The type, location, and extent of injury to the trunk are among the controlling factors in the deficit of pulmonary function in the postoperative patient. The restrictions of function of the chest cage limit ventilation, and if lung mechanics are compromised by direct injury or by preexisting disease, the injured chest cage is less able to do the required added work. Upper abdominal incisions produce pain and muscle spasm compromising postoperative pulmonary function more than lower abdominal incisions, because restriction of motion of upper abdominal muscles compromises chest cage motion more than does restriction of motion of lower abdominal muscles. Likewise, large incisions or operative procedures which require vigorous and prolonged retraction injure more muscles, causing more pain and spasm and leading to greater restriction of chest cage motion postoperatively.

Midline sternotomy injures fewer muscles than does anterolateral thoracotomy, and anterolateral thoracotomy injures fewer muscles than does lateral thoracotomy. Thus, lateral thoracotomy compromises the chest wall most, midline sternotomy least. The degree of compromise by all three incisions depends in large part on the degree to which the rib spreader is opened. The more the incision is spread, the greater the disruption of the chest wall that results.

Postoperatively the compliance of the chest wall is decreased. This is not the result of loss of elasticity but rather is due to muscle spasm, which splints a region of the chest cage and will not allow it to expand. This splinting in effect requires the other areas of the chest to move more to achieve the same increase in volume. The rapid, shallow respirations of postoperative patients represent an adjustment to this decrease in compliance of the chest wall.

In the heavily muscled individual, the effects of muscular spasm are exaggerated because of the larger mass of muscle injured and the greater force it can exert when in spasm. In obese patients the added burden of moving the dead weight of the fat further restricts the freedom of motion of the injured chest cage.

Postoperative Lung Mechanics.   The restrictive pattern of ventilation due to chest wall injury results in deterioration of lung function even if there is no direct injury to the lungs. Shallow breathing results in poor distribution of tidal volume to various areas of lung (Fig. 12-1A). In addition, the sighs or deep breaths taken by normal individuals every few minutes to regenerate the free energy of the surfactant are not taken by the patient who has sustained injury to the chest or abdomen, so progressive collapse of alveoli occurs. This combination of shallow breathing and lack of occasional deep breaths results in decrease in lung compliance and the development of areas of microatelectasis in the lung. It is these areas of microatelectasis—unventilated lung— which cause the depression in arterial pO_2 that does not respond to 100% oxygen therapy.

Breathing of 100% oxygen can differentiate low arterial pO_2 due

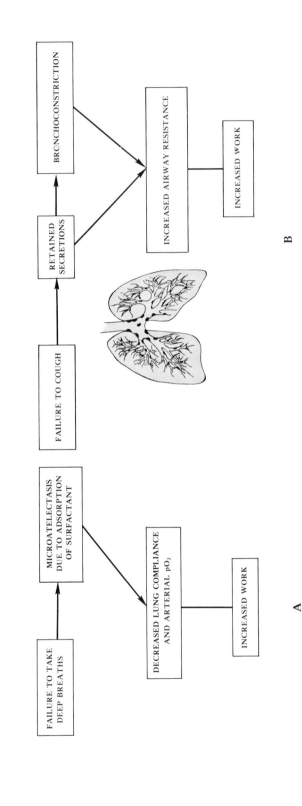

FAILURE TO TAKE DEEP BREATHS → MICROATELECTASIS DUE TO ADSORPTION OF SURFACTANT → DECREASED LUNG COMPLIANCE AND ARTERIAL pO_2 → INCREASED WORK

A

FAILURE TO COUGH → RETAINED SECRETIONS → BRONCHOCONSTRICTION → INCREASED AIRWAY RESISTANCE → INCREASED WORK

B

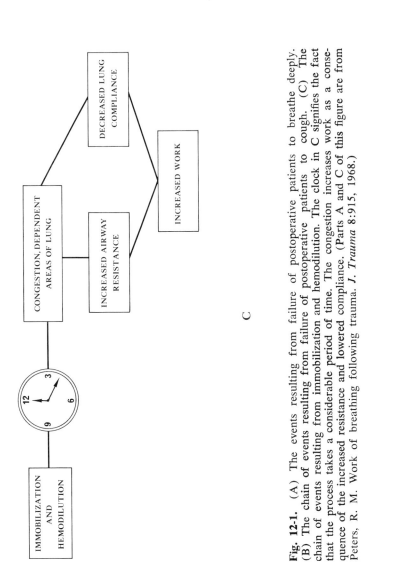

Fig. 12-1. (A) The events resulting from failure of postoperative patients to breathe deeply. (B) The chain of events resulting from failure of postoperative patients to cough. (C) The chain of events resulting from immobilization and hemodilution. The clock in C signifies the fact that the process takes a considerable period of time. The congestion increases work as a consequence of the increased resistance and lowered compliance. (Parts A and C of this figure are from Peters, R. M. Work of breathing following trauma. *J. Trauma* 8:915, 1968.)

to ventilation-perfusion incoordination from that due to shunting, and it has been shown that 80% of the postoperative depression in arterial pO_2 is due to shunt. The remaining 20% is the result of ventilation-perfusion incoordination. After uncomplicated abdominal operations, the arterial pO_2 is around 88 mm. Hg, representing a shunt fraction of 8 to 10%. After aortic valve surgery or lobectomy, the arterial pO_2 is in the range of 65 mm. Hg, a shunt fraction of 15 to 20%.

Postoperative patients fail to cough, which causes retention of secretions and increase in airway resistance (Fig. 12-1B); the retained secretions produce obstruction and induce spasm of the airways. This not only directly increases the work of breathing but indirectly leads to further increase in work by causing ventilation-perfusion incoordination requiring increased alveolar ventilation.

Pain also prevents patients from turning regularly, so they develop congestion in the dependent portions of their lungs (Fig. 12-1C). Congestion aggravates the effects of failure to take deep breaths and failure to cough, because the swelling narrows the small airways and fills some of the alveoli in these dependent, usually posterior, portions of the lungs.

If there is direct injury to the lungs or the mechanical function of the lung is compromised due to preexisting disease, all of the effects of restriction of chest wall motion are exaggerated.

Postoperative Pulmonary Circulation. In the immediate postoperative period, pulmonary vascular resistance is elevated. The elevation is small and probably has little clinical significance in the otherwise normal patient. In patients with preoperative elevation in pulmonary vascular resistance the rise in pulmonary vascular resistance postoperatively may be exaggerated. The exact cause of this rise in pulmonary vascular resistance is unknown. Perhaps the most important effect of operation on the pulmonary vasculature results from the failure of the patient to turn regularly. The prolonged elevation of hydrostatic pressure in the dependent portions of the lungs results in effusion of fluid with congestion and ultimate filling of alveoli with fluid.

Postoperative Respiratory Work. The combined consequences of the restriction of chest motion and the resultant deterioration in lung mechanics are an increase in the work of breathing. Measures of postoperative work per minute done on the lung have varied, and should of course be correlated with the oxygen consumption and the work per unit of ventilation. These studies are difficult to carry out in the immediate postoperative period, and no methods to date are available to permit measurement of work done on the chest wall. The studies done so far indicate that respiratory work is increased postoperatively, as would be predicted from the deterioration in lung and chest wall mechanics.

A consideration of the work required by the postoperative patient to maintain cardiopulmonary function is a good basis for the development of proper treatment. The careful use of narcotics, by reducing the pain enough to permit relaxation of muscle spasm and thus removing some of the inhibition to deep breathing, coughing, and turning, can increase efficiency of the respiratory system. In the injured patient, narcotics may actually increase rather than decrease ventilatory exchange. The use of narcotics prior to performing endotracheal suction, moving the patient, or carrying out other such procedures may make these necessary therapeutic steps both more tolerable to the patient and more effective in restoring lung function.

A regime of good postoperative care requires careful consideration of the interaction of factors which can enhance or decrease effective cardiopulmonary function. The surgeon must evaluate the interplay of these various factors and intervene when necessary to lighten the load on the patient. In the extreme, this means the provision of complete support by ventilation with a respirator.

As in all diseases, prevention is the best form of therapy. Postoperative ventilatory difficulty can often be avoided by proper preoperative preparation. As previously mentioned, elective surgery in obese patients should be delayed until their weight has been reduced, even if this requires hospitalization. Patients who smoke should be required to stop smoking for ten to fourteen days prior to operation to permit regression of the chronic tracheobronchitis inevitably present. A program of graded exercise to increase ventilatory and circulatory reserve is very helpful, particularly in the patient with borderline reserve. Graded postoperative exercise can also speed recovery of ventilatory function, which usually requires a minimum of six weeks to reach its maximum after major upper abdominal or thoracic operations.

INJURIES TO THE CHEST CAGE

Crushing Injuries.   Crushing injuries to the chest destroy the integrity of the chest wall skeleton. Ventilation of the lungs depends on a pressure differential between atmospheric and pleural pressure. In patients with multiple rib fractures, during inspiration, when the intrapleural pressure is lower than atmospheric pressure, the atmospheric pressure will push the disrupted portion of the chest wall inward. During expiration, when the intrathoracic pressure rises to or above atmospheric pressure, the disrupted portion of the chest wall will move outward. The direction of motion in the area of the fractures is the opposite of that in the normal

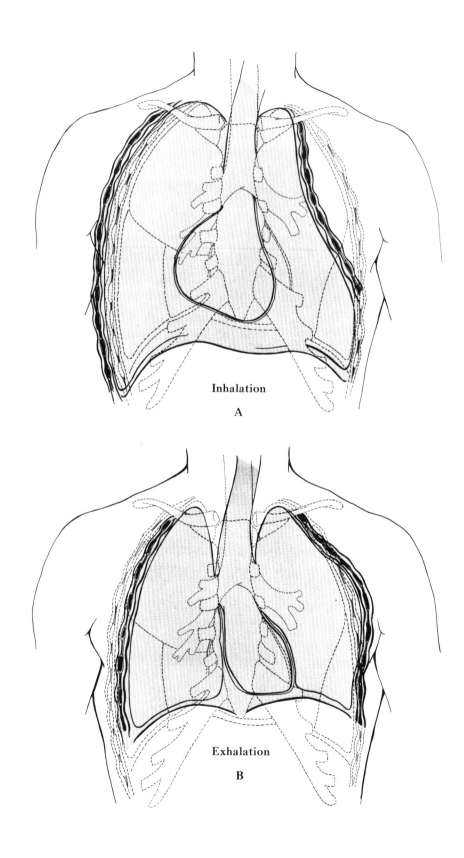

Inhalation

A

Exhalation

B

portions of the chest and has been labeled *paradoxical respiration* (Fig. 12-2). The amount of paradoxical motion depends on the extent of the injury and its location. Paradoxical respiration is most marked when injury occurs in the highly mobile anterolateral portion of the chest, which is poorly protected by the shoulder girdle muscles. This also is the area most likely to be injured in trauma inflicted in vehicle accidents.

Penetration of the Chest Wall.   The mechanical effect of an injury which results in an actual penetration of the chest wall (open pneumothorax) is physiologically the same as the effect of a crushing chest injury (Fig. 12-3). On inspiration, air rushes into the chest; and on expiration, it rushes out again. The proportion of the increase in chest volume which results in ventilation of the lungs or in air rushing through the hole in the chest into the pleural cavity depends on the relative resistance to airflow of the tracheobronchial tree and the compliance of the lungs versus the resistance to airflow through the hole in the chest or the resistance to distortion of the area of crushed chest. A well-conditioned individual with essentially normal lungs can tolerate a larger hole in the chest wall or larger area of paradoxical motion than an individual in poor condition or an individual with compromised lung function.

If the mediastinum was an immobile barrier between the two chests, most patients could tolerate a large opening in the chest wall without difficulty. It is, of course, not an immobile barrier, but rather acts as a thin membrane which moves freely and maintains nearly identical pressures in the two chests. The effect of disruption of the chest wall is transmitted to both lungs. If the chest wall opening is large, the rush of air in and out of the opening is associated with continued back-and-forth motion of the mediastinum. This greatly increased motion, as well as compromising respiratory exchange, compromises venous return to the heart. If the mediastinum is stabilized by manual traction on the ipsilateral hilum during thoracotomy, a patient can maintain spontaneous

---

Fig. 12-2.   Paradoxical respiration. When the stability of the chest wall is disrupted, inhalation (A) causes the pressure in the chest to fall below atmospheric pressure; the disrupted portion of the chest moves inward, rather than out. The intact chest wall permits a more subatmospheric pressure in the uninjured chest, and the heart and mediastinum move toward that side. Some air goes into the injured lung during inspiration, because a subatmospheric pressure must exist in this hemithorax to pull the chest wall in.

During exhalation (B), the elastic recoil of the lung on the injured side expels air. Any forced expiration, which requires elevation of intrapleural pressure above atmospheric level, causes the injured chest to bulge outward and the heart to move toward the injured side.

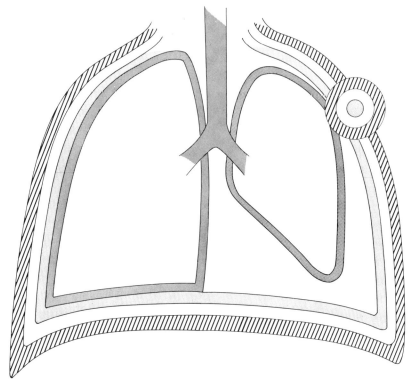

Fig. 12-3. Open pneumothorax. If a hole is made in the chest wall, equal to the small, light-gray dot, to expand the lungs with a tidal volume shown as the dark-gray outline of the trachea and lungs requires an increase in the chest volume by an amount equal to the light and dark gray outlines. If the hole is as big as the white circle, the same tidal volume will require the added chest expansion of the white area between the gray and cross-hatched outlines. If the hole is as big as the cross-hatched circle, to pull the same tidal volume into the lung the chest volume must be expanded by an additional increment equal to the cross-hatched area. Thus, the larger the defect in the chest wall, the greater the change in chest volume required to expand the lungs. If the hole is very large and resistance to flow through it is negligible (open thoracotomy wound), no air will enter the lungs despite maximum effort.

ventilation despite the large open wound. Without such traction, air exchange despite maximum effort is insufficient, and respiratory failure will soon result.

Diaphragmatic Paralysis. Paralysis of a diaphragm has the same effect on air exchange as does crushing of the chest wall. On inspiration, the diaphragm is pulled up by the negative pressure in the chest; and during expiration, it is pushed down. This paradoxical motion of the diaphragm greatly compromises ventilatory function. Paralysis of both diaphragms results in respiratory insufficiency.

Effect on Mechanical Function of the Lungs.   In addition to defects in the chest wall, traumatic or operative injury to the chest wall also results in deterioration of the mechanical function of the lungs. The changes that result from limitation of chest wall motion, outlined in the section Postoperative Respiratory Function, will lead to increased lung stiffness and airway resistance. If, in addition, there is direct trauma to the lung with contusions or lacerations, the mechanics of the lung will be further compromised. Immediately after injury the compromise of lung mechanics may not be serious, but as edema develops in the contused lung and as inability of the patient to cough and take deep breaths leads to fall in lung compliance and elevated airway resistance, the lungs become increasingly more difficult to ventilate. Adequate ventilation under these circumstances requires greater force and thus greater swings in pleural pressure. These greater swings in pleural pressure cause more paradoxical motion of the chest wall and allow more air to rush in and out of the opening in the chest and less air to come through the tracheobronchial tree into the alveoli for any given effort. The continued escalation of ventilatory work leads to progressive fatigue and ultimate respiratory insufficiency.

Rib Resections.   The operative removal of ribs to collapse the lung—thoracoplasty—or to remove tumor-bearing tissue has the same effect as crushing the chest. Removal of posterior portions of ribs is better tolerated than removal of anterior or lateral portions, because the posterior rib cage is less mobile and is better protected by the shoulder girdle. In addition to the effects on ipsilateral chest wall mechanics, partial resection of ribs on one side of the chest also restricts the motion of the contralateral side. This is particularly true following removal of the first rib or the anterior portions of ribs.

Use of a Respirator in Open Pneumothorax.   Intermittent positive-pressure ventilation with a respirator is the best form of therapy for open pneumothorax or paradoxical chest wall motion. It stops motion of the crushed chest wall and acts like balanced traction. In an open pneumothorax it inflates the lungs by raising alveolar pressure above atmospheric, thus preventing air from rushing into the chest. When an open pneumothorax is present, it is best not to let the end-tidal pressure fall to zero, since this results in a lower than normal end-tidal volume (see Chapter 13, "Respirators," pp. 294–296) and collapse of alveoli with intrapulmonary shunt of blood.

Pendelluft. There has been considerable speculation over whether with paradoxical respiration air goes from one lung to the other during the respiratory cycle—the condition called *Pendelluft.* If during inspiration the chest wall on the injured side is to be pulled in, the pleural pressure on the injured side must decrease, and this will cause its lung to expand. The movement of the mediastinum toward the uninjured side will also result in expansion of the lung on the injured side. The reverse will be true during expiration. Thus air must move into both lungs during inspiration and out of both lungs during expiration, not from one to the other. During pauses in respiration air may redistribute itself between the two lungs, depending on the resistance and compliance of each and their respective time constants (see pp. 159–164 in Chapter 7, "Coordination of Ventilation and Perfusion"). This redistribution is quantitatively negligible. Pendelluft is not of any consequence in patients with open pneumothoraxes or paradoxical chest wall motion; it is rather a theoretically possible but practically unimportant concept.

INTRATHORACIC COMPLICATIONS OF INJURIES AND INFECTION

CLOSED PNEUMOTHORAX

Fractured ribs or penetrating injuries to the chest can cause lacerations of the lung. During inspiration these lacerations are pulled open by the negative pleural pressure, and air rushes out of the lung into the pleural cavity. During expiration the edges of the lacerations collapse together, and the air in the pleural cavity cannot escape. The same mechanism operates when a bleb on the lung bursts due to excessive tension. Air escapes through the defect during inspiration and is trapped in the pleural cavity during expiration.

The air in the pleural space occupies chest volume and compresses lung expansion. To maintain normal expansion of the lung, the chest volume would have to be increased proportionate to the volume of air trapped in the pleural cavity, but this is not what actually occurs. Patients do not increase chest volume to equal the volume of the pneumothorax. Instead, the lung on the affected side loses volume. It has been estimated that lung volume is decreased by about one-half the amount of intrapleural air. Consequently, half the pneumothorax volume collapses the lung, and half is taken up by increased chest volume.

The diagnosis of pneumothorax by physical examination, particularly if there is associated injury to the chest wall, is often impossible. The difference in the percussion note between air and aerated lungs is slight, and if there is any increase in breath sounds, the transmission of the sound through the pneumothorax may be at normal levels, making auscultation equally unreliable. A chest x-ray is the modern way to make this diagnosis. The film should be taken in the upright position; otherwise, the superimposition of fluid, air, and lung may obscure one another. Even using x-ray examinations, the volume of pneumothoraxes is usually underestimated. Routine chest films are taken at maximum inspiration, when chest volume is greatest, which makes the pneumothorax appear smaller relative to lung volume. By taking a film in expiration, the volume of the pneumothorax relative to the lung is exaggerated, and a small pneumothorax can be identified more easily. The most accurate assessment of pneumothorax volume can be made from a film taken at normal end-tidal volume. In addition to the error introduced by the disproportion at full inspiration, a further error is often added in x-ray interpretations due to failure to remember that the chest is three-dimensional and that the outer one inch contains approximately 30% of the total volume.

Since the mediastinum is mobile, air can continue to escape even after complete collapse of one lung, with the result that a volume is trapped in the chest which is greater than the volume of the affected hemithorax. The continued accumulation of air can cause complete collapse of the ipsilateral lung and compression of the contralateral lung by displacement of the mediastinum. A patient in such a situation may develop a markedly positive pleural pressure during expiration—a tension pneumothorax. In a patient with a tension pneumothorax, pleural pressure must drop below atmospheric during inspiration or no air will enter his lungs. The patient achieves this drop in pleural pressure by breathing with maximum effort to hyperexpand the thoracic volume. A patient with a tension pneumothorax is in severe respiratory distress and must have immediate relief to allow air to escape from the pleural cavity.

The size of pneumothorax tolerated depends on the respiratory reserve and the physical condition of the patient. In patients with crushed chest injuries, a relatively small associated pneumothorax may cause respiratory failure because of the compromised chest wall function. Likewise, when a lung bleb ruptures in patients with an obstructive lung disease such as bullous emphysema, and when there is restriction in pulmonary function, respiratory insufficiency may develop when only a relatively small pneumothorax is present.

If there is a laceration in the parietal as well as the visceral pleura—

the case in all penetrating wounds and crushed chest injuries associated with pneumothorax—air may escape from the chest into the subcutaneous tissue to partially decompress the chest. This escape is exaggerated when the patient raises intrapleural pressure with cough. This subcutaneous emphysema can be massive, spreading from head to groin, or only local. It rarely, if ever, has deleterious effects on either respiratory or circulatory function. Its principal effects are to cause marked discomfort for the patient and to frighten both patient and family.

RUPTURE OF A BRONCHUS

Traumatic lacerations of a major bronchus can result from compression injuries to the chest, such as occur when the chest is run over by the wheel of a car. They are the result of explosive disruption of the bronchus or trachea from excessive transmural pressure. These lacerations rarely result in tension pneumothorax, because air can move freely through them during both phases of respiration. If they are large, so much air may escape through them that little air reaches the alveoli. Their presence is suggested by a large, continuous leak from a chest cavity after insertion of a chest tube.

RUPTURE OF THE ESOPHAGUS

Rupture of the esophagus can also lead to large accumulations of mediastinal or pleural air as a result of the patient's swallowing. If the mediastinal pleura is intact, the air stays confined to the mediastinum and escapes into the neck (a lateral cervical spine film showing air between the spine and posterior pharynx gives the earliest indication of injury to the upper half of the esophagus). If the pleura is perforated, a pneumothorax will develop. These patients, in addition, have all the toxic symptoms resulting from the pouring out of the highly infectious esophageal and mouth organisms into the chest and mediastinum. This injury requires prompt drainage or surgical repair and massive antibiotic therapy.

HEMOTHORAX, HYDROTHORAX, AND PYOTHORAX

Pneumothorax is frequently complicated by hemo- or hydrothorax. When fractured ribs or penetrating chest injuries result in laceration of the lung, some bleeding does occur from the cut lung surface. However, since the pulmonary artery pressure is low and the associated pneumohemothorax collapses the lung, bleeding from the lung is usually of minor significance. Severe bleeding from the lung results only from hilar injuries. However, there is frequently very significant bleeding from the chest wall from lacerated intercostal or internal mammary arteries.

Some patients who develop spontaneous pneumothoraxes may tear an adhesion from the chest wall, causing steady, slow bleeding from the chest wall that can result in accumulation of more than a liter of blood in the chest. With most chest injuries bleeding is not massive, and the conservative therapy of chest drainage and transfusion is adequate.

If infection occurs in the pleural cavity, either from contamination through a bronchopleural fistula or secondary to intrapulmonary infection, large amounts of fluid or frank pus can accumulate in the chest. Accumulations of fluid or blood in the chest compromise pulmonary function, just as does accumulation of air. The volume available for lung expansion is limited.

The obvious goal of treatment of these diseases of the pleural cavity—hemothorax, hydrothorax, and pyothorax—is to evacuate completely all the air and fluid as promptly as possible. A drainage system must be devised which will allow fluid and air to escape but will not permit air to be sucked into the chest when pleural pressure is below atmospheric pressure. Therefore, some kind of one-way drainage must be devised, since open drainage would result in a sucking chest wound. The simple, commonly used system is underwater sealed drainage. A drainage tube is inserted into the chest and connected to a tube which leads down into a bottle on floor level beside the patient's bed. The tube extends to the bottom of the bottle, and the end of the tube is covered with a few centimeters of water. Air can escape when the pleural pressure rises above atmospheric and exceeds a pressure equivalent to the number of centimeters the tube is below the fluid surface. This occurs during cough, straining, or when there is a tension pneumothorax. If only fluid is present in the chest, it is sucked out by a pressure equivalent to the distance from the patient's chest to the top of the fluid level in the bottle. For example, if a patient with a large hydrothorax is connected to a water-seal drainage bottle placed on the floor, the negative pressure sucking fluid out of the chest is 100 cm. H_2O, or the height of the column of fluid extending from the patient to the drainage bottle.

If the lung on the side of the hydrothorax cannot expand promptly to fill the space as the fluid is drained out, the mediastinum will be pulled into the affected chest; severe discomfort and respiratory distress may result. In such patients the bottle should not be placed on the floor but at a level 10 to 20 cm. below the patient. This will slow the egress of fluid and assure that too great a negative pressure is not applied to the chest cavity.

If there is a large air leak in the lung, the chest tube may not serve to keep the chest cavity free of air because the egress route through the tube is smaller than the leak in the lung. Under these circumstances a

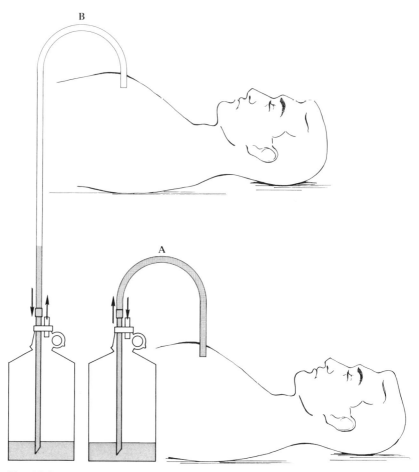

Fig. 12-4. Closed chest drainage. The chest drainage bottle has a long tube extending to the bottom of the bottle which is filled with sterile water to a level 1 cm. above the end of the long tube. The long tube is connected to the catheter in the chest; the short tube opens the bottle to air. If the bottle is at the level of the patient (A), the negative pressure in the chest can lift the water from the bottle and it will enter the chest. In (B), the bottle is on the floor, below the patient's chest, and the subatmospheric intrapleural pressure cannot create enough force to pull fluid from the bottle into the chest. Any positive intrapleural pressure of more than 1 cm. H_2O—such as is created by a cough—will push air out of the chest. Fluid can also escape through this tube and is sucked out with a force equal to the height of the column of fluid above the floor.

controlled negative pressure of 10 to 30 cm. H_2O can be applied to the chest bottle. This negative pressure speeds the evacuation of fluid.

To drain fluid from the chest adequately, the tube should be placed in a dependent portion of the chest cavity to which the fluid gravitates, usually the fifth or sixth interspace in the posterior axillary line. This is not the best site for the evacuation of air, which goes to the anterior superior portions of the chest. To evacuate air, the tube should be placed in the second anterior interspace. If air and fluid are both present, two tubes are advisable, one placed posteriorly to drain fluid and one placed anteriorly to evacuate air. A single posterior tube is apt to become occluded with fibrin clots, which, if an air leak is also present, will result in recurrence of pneumothorax. Likewise, an anterior tube fails to completely evacuate the fluid, since the fluid must be pushed up to the level of the tube before it can drain out of the chest.

Anything which causes the patient to increase pleural pressure will aid in the evacuation of air and fluid from the chest by providing a positive force to pump fluid out of the pleural cavity. The pleural pressure can be increased by having the patient turn, which causes him to strain; by having him do Valsalva maneuvers; or by having him use blow bottles. The most important factor is frequent, effective coughing. This markedly elevates pleural pressure to evacuate fluid and air and also clears the airways so the lung can reexpand to fill the chest cavity.

If blood is not promptly evacuated from the pleural cavity or cannot be effectively evacuated due to clotting, a number of complications may occur. Fortunately, in about a third of the patients the blood will liquefy and be reabsorbed in four to six weeks, while in another third it will liquefy in ten days to two weeks after injury and at that time can be aspirated or drained. In the remaining 20 to 30% of patients the blood organizes into a fibrinous and then fibrous peel that traps the lung in a partially collapsed position. Trapping of the lung in such a collapsed position diminishes both ventilation and perfusion. The fibrothorax may restrict the chest wall and diaphragmatic motion by obliterating the costophrenic angle. Such a fibrothorax decreases perfusion to the area of lung with restricted motion much more than it lowers ventilation. A basal fibrothorax that obliterates the costophrenic angle may result in a ventilation-perfusion ratio to the basal region of the lung on the affected side that is two to ten times normal. No good explanation has been made for the relatively greater decrease in perfusion than ventilation to trapped portions of the lung.

If hemothorax does not liquefy or resorb in six weeks, operative removal of the peel is advisable. This frees the lung, and if vigorous physiotherapy is instituted before and after operation, most of the lost pulmonary function can be restored.

While a fibrothorax that traps the lung and restricts its expansion does limit ventilatory function, the obliteration of the pleural space by light, filmy adhesions has very little effect. In patients who develop repeated, spontaneous pneumothoraxes, irritation of the pleura by vigorous rubbing with a dry sponge causes the development of such adhesions and prevents the development of subsequent pneumothoraxes. More radical operative procedures, such as parietal pleurectomy, are unnecessary and contraindicated, since they cause such heavy scarring between lung and chest wall that function is limited.

If pleural fluid becomes infected, it must be promptly evacuated, just as must any collection of infected fluid. Attempts to control empyemas by repeated thoracenteses and injections of antibiotics are rarely effective and usually prolong and complicate therapy. An acute empyema requires closed drainage using a water-seal bottle to prevent lung collapse. When the pleural fluid becomes thick and frank pus develops, adhesions will already have formed between the lungs and chest wall which prevent collapse of the lung. At this stage of the disease a large, open drainage tube can be inserted for more effective drainage of thick pus and detritus. An open drain must not be used until adequate adhesions have formed, or an iatrogenic and potentially fatal sucking chest wound will have been inflicted. Many young men died in World War I until this principle was enunciated by the precise work of Dr. Evarts Graham.

ATELECTASIS AND PULMONARY INFECTIONS

Atelectasis. Lack of gas within the lung and, more particularly, within the alveoli, is atelectasis. Obstruction of a lobar main-stem bronchus results in reabsorbtion of air from the lobe or lung and the development of atelectasis. This reabsorption may take a period of hours if, at the time the obstruction occurs, the patient is breathing air or less than 50% oxygen in nitrogen. If the patient is breathing 100% oxygen at the time obstruction occurs, complete collapse can develop in just a few minutes, as the venous blood sucks the oxygen out of the alveoli. The total collapse of lung that occurs under anesthesia is the result of acute obstruction in patients breathing very high oxygen mixtures.

In an otherwise normal individual, the complete collapse of one lung is tolerated unless severe exertion is required. Such collapse results in decreased lung compliance and increased resistance. A collapsed portion of lung is not ventilated, so there is no gas exchange with the blood flowing to the area of collapse. This results in a shunt. Fortunately, when an area of lung collapses, the blood flow through it also diminishes, decreasing the shunt effect.

There is some controversy about the time interval between lung collapse and decrease in flow. Some investigators have found that flow falls to low levels in a few minutes, others that hours are required to decrease the shunt significantly. These differences may depend on the completeness of collapse, the position of the subjects, and the manner in which the subjects were ventilated.

Obstruction of a segmental bronchus may not result in atelectasis, because there are microscopic collateral connections at the alveolar levels which permit some air to cross from one segment to another. Following obstruction of subsegmental bronchi, these collaterals may be very effective in maintaining aeration of the obstructed area of lung. The maintenance of aeration through these collaterals insures that air is present, so a pressure head of air can be developed behind the obstruction during coughing which aids in expulsion of the obstructing agent.

Microatelectasis as well as gross atelectasis can occur throughout the lung. This is discussed in detail in the section on the shock lung syndrome (pp. 271–279).

After an obstruction is relieved, a collapsed alveolus will not reopen during normal quiet breathing, which does not provide a high enough opening pressure. Coughing serves to force out the obstruction; prior to opening the glottis, pressures in the hyperinflated lungs are elevated well above the opening pressures of the collapsed alveoli. However, the opening of these alveoli depends on air shifting from expanded alveoli into areas of collapse. This transfer takes time and often cannot occur during the short period of high intrapleural pressure during a cough. A prolonged hyperinflation with the maintenance of high intratracheal pressure is more effective. This can be achieved by having the patient hyperinflate his lungs and blow out against a resistance such as blow bottles.

Lobar Pneumonia. Lobar pneumonia affects pulmonary function in almost exactly the same manner as does atelectasis. The consolidated area of lung is not ventilated, and so ventilatory reserve is proportionately reduced. It has been clearly demonstrated that blood flow to the consolidated area of lung is also reduced, so the shunt effect is diminished. With pneumonia, the infection greatly increases metabolic rate and thus the demands for gas exchange. The inflammation also often leads to chest pain and general lassitude, which further restrict the respiratory reserve.

With modern antibiotics, lobar pneumonia can be controlled if the patient can maintain adequate gas exchange for 48 to 72 hours. If the pneumonia is extensive or the respiratory reserve is limited by previous disease, artificial respiration may be indicated. The use of respiratory support is widely accepted for the patient in whom pneumonia complicates preexisting chronic respiratory disease. Unfortunately, it is not used frequently enough in otherwise healthy individuals with extensive bilateral pneumonia. Many such patients die of progressive fatigue from attempts to maintain maximum respiratory effort in the face of massive infection. Relieved of the respiratory work they can cope with the infection.

Patients who recover from pneumococcal lobar pneumonia are usually left with no residual effects. The same may be the case following staphyloccal pneumonia, though often, as with *Aerobacter* pneumonia, staphylococcal infection causes disruption and destruction of the normal lung structure. Tuberculosis also leads to such destruction. These diseases destroy both the alveoli and the vessels supplying them. For this reason, such lesions result in a restriction of function proportional to the areas of lung destroyed and there is no shunt effect. Tuberculosis, which is usually confined to the upper portions of the lung, affects the least perfused and thus the least used part of the lungs in man. There has been much speculation but no good evidence connecting the predilection of tuberculosis for the upper lobes to the decreased blood flow to these areas of lung.

Bronchiectasis. This disease, which mainly affects the lower half of the lungs, is disappearing in areas of the world where pertussis and measles vaccines and adequate antibiotic therapy are available. While there is still some controversy about the mechanism of development of bronchiectasis, it seems to result from the combination of airway obstruction with acute bacterial infection. In infants and children with small airways, pertussis or measles complicated by bacterial infection frequently provides the combination necessary to produce the disease. Aspiration of foreign bodies, tumor, or obstruction of a central bronchus by compression from an inflamed lymph node are other initiating causes. With increased skill in endoscopic removal of foreign bodies and antibiotics to control secondary infection, bronchiectasis due to aspiration is becoming a rarity.

Despite the fact that this disease is disappearing, it deserves brief discussion because of its interesting late pathophysiology. These patients all have severe, chronic infection of the tracheobronchial tree with destruction of large areas of the functioning alveoli. However, they still have some pulmonary blood flow to the affected regions of lung. Characteristic of this disease is a marked increase in size of vessels and in blood flow through the bronchial arterial system. Injection studies of such lungs show extensive anastomosis between these bronchial collaterals and the pulmonary arterial system. Angiographic and oxygen saturation studies of the pulmonary artery demonstrate that blood flows from these collaterals into the pulmonary arterial system to produce a systemic pulmonary shunt. In severe bronchiectasis this shunt can amount to 15% of left heart output. The same type of picture is found in experimental animals following ligation of a pulmonary artery. No such bronchial collateral develops following experimental or traumatic interruption of a main-stem bronchus unless there is associated infection.

The clinical significance of the left-to-right shunt is largely surgical. Resection of such lobes is difficult and frequently associated with considerable blood loss. Great care should be taken to insure ligation of all bronchial collaterals.

Some investigators have attributed considerable physiological significance to the bronchial collateral circulation. It has been considered to be the mechanism by which blood flow to unventilated lung is prevented. However, the decrease or absence of bronchial collateral circulation in chronic atelectasis uncomplicated by infection and in scarred, contracted, burned-out areas of tuberculosis, to which pulmonary blood flow may be almost negligible, does not support this contention. The development of bronchial collateral circulation is more likely a response to decreased blood flow or chronic, active infection and does not serve to diminish pulmonary artery blood flow to functionless lung.

Because it is a destructive process associated with chronic endobronchial infection, bronchiectasis leads to restrictive pulmonary disease. If not treated early in life, it can also result in obstructive disease due to the constant flooding of the tracheobronchial tree with infected material from the diseased area. If bronchiectasis develops in early childhood, there is some evidence that the unaffected portions of the lung may hypertrophy and compensate for the decrease in effective lung tissue. Early resection of the diseased areas of lung is the treatment of choice, but it should be undertaken only after maximum cleanup of bronchial secretions by vigorous antibiotic therapy and postural drainage.

PULMONARY RESECTION

Resection of a portion of lung reduces the total alveolar, bronchial, and vascular mass. The reduction is directly related to the relative weight of the region of lung resected. Table 12-1 gives these relative weights for adults. Since cardiac output must be maintained at approximately the same level regardless of the total amount of lung present, the perfusion to the remaining lung increases following pulmonary resection. The absolute anatomical dead space decreases by an amount equal to the amount of anatomical dead space removed. The tidal volume is maintained unless such a massive amount of lung is resected as to lead to

Table 12-1. Relative Weights of Lung Segments in Adults

Right upper lobe	20%	Left upper lobe	22%
Right middle lobe	8%	Left lower lobe	25%
Right lower lobe	25%		
Right lung	53%	Left lung	47%

severe restriction. The reduction in ventilation and maintenance of tidal volume result in a decrease in the proportion of the tidal volume that ventilates the dead space.

Resection reduces the diffusion surface and therefore the diffusion capacity. However, one would anticipate that the diffusion capacity would not be reduced as much as predicted from the mass of lung resected. The increased perfusion and ventilation of the remaining lung should increase its diffusion capacity, just as the increased ventilation and perfusion induced by exercise increases the diffusion capacity of normal individuals.

Studies of postoperative patients have shown, however, that the reduction in diffusing capacity is proportionate to the number of segments resected, as is the reduction in lung compliance. Postoperative bronchospirometric studies have shown that the decrement in function following segmental resection and lobectomy is greater than would be predicted from the mass of lung resected. The loss of function following lower lobectomy is proportionately greater than following upper lobectomy. Following pneumonectomy, the loss is more nearly equal to the volume of lung resected. The greater loss following segmental resection and lobectomy is related to the operative damage to the remaining lung, chest, and pleural space, which restricts motion of the lung.

In the early postoperative period, the deficits in function due to lung volume loss are all aggravated by the effects of thoracotomy on pulmonary function (see section entitled Postoperative Respiratory Function, p. 248). The lung remaining in the ipsilateral chest following thoracotomy also must recover from the effects of the trauma inflicted on it during the operation. These acute effects of trauma may result in such severe compromise of pulmonary function that respiratory decompensation results. In studies done in our laboratories, we have found that the elevation in work that must be done to ventilate the lung following pulmonary resection take seven to fourteen days to return to near-normal levels. If tracheal toilet, position change, and the need for deep breathing are not carefully monitored, even patients with good respiratory reserve can develop respiratory decompensation after pulmonary resection. If respiratory function is borderline, assisted ventilation may be required to help the patients through the postoperative period. Frequent determinations of blood gases are indicated in the patient with limited reserve; if pCO_2 rises or pO_2 falls significantly on 50% oxygen breathing, respiratory assistance is indicated.

The amount of lung that can be resected depends on the respiratory reserve of the patient. Studies have indicated that the limiting factor is the vascular bed and that reduction of this bed by 65 to 70% is the maximum that is tolerable for any level of useful function. Since the size of the vascular bed decreases with aging, the limits of resection are reduced in the elderly. In patients with emphysema and destruction of the capillary bed, the amount of lung that can be removed may be very limited.

No completely satisfactory test has been devised to predict the amount of lung that can be resected in individual patients. A maximum breathing capacity below 50% is associated with increased operative mortality. If the pulmonary artery pressure at rest is above 36 mm. Hg, the mortality is increased tenfold.

To further determine the amount of lung that can be resected, i.e., to answer the question whether the individual can tolerate a pneumonectomy, cardiac catheterization with balloon occlusion of the artery to the diseased lung has proved helpful. Since the amount of resection tolerated is related to the amount of vascular bed available, the occlusion of the affected vascular bed aids in the prediction of the tolerable limits of resection. If pulmonary artery pressure proximal to the occluding balloon rises at rest, it is apparent that the vascular bed in the remaining lung is limited and that increases in cardiac output with exercise will result in large rises in pulmonary artery pressure.

Arterial oxygen desaturation at rest may be the result of an intrapulmonary shunt in the diseased area of lung. If the presence of a shunt can be confirmed, such desaturation is not a contraindication to resection. If arterial oxygen desaturation or elevation of arterial pCO_2 occurs with exercise, it indicates a lack of functional reserve, and pulmonary resection is usually contraindicated.

To fill the intrapleural space left by pneumonectomy, the mediastinum shifts toward the side of resection, the diaphragm is elevated, and the intercostal spaces are narrowed, all of which decrease the volume of the hemithorax. The space which remains after these accommodations is filled with fluid or by hyperexpansion of the remaining lung. The hyperexpansion occurs largely across the anterior mediastinum, where the lung may occupy most of the anterior portion of the chest, thereby rotating the heart posteriorly into the hemithorax of the resected lung. These late shifts following pneumonectomy can be so marked in young patients that the hemithorax of the resected lung contains as much as one-third of the apparent lung volume.

Following lobectomy, the adjustments are less extreme. In young people in whom the remaining lung is undamaged, the only radiographic evidence of resection may be hyperlucency of the resected lung. If the lung volume is inadequate to fill the remaining hemithorax following lower lobectomy, the diaphragm is elevated and partially immobilized.

Following upper lobectomy, there may be a persistent air and/or fluid collection in the apex of the chest. These apical collections of fluid and/or air may become infected, but more often they remain for years without significant complications.

A postresection hemothorax or empyema can result in restriction of the motion of the chest wall and decreased expansion of the lung remaining in the hemithorax in which lobectomy was performed. Such pleural complications trap the ipsilateral remaining lung in critical scar, reducing its function to near zero. The crippling nature of such pleural scars should be kept in mind when judgment must be made regarding reexploration for postoperative bleeding.

The pulmonary function can be improved and the level of activity possible without dyspnea increased by postoperative physical training. These changes can be dramatic if a careful program of breathing exercise and graded exercise is set up. Much of the early postoperative decrease in function results from the painful, stiff chest wall and wasting of the trunk muscles from inactivity. One evidence of the importance of an exercise regime is its effectiveness in relieving wound pain. Immobility aggravates, while exercise alleviates, postoperative chest pain.

Pulmonary resection in children requires some special consideration. Infants and children through 2 to 3 years of age have considerably less respiratory reserve than do older children and adults. These younger children therefore tolerate resection less well. There is considerable controversy over whether in children the remaining lung hypertrophies following resection or just hyperexpands, as happens in the adult. Unfortunately, adequate studies of the actual volume of the capillary bed and of the alveolar diffusing surface have not been made. Studies in our laboratories show that children who undergo resection prior to the adolescent growth spurt seem to have better function than those that have resection after the adolescent growth spurt.

The ultimate functional capacity in children after resection appears to be related to the amount of physical activity. Those children who are not allowed activity have relatively poor function, while those who are actively trained have amazingly good function. This question may be finally resolved with new techniques of microradiography, by determination of diffusion capacity, and by careful pathological examination of lungs of young adults dying of trauma who have had lung resection as children. While only such studies can resolve the question of true hypertrophy versus hyperexpansion of the same number of pulmonary units, there can be no doubt that if children will exercise strenuously following pulmonary resection, their functional capacity will increase to a point nearly equal to that of normal children.

THE SHOCK LUNG SYNDROME

Each time the tragedy of serious injury to large numbers of young, healthy men in war takes place, new problems in medical care of the injured arise. In World War II, shock and infection were intensively studied and their treatment improved; in the Korean war, it was renal failure that received priority. In Vietnam fast evacuation by helicopter and resuscitation with electrolyte solution and carefully matched whole blood have saved the lives of many men with massive injuries who in previous wars would never have survived. Unfortunately, a portion of these individuals within hours to days after resuscitation develop respiratory failure, the so-called shock lung syndrome. This same syndrome is seen as the postperfusion lung syndrome in patients who have had a long period of extracorporeal perfusion for the performance of complicated intracardiac surgery. It is also seen following septic shock.

This syndrome is the subject of intense investigation and controversy at this time, and there is disagreement on every aspect of the problem. Of necessity, this section can only review the highlights of this syndrome and present the author's viewpoint.

CLINICAL COURSE

Hypovolemic shock causes decrease in cardiac output and lowered systemic and pulmonary artery pressures. The decreased tissue perfusion results in lactacidemia and metabolic acidosis due to tissue hypoxia. These acid-base changes cause the injured subject to hyperventilate to restore arterial pH to normal. Resuscitation by blood and fluid replacement can restore blood pressure and pulse, but the hyperventilation persists, sometimes even after the lactacidemia has decreased. This persistent hyperventilation results in a paradoxical post-resuscitation alkalosis.

Only a small percentage of patients resuscitated from the circulatory insufficiency due to hypovolemia develop respiratory complications. The patients that develop such complications have apparent restoration of circulatory dynamics to provide adequate tissue perfusion and renal function, but, despite this, they begin to manifest some mild respiratory distress. At this stage the cardiac output is increased over normal resting levels and the patients have persistent hyperventilation and hypocapnia. The arterial pO_2 is slightly depressed. The administration of oxygen does not correct this depression—evidence of an intrapulmonary shunt. The alveolar–arterial oxygen difference may continue to widen, with a resulting persistence in significant arterial desaturation despite inhalation of gas with high oxygen concentrations.

In some of these patients, when judicious use of oxygen to keep arterial pO_2 between 80 and 100 mm. Hg, frequent turning, and encouragement of deep breathing are instituted, the process reverses itself and recovery occurs. In others who go on to develop progressive respiratory distress, insufficiency manifests itself as a steady fall in arterial pO_2 despite a progressive increase in inspired oxygen concentration. These patients may develop rales and rhonchi, and patchy areas of consolidation are apparent on chest x-ray examination. Lactacidemia recurs as a result of inadequate tissue oxygen from the low arterial pO_2. In patients who reach this stage of disease, all therapy is to no avail. They develop persistent, severe hypoxemia, rapidly rising lactate, fall in bicarbonate and pH, and rising arterial pCO_2. Death is preceded by bradycardia.

EXPERIMENTAL STUDIES

Many experimental studies have been made to elucidate the effects of shock on the lung. The most frequently used shock model is that of Wiggers, in which dogs or primates are bled until blood pressure drops to 50 mm. Hg, maintained at this level for two hours, and then the shed blood restored with or without added electrolyte solution. This is the so-called standard shock model, but it certainly is not similar to any clinical situation. The final definition of the human shock syndrome may require a model closer to the true clinical situation.

Investigators using the standard Wiggers model have found that pulmonary artery pressure falls right after bleeding, when cardiac output is 33% of control. By the end of the two-hour shock period, the pulmonary artery pressure rises to 140% of control, despite a continued low cardiac output. After reinfusion of shed blood, the pulmonary artery pressure rises to more than 200% of control and then slowly falls back to normal over a period of hours. The cardiac output is only 50 to 60% of normal when pulmonary artery pressure is 200% of normal, evidence of a large increase in pulmonary vascular resistance. There is marked widening of the arteriovenous oxygen difference, due to the low cardiac output, and there is an increasing alveolar–arterial oxygen difference, the result of ventilation of unperfused alveoli.

The pathological changes in these experimental animals vary from severe to mild. In the lungs with severe changes, there are large, confluent areas of hemorrhagic consolidation with frothy, bloody secretions, and the areas of extravasation of red blood cells throughout the lungs take on the appearance of liver. In the mild cases, there are areas of punctate hemorrhage which appear similar to small infarcts. These areas of punctate hemorrhage are distributed throughout all areas of the lung and are not any more apparent in the dependent than they are in the superior portions of the lungs. These hemorrhagic areas readily collapse on relief of the inflating pressure and can be reinflated only with difficulty.

The hemorrhagic areas occur first around arteries less than 50 μ in diameter. Next to the areas of hemorrhage are seen some hyperinflated alveoli. In the posterior portions of the lungs, some edema may be present. Ultrastructure studies have shown some opening of pores present between endothelial cells and necrosis of capillary walls. In addition to the hemorrhagic changes, there is often some thickening of the alveolar walls by a protein-containing exudate lining the surface of the alveoli, a picture similar to that seen in infants with the respiratory distress syndrome. Much controversy has been raised as to the relative role these changes play in the production of the shock lung syndrome and whether these changes are the result of changes in surfactant. At this time it seems likely that surfactant changes are one of the causes of the shock lung syndrome.

HUMAN SHOCK LUNG

In human beings, shock obviously is not produced in a standard manner by bleeding patients to lower blood pressure to 50 mm. Hg for two hours, nor is treatment the same as that used in animals. In human beings, homologous rather than heterologous blood is used, and electrolyte solution in large quantities is usually administered, which results in significant hemodilution. In addition, most human patients have suffered operative or accidental trauma to the trunk and have the changes in respiratory pattern consequent to such injuries.

Following trunk injury, even without shock, an intrapulmonary shunt develops due to areas of microatelectasis and the patient's failure to turn or take deep breaths (see p. 249). Injuries to the extremities can lead to fat embolism, which has been indicated by some as the primary cause of shock lung.

It is apparrent that the great variability in the clinical appearance of the human shock lung syndrome can be related to the effects of the injuries which caused hypovolemia. Another factor in this varied picture is the number of methods used to restore circulatory volume. If large quantities of balanced salt solution or Ringer's lactate are used, the hemodilution will lower the oncotic pressure of proteins and lead to loss of fluid into the lungs. On the other hand, the administration of large quantities of homologous blood, particularly if matching is poor, is known to result in many of the clinical and pathological changes seen in the shock lung. In fact, one of the most precise models of the human "shock lung" is the postoperative "artificial perfusion lung," a syndrome which many investigators think can be alleviated by the use of hemodilution rather than large quantities of homologous blood to prime the pump.

In contrast to the experimental animals, which have a low cardiac output after replacement of shed blood, human patients develop a higher than normal cardiac output in the postresuscitation period. It is during this postresuscitation period of high cardiac output that the shock lung develops.

In human lungs, in addition to the picture described in animal lungs, there are often evidences of transudation of fluid in the dependent portion of the lung despite low central venous and left heart pressures. Transudation of fluid with associated hypoxia, high cardiac output, moderate pulmonary hypertension, and low left heart pressure produce a clinical picture similar to that seen in the acute pulmonary edema developed by some individuals going to high altitudes. Because of the severe nature of this illness, few good studies of the pulmonary circulatory dynamics of the high-output period have been made, so its significance is not clear. It is intriguing to speculate that the mechanism of development of fluid transudation into the lungs may be similar to that of mountain sickness.

In the experimental animal the model is pure, and the changes in the lung appear to be due to the changes in circulatory dynamics. If the lung is excluded from the circulation and rendered entirely ischemic during the period of shock, the changes are not seen. Experiments in our laboratories also show that when the pulmonary flow is maintained by artificial perfusion during the period of shock, no changes are found in the lungs. These experiments seem to exclude either ischemia or a toxin as the causative agent, so even in the simple laboratory model there is much to be learned about the nature of the injuring agent.

In the human being the problems of identification of etiology are compounded. All human victims of shock have severe associated trauma or disease. With present modes of therapy, all receive massive amounts of homologous blood and electrolyte solutions. In many of the Vietnam war casualties, resuscitation is first carried out with electrolyte solution while typing and cross-matching are accomplished. These casualties may have dilution of the hematocrit to less than 20% for a period of time. Of those reported, many are the victims of injuries by land mines which result in loss of both lower extremities and in which some blast injury is likely. All have significant injury to the trunk. Some of these patients may have had greater quantities of fluid than were absolutely essential, though they did not evidence a rise in venous pressure. In animals, quantities of fluid of the order of magnitude of those given to resuscitate some of these patients can result in marked transudation of fluid in the lungs. This complication of fluid therapy has been seen in patients as the result of overenthusiasm for the use of fluids during extensive operative procedures. The clinical picture is one of pulmonary edema, not that seen with the shock lung. It seems unlikely that overzealous use of fluids is the primary causative factor of the shock lung syndrome, although this undoubtedly can complicate the condition further.

Many of these patients receive gases containing very high concentrations of oxygen, in the range of 70 to 100%. Many of the pathological changes described in the lungs can result from the administration of high concentrations of oxygen (see pp. 299–300). Finally, in some patients, particularly those in the older age group or those suffering extensive trauma, evidence appears of cardiac failure with low blood pressure and high venous pressure.

PULMONARY MECHANICS

Pathological changes such as those seen in patients or animals with the shock lung syndrome would be expected to be associated with changes in lung mechanics. Few careful studies of lung mechanics have been made in shocked animals, and virtually none in human beings. The results of the few studies compiled have shown a slight rise in lung compliance during the shock period, followed by a fall after reinfusion of shed fluid. If additional balanced salt solution is given, a further fall in compliance may result. The changes shown in compliance are much less than would be predicted from the pathological changes in the lungs. This discrepancy is most likely the result of the method of measurement used in the studies to date.

Areas of lung may become collapsed and completely nonaerated by the tidal volume, which is distributed only to the intact alveoli. These intact areas of lung have a near-normal compliance (see Fig. 12-5). Only on deep inflation is it apparent that the small change in slope is not indicative of the amount of lung that is ventilated or that can be expanded at normal transpulmonary pressures. In most of the studies of lung mechanics, the compliance is measured by relating the difference between end-inspiratory and end-expiratory pressures to tidal volume.

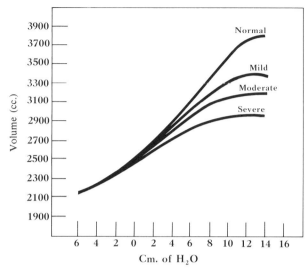

Fig. 12-5. The theoretical comparative effects of loss of volume and fall in compliance in shock lung. Each curve represents a volume-pressure curve for a degree of severity of the shock lung syndrome. The slope of the midpoint, around 2,500 cc. residual volume, is not markedly changed. However, on full inflation there is a significant change in compliance, and the flat portion of the curve is reached at a lower volume.

This method measures compliance only on a small portion of the straight segment of the curve, and it does not identify the fact that this portion is foreshortened. That there is a low arterial pO_2 supports the contention that some areas of lung are completely collapsed, despite the small change in compliance.

Studies have also shown an increase in resistance of the lungs in shock. This increase in resistance could be the result of ventilation of fewer portions of the lung, retention of secretions, airway constriction, or edema of the small airways. To date, studies of resistive changes in patients with shock lung are so few that no differentiation between the possible causes can be made. Some patients with the shock lung syndrome manifest evidence of acute, severe change in respiratory mechanics. They have wheezes and rhonchi throughout the chest as well as severe retraction, and there is much evidence of an acute rise in required inflation pressures. If the patients are being ventilated by the anesthetist, it is apparent that greatly increased pressures are required to inflate the lungs. These patients usually die in a very short period of time. In other patients, as the syndrome progresses, the effort required to breathe steadily increases. If the patients are being ventilated with a respirator, the inflation pressure must be steadily increased to maintain an adequate tidal volume. These clinical observations are the principal available observations of changes in lung mechanics in these patients. The changes in inflation pressure are probably the result of both decrease in compliance and increase in airway resistance.

Since patients in shock must hyperventilate in order to lower the arterial pCO_2 in an attempt to compensate for the severe metabolic acidosis, respiratory work per breath and per liter is increased. If the mechanical changes are present also, the work is increased both by the hyperventilation and the mechanical changes. The persistent hyperventilation after the restoration of circulatory dynamics and with the development of intrapulmonary shunting and low arterial pO_2 keeps the energy cost of breathing at very high levels.

TREATMENT

In the human shock lung syndrome, therapy or prevention requires consideration of (1) the damage to the lung that can occur as a result of hypovolemic shock, (2) the effects on lung function of the fluids and blood used for resuscitation, (3) the consequences to respiratory mechanisms of the trauma causing shock, (4) deleterious effects of administration of gases with high oxygen concentration, (5) the ability of the patient to perform the added work required to hyperventilate mechanically disrupted lungs, (6) the cardiac reserve of the patient, and (7) the effect of the pattern of ventilation on the preservation of lung function. Like all diseases, the best treatment of this syndrome is prevention, but the obvious goal of preventing shock is unlikely in our complex, mechanized society. Unfortunately, prevention or prompt treatment to decrease the incidence or severity of the syndrome, once shock develops, depends on an understanding of the etiology, a goal still of the future. Since it is likely that the full-blown shock lung syndrome has multiple etiologies, treatment designed with the seven points above in mind may decrease the incidence and severity of the injury to the lung. Prompt and effective resuscitation to shorten the period of hypovolemic shock is obviously the most important preventive and therapeutic measure. The likelihood of developing the shock lung syndrome seems directly related to the severity and duration of shock.

With the addition of electrolyte solutions to the treatment regime of patients in severe shock—typically, the infusion of four to six liters of balanced salt—there has been a great improvement in recovery, and problems with renal function have become rare. Unfortunately, the concepts of the originators of this form of therapy have been abused, and excessive amounts of fluid are often administered. Severe hemodilution will inevitably result in loss of fluid from the vascular volume. Fluids containing no colloids are distributed one-fourth in the vascular bed and three-fourths in the extravascular space. Excessive use of noncolloidal solutions can only result in transudation of fluids into all tissues, including the lung.

On first inspection, measurement of blood volume would seem to be an effective means of determining whether therapy has been effective. Further study shows that even in the normal subject, the variation of blood volume is so great that therapy cannot be based on restoring volume to a statistically normal level. Even if the individual's volume was known before injury, restoration to preinjury levels may also be inadequate, since venous pooling often occurs after injury. The same may be the case if cardiac output can be determined; the normal range is great, and much evidence is available that recovery from injury is dependent on an increased cardiac output.

Some studies of shock patients have suggested that changes in central venous pressure do not reflect changes in left atrial pressure. When central venous pressure is normal, left atrial pressure may be elevated. Pulmonary artery pressure has been advocated as a better measure of the changes in left atrial pressure. In fact, except in investigative shock units, such measurements are impractical, and, in any case, may dangerously delay therapy.

The best criteria for adequate fluid replacement remain systemic blood pressure, central venous pressure, clinical assessment of peripheral perfusion, and the adequacy of urine output. In resuscitation of previously normotensive patients, restoration of blood systolic pressure to between 95 and 100 mm. Hg seems adequate. Attempts to raise it above these levels result in the administration of excessive amounts of fluid. A combination of Ringer's lactate or balanced salt solution and homologous blood seem to be the most effective agents for restoring vascular volume. Mannitol should be given after volume replacement if urine output is depressed.

Many of these patients have severe metabolic acidosis, which should be treated by the administration of sodium bicarbonate. Correction need not be complete, as restoration of adequate circulation will lead to reduction of lactacidemia and endogenous correction. Excessive amounts of alkali can result in a late alkalosis of serious degree.

In summary, it should be emphasized that resuscitation of patients with hypovolemic shock depends on prompt, effective replacement of blood volume. Failure to adequately replace volume is more dangerous than some hyperexpansion. However, this principle does not justify complete disregard of what are reasonable quantities of administered fluids.

During and following the period of resuscitation, careful attention should be paid to tracheal toilet. The patient's position should be changed from the usual supine posture as soon as possible, and a regimen of regular turning should be instituted. If anesthesia is required, the lungs should be inflated to a large volume at frequent intervals during its administration. The concentration of inspired oxygen should not exceed a maximum of 50% except for short periods of time. Only enough oxygen should be added to the inspired mixture to maintain arterial pO_2 between 85 and 90 mm. Hg; it is not necessary or usually feasible to get it above this level.

The great effort involved in hyperventilating the mechanically deranged lungs and chest wall may exceed the ability of the injured patient to provide the added cardiac output and gas exchange necessary to do the added work. Such patients require intermittent positive-pressure ventilation. The maintenance of an end-expiratory pressure as much as 10 to 20 cm. H_2O above atmospheric, while using a volume-cycled respirator that can deliver an adequate tidal volume at the increased pressures required, has been shown to stop progression of the shock lung syndrome.

This clinical finding suggests one etiology of the progression of the disease. If, as has been postulated, during voluntary ventilation the muscles of the chest wall are completely relaxed at end-expiratory volume, a fall in lung compliance results in a decrease in the end-expiratory intrapulmonary volume. The fall in compliance and end-expiratory volume results in an increase in the number of alveoli reaching the critical volume at which they collapse. This phenomenon is that seen on pathological study of lungs in which on release of inflation pressure, areas of alveoli collapse and cannot be reexpanded except with greatly increased inflation pressure. (The theoretical basis for the loss of lung volume with fall in compliance is presented in Chapter 13, pp. 294–296.)

Once alveoli have become airless as a result of inadequate inflation pressure, it may require pressures as high as 50 to 70 cm. H_2O to reexpand them. Studies must be made to see if such vigorous inflation efforts can correct severe shock lung syndrome. In any event, the treatment of this serious complication of shock requires skillful coordination of restoration of circulatory dynamics with support of the respiratory system.

13. RESPIRATORS

THE lethal nature of an open chest wound and the importance of its prompt closure were recognized in ancient times. Vesalius is the first physiologist known to have used positive pressure to inflate the lungs. In 1543 he bilaterally incised the pleura in rabbits and noted the collapse of the lungs and cessation of the heartbeat. By breathing through a reed inserted into the trachea he restored life to the rabbits. The full significance of this work was not recognized until after the first quarter of the twentieth century. In 1924 Bunnell was the first surgeon to give positive-pressure anesthesia through an endotracheal tube, though Meltzer had insufflated anesthetic gases through a rubber tube 15 years earlier. Before this, the surgical profession had gone through the cumbersome period of the negative-pressure operating rooms designed by Sauerbruch and Meyer.

In retrospect it seems surprising that it took so long to recognize that positive-pressure insufflation of air into the lungs is the normal method of inflating the lungs. It is not the "negative" pressure in the pleura that pulls air into the lungs but the fact that the pressure at the mouth is greater than that in the pleura. In Sauerbruch's room or the Drinker-type respirator, the relative increase in pressure at the airway opening is achieved by decreasing the atmospheric pressure around the patient, a cumbersome way of increasing the relative airway pressure at the mouth. Such cumbersome methods of respiratory support have gone out of use in favor of intermittent positive pressure in the airway opening. This change in the technology of respiratory assistance was mandatory for the proper adaptation of respirators to surgical patients. Tank respirators were impractical for surgical patients and may be considered obsolete for all but those patients with permanent neuromuscular paralysis.

INDICATIONS FOR VENTILATORY SUPPORT

The treatment of acute respiratory insufficiency by employing intermittent positive-pressure respirators is now a commonly used therapeutic regimen. With increasing knowledge of the pathophysiology of respiratory disease, the indications for use of respirators and the management of patients requiring respiratory support assumes great importance in the treatment of postinjury, postoperative patients and patients with cardiac and pulmonary disease. While failure to use a respirator properly where it is indicated can lead to death of a patient, artificial support of respiration can lead to serious complications such as infection, tracheal stenosis, and convulsions, so that its promiscuous use can be dangerous.

Since the purpose of lung function is to supply adequate oxygen to the blood and to remove carbon dioxide from it, determinations of arterial pO_2 and pCO_2 are the critical laboratory procedures for measurement of the adequacy of gas exchange. Elevation of the arterial pCO_2 is a direct indication of inadequate ventilation. The inadequate ventilation may be due to central nervous system depression or to mechanical derangements of the lungs or chest wall which have escalated the work of ventilation to a level which is impossible for the patient to accomplish.

Depression of arterial pO_2 can result from ventilation-perfusion incoordination, intrapulmonary shunts, or diffusion defects as well as from central nervous system depression and mechanical derangements; therefore, arterial pO_2 can be depressed without elevation of arterial pCO_2. Unless inspired air has an increased concentration of oxygen, elevated arterial pCO_2 will always be associated with depressed arterial pO_2, since a ventilatory exchange that is insufficient to remove carbon dioxide will also be inadequate to supply oxygen.

CENTRAL NERVOUS SYSTEM NEUROMUSCULAR DYSFUNCTION

In patients with neurological dysfunction, artificial respiration is indicated when the central control mechanism fails to stimulate the respiratory muscles adequately or when paralysis or weakness prevents the muscles from providing adequate contraction to ventilate the lungs. Inadequacy of function is indicated by an elevated arterial pCO_2 and a depressed arterial pO_2. If arterial pCO_2 is elevated, respiratory support is indicated; if only arterial pO_2 is depressed, oxygen therapy is indicated.

Historically the early effective use of respirators to support ventilation was in patients with motor nerve paralysis as a consequence of poliomyelitis. These patients usually had normal lung and chest wall mechanics. Patients with dysfunction due to central nervous system depression resulting from drug overdosage or head injury also most often have normal lung and chest wall mechanics. (Parenthetically it should be emphasized that in patients suffering head injuries in association with injuries to the chest cage, the development of relative respiratory insufficiency with hypoxia or hypercarbia will add further insult to an already injured brain. Prompt cardiorespiratory resuscitation and support are among the specific treatments of head injury in patients with multiple injuries [Fig. 13-1].)

MECHANICAL DYSFUNCTION

The indications for use of artificial respiration in patients with mechanical dysfunction of the lungs and/or chest wall are complex, as is the proper operation of the ventilator. The general indications are elevation of arterial pCO_2 and clinical evidence that the effort needed to maintain ventilation is excessive. Mechanical dysfunction which increases respiratory muscle work can lead to fatigue just as can excessive work demands made on other muscle groups.

It is most difficult to assess the need for artificial ventilation in those patients with some cardiopulmonary limitations who are reasonably

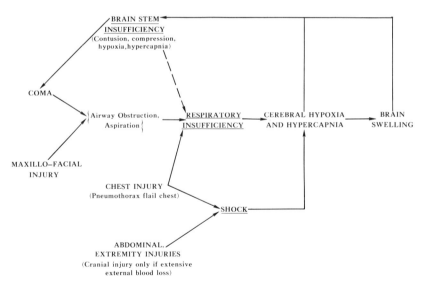

Fig. 13-1. Depicts interaction between the effects of trauma to the head, and injuries which cause shock and compromise pulmonary function. In many patients a traumatic injury to the brain from which complete recovery would be possible becomes irreversible when added insult is inflicted by cerebral hypoxia and hypercapnia resulting from respiratory insufficiency and shock.

well compensated until operation, injury, or acute medical illness makes excessive metabolic demands or acutely increases the work of breathing. Such patients fall in four general groups: (1) those with skeletal and chest wall abnormalities, (2) those with chronic lung disease, (3) those with heart disease, and (4) those with massive infection.

Operation, traumatic injury, or moderate infection can cause acute respiratory decompensation in patients with malfunction of the chest bellows because of skeletal or chest wall abnormalities. Examples of such persons are those with chest deformity, excessive obesity, or abdominal distension. The evolution of respiratory failure is not dramatic. These patients slowly accumulate carbon dioxide and develop progressive hypoxemia because of an inadequate ventilatory volume. An index of suspicion is important. To make the diagnosis, blood gas concentrations must be determined to confirm the presence or absence of respiratory insufficiency; if the arterial pCO_2 is found to be elevated, respiratory assistance is indicated.

Patients with chronic lung disease may develop acute respiratory decompensation from a relatively mild pulmonary infection or from a traumatic injury. In these patients conservative treatment with bronchodilators, breathing exercises, etc., should be tried for minor infections or injuries. For severe infections, respiratory assistance is mandatory, because these patients are at the limit of their respiratory work ability prior to the damage created by infection. Elevation of arterial pCO_2 above 50 to 55 mm. Hg usually is an indication for respiratory assistance during the acute illness. An arterial pCO_2 below 50 to 55 mm. Hg is not an indication if there is no complicating acute injury or infection.

The use of respirators in postoperative cardiac patients has been a very important and lifesaving innovation. Many such patients with borderline cardiac reserve cannot support the effort of breathing without developing cardiac failure. If cardiac failure does develop, the lung mechanics deteriorate as pulmonary edema develops and ventilatory work rises, requiring an increase in work to exchange gas which in turn requires a higher cardiac output. If the cardiac output cannot be increased, metabolic acidosis results and the fall in pH stimulates respiration further, setting up a vicious cycle (Fig. 13-2). If respiratory assistance is provided at this point, respiratory work is diminished and the depressed cardiac output may be adequate when the muscular effort of breathing is no longer required. This can lead to correction of the metabolic acidosis and clearing of the pulmonary edema. The use of respirators should be as helpful in coronary infarction patients who develop shock or pulmonary edema as it is for the postcardiotomy patient.

In patients with overwhelming infections, metabolic rate is greatly

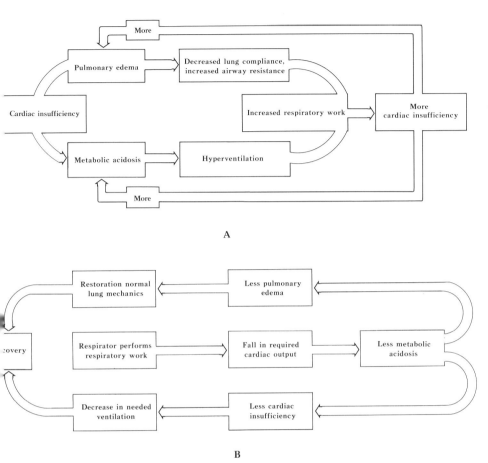

Fig. 13-2. (A) The cycle of deterioration in uncontrolled cardiac failure. (B) Interruption of the escalation of cardiac insufficiency by the use of artificial ventilation.

increased. Peritonitis, which elevates and fixes the diaphragms, and pneumonia, which reduces lung volume, compromise respiratory function; at the same time, these conditions increase the metabolic rate, requiring an increase in gas exchange. In these patients respiratory insufficiency may develop quickly, as manifested by a fall in arterial pO_2 and later by a rise in arterial pCO_2. A respirator can ventilate the inefficient lungs or chest bellows system without any muscular effort on the part of the patient. The respirator relieves the fatigued, toxic patient of the effort of breathing and permits the patient to survive until specific antibacterial therapy can arrest the infection.

The respiratory acidosis due to respiratory insufficiency and metabolic

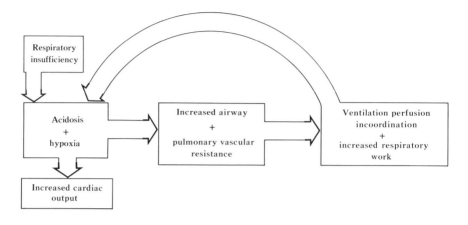

A

B

Fig..13-3. The manner in which respiratory insufficiency (A), metabolic acidosis (B), and mixed acidosis (C) can result in a feedback that, rather than being protective, is destructive. Treatment (D) with a ventilator and bicarbonate can interrupt this disruptive feedback.

acidosis which results from cardiac insufficiency cause increased demands on the cardiorespiratory system at a time when it cannot respond. The hypercapnia and hypoxia increase the demand for ventilation and also increase airway and pulmonary vascular resistance. The metabolic acidosis causes hyperventilation and decreases myocardial efficiency (see Fig. 13-3A, B). If mixed acidosis is present, the deleterious effects are

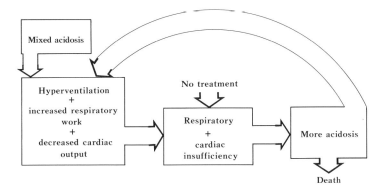

C

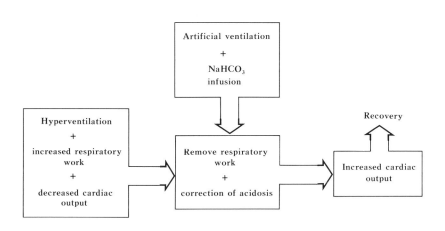

D

additive (see Fig. 13-3C). Treatment of the acidosis and artificial respiration (Fig. 13-3D) are often life saving and are commonly required in the immediate postoperative period after cardiac surgery.

TRAUMATIC INJURIES

Most serious injuries of the chest cage are complicated by pneumothorax, and it is imperative that this complication be treated with proper closed drainage. If an intermittent positive-pressure respirator is used without an effective means of evacuating air accumulated in the pleural cavity, a tension pneumothorax and collapse of the lungs are certain (see Complications of Artificial Ventilation, pp. 298–301).

Shortly after injury a patient with multiple rib fractures may evidence little respiratory distress and little paradoxical motion of the chest cage once the pneumohemothorax is evacuated by closed chest drainage. Over the course of hours, as edema stiffens the traumatized lung and failure to cough up secretions leads to blockage of the bronchi, the lung becomes increasingly difficult to ventilate, requiring greater force and thus greater swings in pleural pressure to exchange the tidal air. The greater pressure swings increase the paradoxical motion of the chest wall. After simple observation of the patient, it is usually apparent that the patient is suffering fatigue, and arterial blood gas analyses may show evidence of elevation in pCO_2 and depression of pO_2. If such a patient appears to be doing excessive work to breathe, the respirator should be employed even though the arterial pCO_2 is not elevated. In patients with multiple fractured ribs and paradoxical respiration, positive-pressure respiration splints the chest as balanced traction splints other fractures while continued spontaneous respiration may be likened to walking on a broken leg.

Some injured patients may suffer compromise in lung function as a result of the posttraumatic lung syndrome. The escalating alveolar–arterial oxygen differences these patients develop is due to a progressive microatelectasis. Ventilatory support is essential to halt the progressive collapse of alveoli. Special consideration of this problem is detailed in the section on special problems in artificial ventilation.

In summary, artificial ventilation is indicated for inadequate ventilation due to neuromuscular disease or to deranged lung and chest wall mechanics, or when deranged lung and chest wall mechanics require a level of respiratory work the patient cannot maintain. The chemical indexes of such decompensation are elevated arterial pCO_2 and depressed arterial pO_2.

RESPIRATORS

TYPES OF RESPIRATORS

Respirators inflate a patient's lung by creating a higher pressure at the entrance of the airway than is present in the alveoli. In the Drinker tank respirator this is accomplished by lowering the pressure about the patient's body below ambient atmospheric pressure, i.e., to 735 mm. Hg, while in the positive-pressure ventilator this is accomplished by raising the pressure at the mouth above atmospheric pressure, i.e., to 785 mm. Hg. With both types of respirator the higher pressure at the mouth than on the surface of the body exerts a force on the system which drives air through the resistance system, the airways, and into the lungs, stretching the lungs and chest wall until at end-inspiration the pressure difference between mouth and body surface is equal to the recoil force of the stretched lungs and chest wall. When the valve opens to release the pressure at the start of expiration, the potential energy stored in the stretched lungs and chest wall provides the force for exhaling.

In patients with neurological disorders in whom respiratory mechanics are normal, peak pressures across the system of 20 cm. H_2O are adequate for ventilation and any type of ventilator can be made to function adequately. This is not the case in patients with abnormal pulmonary or chest wall mechanics. In these patients high inspiratory pressures may be needed to inflate the lungs, and care must be taken to assure that the recoil force is adequate to deflate the lungs.

The simplest problem in artificial respiration is to provide ventilation for a patient with complete apnea because of neuromuscular depression but with normal airways, lungs, and thorax. The most difficult problem is to provide adequate ventilation for a patient with spontaneous but inadequate breathing who also has serious abnormalities in distribution of inspired gas and pulmonary capillary blood flow, impaired alveolar capillary diffusion, or mechanical restrictions to breathing in or out.*

Ventilators were originally used for the treatment of patients with respiratory insufficiency due to neuromuscular dysfunction, such as is found in poliomyelitis, and the design criteria were those suitable for such patients; these respirators are inadequate for use in patients with mechanical derangements of lung and chest wall. To create high pressures the bellows of these tank-type respirators must be very large, and the need to maintain a closed tank prevents adequate care of the patient. For acutely ill, traumatized, and postoperative patients the tank-type respirators are no longer used. The ventilators that are commonly used are of two types, pressure-controlled and volume-controlled respirators.

Pressure-Controlled Respirators. These respirators are driven by an air or oxygen source, and a peak pressure is set by a valving mechanism. Gas is forced into the patient's lungs until this peak pressure is reached, when the expiratory valve opens and the inspiratory valve closes. The amount of air forced into the patient is a function of the forces opposing the applied pressure.

Volume-Controlled Respirators. In this type of respirator air is pumped into the patient with a piston pump. The amount of gas forced into the patient is determined by setting the stroke volume of the piston,

*J. H. Comroe, Jr., "Respiratory Gas Exchange." In J. L. Whittenberger (Ed.), *Artificial Respiration.* New York: Hoeber Med. Div., Harper & Row, 1962. P. 11.

and the resultant peak pressure is dependent on the mechanical properties of the lungs and chest wall.

PRINCIPLES OF OPERATION

To make an intelligent choice of the type of respirator needed, it is essential to know what determines the ventilatory requirements of the
patient and how these requirements can be met with an artificial ventilator. The gas exchange requirements of the patient are determined by
his metabolic rate, which can be altered by disease, fever, etc. Since only
the air that reaches the alveoli can exchange gas with blood, the patient's
alveolar ventilation will determine the amount of gas available for exchange. The needed tidal volume, therefore, is affected by the amount
of dead space in the patient's airways and in the valves and tubing of
the ventilator. Because all patients on ventilators have an endotracheal
tube or tracheostomy tube inserted, the patient's airway dead space is
small. However, the respirator dead space may be large and must be included in the dead space calculation. To help in determining the ventilatory requirements, a number of nomograms have been made up which
are useful in estimating basal tidal volume and rate if dead space is
normal. To all these nomograms must be added any dead space inherent
in the ventilator which is being used.

After an initial determination of a patient's ventilatory requirements
has been made, several further factors must be considered. Since all
ventilators have some leaks in their valving mechanism, the volume
setting of the ventilator cannot be trusted; therefore, some other means
of monitoring tidal volume is necessary. The most satisfactory method
is to measure expired volume with a gas meter or spirometer. Even if
the tidal volume is measured accurately and appears to be adequate, abnormalities of ventilation and perfusion or a high metabolic rate could
make the calculated alveolar ventilation inadequate. For this reason it
is imperative to measure the arterial blood gases frequently during the
early stages of ventilatory support until the patient is stabilized. Throughout treatment arterial blood gases should be measured at regular intervals, usually at least once a day. When the arterial pCO_2 is elevated,
alveolar ventilation should be increased; when it is depressed, alveolar
ventilation should be decreased, either by decreasing the tidal volume
and/or rate or by increasing the respirator dead space. If the arterial
pO_2 is depressed when arterial pCO_2 is normal or decreased, up to 50%
oxygen should be used as the ventilatory gas mixture to raise the arterial
pO_2 to 90 to 110 mm. Hg but not above. Increased concentrations of
oxygen can correct an arterial pO_2 which is low due to ventilation-perfusion incoordination, but they will not correct the low arterial pO_2 found

in the postoperative patient with microatelectasis or in the patient with posttraumatic lung syndrome.

The use of respirators would be relatively simple if the only requirements for their proper use were the provision of an adequate tidal volume and rate and the appropriate concentration of oxygen in the inspired air. Just as the respiratory center of the spontaneously breathing subject uses information about the blood gases and proprioceptive and other neural information about the integrity of the cardiorespiratory apparatus, so the physician using an artificial ventilator must use all the information available. In particular, the physician must consider the mechanical abnormalities of the lung and chest wall and the effects of intrapleural pressure changes on cardiac function and bronchial air flow.

In operating a respirator, a tidal volume and rate are chosen which will achieve the desired minute alveolar ventilation. The amount of force or pressure that must be developed by the respirator to force the tidal volume into the patient depends on the resistance of the airways and tubing and the stiffness of the lungs and chest wall. If the lungs and/

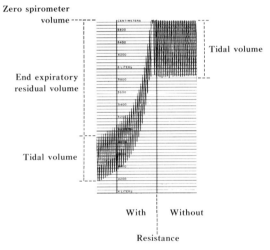

Fig. 13-4. Spirometer kymograph tracing of a mechanical analog of the lungs to illustrate the effect of increased resistance on functional residual volume. When elastic recoil is inadequate to expel all the air in the time available for expiration, air accumulates in the spirometer equivalent to the accumulation of air in the lungs when the elastic recoil of lungs and chest wall is inadequate. The right side of the tracing shows no added resistance. Tidal volume is 900 cc. and there is no air left in the spirometer at the end of the expiratory phase. On the left, after resistance is added, the end-expiratory residual volume progressively rises until recoil force (pressure) is high enough to overcome the added resistance. At equilibrium, tidal volume has fallen to 750 cc. and end-expiratory volume has risen to 1,850 cc. (From R. M. Peters and P. Hutchin, Adequacy of available respirators. *Ann. Thorac. Surg.* 3:421, 1967.)

or chest wall are stiff, the force required to stretch them is increased and the potential elastic energy stored in lungs and chest wall for expelling the air is increased. If the airway resistance is increased, both the inspiratory and expiratory force necessary to drive air past this resistance must rise (transairway pressure increase) or the time over which the force acts must be prolonged. The inspiratory pressure can be raised in a pressure-operated respirator by resetting the pressure control. In a volume-operated respirator the inspiratory pressure increases automatically in response to increased resistance. The maximum expiratory force or pressure is dependent on the amount of stretch imparted to the lungs and chest wall during inspiration. If this pressure is inadequate to force all the air pumped in during inspiration out during the expiratory phase of the cycle, some of the inspired air will remain in the lung (Fig. 13-4). Air will continue to accumulate in the lungs until the lungs and chest wall are stretched enough to provide an adequate recoil force to expel the inspired tidal volume.

At a given tidal volume the amount of added functional residual volume needed to provide the force for a system with a given compliance and resistance can be expressed by the following equation:

$$V_E^N = (V_E^O + \Delta V) \left(\frac{1}{e^{t/RC} - 1} \right) + V_E^O$$

where V_E^N = new functional residual capacity (FRC)
 V_E^O = original FRC
 ΔV = tidal volume
 t = time of expiration
 R = resistance
 C = compliance

This equation provides an answer for a means of limiting the increase in functional residual capacity needed to provide elastic recoil. This is to control the expiratory time. As t increases, t/RC gets larger and the fraction $1/(e^{t/RC} - 1)$ gets smaller, thus decreasing V_E^N. This can be shown in another manner by considering the pressure needed to expel the air. If the duration of expiration can be prolonged, then the same amount of air can be expelled with a lower pressure.

Since $$R = \frac{P}{F}$$ (1)

then, transposing, $$P = R \times F$$ (2)

and $$F = \frac{V}{t}$$ (3)

If a given tidal volume must be expelled by elastic recoil, the flow rate F will be less if the time t is prolonged. From Equation 2, if F is smaller, P will be smaller. In simple, practical terms, if the airway resistance is elevated, air trapping can be minimized by increasing the duration of expiration. For this reason it is important for a respirator to have a provision for changing the ratio of inspiratory time over expiratory time, so that when airway resistance is elevated, expiratory time can be increased.

If airway resistance is increased and lung compliance is normal or high, as in obstructive emphysema, positive intrapleural pressure will occur during expiration. Despite the more compliant lungs, inflation pressure is elevated to overcome resistance to airflow during inspiration and remains up during expiration because end-tidal volume must be raised to provide the elastic recoil necessary to force air through the narrowed airways. This combination of high lung compliance and high airway resistance can lead to progressive inflation of the lungs and chest wall. Chest wall and lung hyperinflation are not the only deleterious effects of increase in intrathoracic pressure. Elevation of intrapleural pressure associated with hyperinflation can limit venous return to the right heart.

Even without increase in lung volume or airway resistance, if the chest cage is deformed or if the patient is excessively obese, a greater force is required to expand the chest cage or lift the dead weight of fat. To achieve this greater force, the respirator must create a higher positive pleural pressure during inspiration. The increase in pleural pressure raises the pressure in the right atrium and the intrathoracic portion of the great veins and thus decreases filling of the right heart and in turn decreases cardiac output.

The amount of decrease in filling depends on the height to which pleural pressure must be raised, the time that the pressure is maintained above atmospheric, and the venous pressure. The pressure rises above atmospheric during inspiration and falls below it during expiration if lung mechanics are normal. If the expiratory phase of respiration is equal to the inspiratory phase in an individual with normal lung and chest wall mechanics, cardiac output will not be seriously compromised by the positive intrapleural pressure that occurs during inspiration. However, in a patient with a diminished blood volume and low venous pressure, positive intrapleural inflation pressure can dangerously diminish venous return.

For patients on a ventilator who may have compromised chest wall bellows it is imperative to measure central venous pressure and to raise it if necessary by expanding the blood volume enough to insure adequate right heart filling. When the portion of the cycle devoted to expiration is lengthened, the mean intrapleural pressure during the cycle is lowered, just as it is when expiratory time is increased to lessen air trapping when the airway resistance is elevated. The long expiratory period allows filling of the atrium without marked elevation in venous pressure.

A special type of chest wall abnormality that affects artificial respiration is created by widely opening the pleura, as is done in thoracotomy; this removes the elastic force of the chest wall as a factor in ventilation. When the chest is opened, the danger of shutting off venous return as a result of positive intrapleural pressure no longer exists. During inflation, the ventilator must overcome only the elastic recoil of the lungs; however, during exhalation, only the elastic recoil of the lungs is available to force air out. Since when the chest is closed the lungs are held partially inflated by the outward recoil of the chest wall, the end-expiratory volume of the lungs is larger than when the chest is opened. The fall in the functional residual capacity of the lungs when the chest is open leads to progressive collapse of alveoli with an associated fall in arterial pO_2 as an increasing intrapulmonary shunt develops. This collapse can be prevented if the lungs are periodically inflated or if the end-expiratory airway pressure is maintained about 4 to 5 cm. H_2O above atmospheric.

The phenomenon of progressive collapse of a lung which can occur when the chest is widely opened also develops if the compliance of the lungs decreases. At the end of expiration there is virtually complete relaxation of all respiratory muscles, so the end-expiratory volume is determined by the opposing outward elastic recoil of the chest wall and inward recoil of the lungs. If the lung becomes stiffer, the inward elastic recoil of the lung will increase and exert a greater force to pull in the chest wall, thus decreasing the end-expiratory volume. The decrease in end-expiratory volume permits progressive collapse of alveoli and further fall in lung compliance. This fall can be prevented by raising the pressure at the airway exit to balance the effect of the decreased lung compliance. The needed increase in pressure can be expressed by the following equation:

$$\Delta P_A = \frac{1}{C_L{}^2} \left(\frac{V_E{}^0}{C_W} - D \right) \Delta C_L$$

where $V_E{}^0 =$ original functional residual volume
               $\Delta P_A =$ end-expiratory mouth pressure
               $C_L =$ lung compliance
               $C_W =$ chest wall compliance
               $D =$ anatomical dead space
             $\Delta C_L =$ change in lung compliance

This added pressure can be provided by imposing an artificial expiratory resistance which requires greater recoil force to expel the air. This resistance causes the functional residual volume to rise to normal levels, as the lungs must be stretched more to provide adequate recoil force to expel the air against the added resistance. The added end-expiratory pressure also can be provided by putting a water trap on the expiratory egress tube.

The important prediction of the above equation is that if compliance is falling and end-expiratory pressure is not raised, an escalation of the pressure to maintain lung volume will be needed or a fast progression of collapse will result (Fig. 13-5). If these conditions have occurred, forceful inspirations using up to 70 cm. H_2O pressure may be required to reopen enough of the collapsed alveoli to reduce the intrapulmonary shunt and provide adequate levels of arterial pO_2.

This dangerous, progressive fall in compliance can begin for several reasons. It is probable that during spontaneous respiration there never

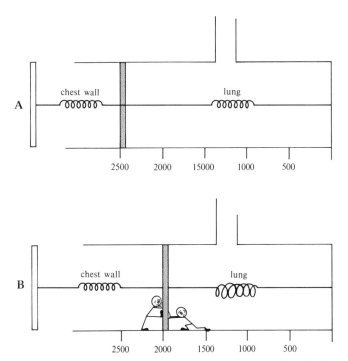

Fig. 13-5. (A) The end-expiratory lung volume (functional residual volume) is determined by the balance of forces exerted by the elasticity of the lung and the chest wall (*springs*). (B) The lung has become less compliant, increasing its elastic recoil so that the end-expiratory lung volume is decreased (*larger spring*). If there is spasm of the chest wall muscles, the volume is less (*man on chest wall side of piston*). If the end-expiratory pressure is above the atmospheric pressure, the end-expiratory volume is larger (*man on lung side of piston*).

is complete relaxation of the chest wall musculature, since chest wall compliance of a normal individual who has been given muscle relaxant is much less than that of an untreated patient. During artificial respiration, patients who have been given muscle relaxants develop findings of increased shunt and lung collapse, presumably due to increased chest wall compliance which has the same effect as decreased lung compliance in lowering the end-expiratory lung volume. Even in a normal individual progressive fall in lung compliance can be initiated if there is failure to take periodic deep breaths to inflate all the alveoli and reactivate the surfactant. It is imperative, therefore, to have a means of periodically hyperinflating the lungs of a patient who is on a respirator. The respirator should have a mechanical yawn; when it does not, this occasional deep breath should be provided periodically by some other means. Another reason for loss of compliance when a patient is receiving artificial ventilation is the all-too-frequent failure to turn the patient; as pointed out in Chapter 5, this alone can lead to edema in the dependent lung with fall in compliance and alveolar collapse.

The phenomenon of progressive collapse described is also encountered in the shock lung, in which measures to increase expansion may also be needed. However, it must be remembered that the use of positive end-tidal pressures, increased expiratory resistance, or high inflation pressures can all cut down the venous return, particularly if the venous pressure is depressed due to hypovolemia. Therefore venous and arterial blood pressures should be carefully monitored.

Although increase in pleural pressure does decrease venous return and thus cardiac output, increases in airway and alveolar pressures do not seem to affect pulmonary blood flow unless the pressures reach extreme levels. In patients with decreased lung compliance it is safe to provide high inflation pressures and to maintain levels of end-expiratory pressure above atmospheric pressure, since the increased pressure is not transmitted to the pleural space and thus the great veins. However, if chest wall compliance is decreased due to injury, deformity, or obesity, the increased inflation pressure is transmitted to the pleural cavity and will diminish venous return. It is mandatory, therefore, to monitor venous and arterial pressure frequently, or continuously, if possible, when artificial ventilation is required to reverse the progressive collapse that results from decreased lung or chest wall compliance.

SPECIAL CONSIDERATIONS FOR INFANTS AND CHILDREN

Infants and children have small chest cavities, small airways, and small lungs. The small chest requires a greater pressure per unit of volume change than the adult chest. The pressure required to create a given tension in the chest wall increases as the radius of the chest decreases (La Place; see text p. 81 and Appendix p. 335). The lung has fewer compliance units, so it requires a greater force per unit of volume change. The smaller airways also have a higher resistance.

The tidal volumes of the infant and of the child are less than those of the adult. The relationship between tidal volume and lung mechanics is such that the pressures required to inflate an infant's or child's lungs are the same as those for an adult. Failure to remember that infants and children have a lower chest wall and lung compliance and higher airway resistance often results in the respirator's delivering an inadequate tidal volume because the pressure maxima of the respirator are set too low.

LIMITATIONS OF AVAILABLE RESPIRATORS

The quality of available respirators leaves much to be desired; their mechanical imperfections result in potentially dangerous complications. The pressure-driven respirators have the primary defects of uncertainty of volume delivered and inadequate maximum pressure for patients with severe derangements of lung mechanics. In addition, when these respirators are driven by oxygen as the pressure source, excessive concentrations of oxygen frequently occur, especially if the required inflation pressure is high. It is mandatory if this type of respirator is used that it be driven by a source of medical-grade, clean, oil-droplet-free compressed air, *not oxygen*. Also, a method of measuring the expired tidal volume is mandatory, since such measurement is the only way to be certain tidal exchange is adequate. The volume-cycled or piston respirators likewise are imperfect. Their particular weaknesses are the valving system and the leaks within the respirator. The valves all leak and can stick. If the expiratory valve sticks, the patient is unable to expire, and effective respiration is prevented. The leaks make it impossible to count on the volume settings of the respirator to indicate inspired volume. In addition, these respirators have large volumes of gas in their tubing and cylinders. When a high inflation pressure is required, this gas is compressed, and, when expired volume is measured with a gas meter, the measured expired volume can include the volume stored by compression of gas in the respirator. This results in a falsely high indicated inspired volume and measured expired volume.

An important mechanical property required of any type of respirator is an easy and effective way of setting the rate and the ratio of inspiratory to expiratory time. In pressure-cycled respirators the rate and ratio are in large part dependent on tidal volume and the pressure opposing the respirators. For this reason the settings can be difficult and will change if the force opposing the respirator changes. In many volume-cycled respirators the ratio between inspiratory and expiratory time is fixed, usually near a one-to-one ratio. This is a very serious shortcoming. Even on the better available volume-cycled respirators, the inspiration-expiration settings are not absolute; and the operator must count the respiratory rate and measure the ratio of the duration of inspiration to expiration.

A problem common to all ventilators is the danger of contamination. The difficulties of cleaning vary, but since in all ventilators there are humidifiers and the moisture content and air temperatures are high, dangerously high bacterial counts of gram-negative organisms, in particular *Pseudomonas*, frequently develop.

COMPLICATIONS OF ARTIFICIAL VENTILATION

INFECTION

While the respirator can be a source of infection, the more serious sources are the humidifiers and the patient attendants. A fetish has developed among many doctors that only if a mist can be seen emerging from the respirator is humidification adequate. Since water vapor is invisible, this mist is not evidence of high humidity, but rather is an iatrogenic smog usually heavily laden with bacteria. While dry, cold air does thicken secretions and irritate the airway when blown directly into it, the airway is no better off if a contaminated smog is blown into it.

Another source of infection is careless care of the airway by the attendants. A patient with an endotracheal or tracheostomy tube in place does not have the protection of the bacterial filters of the nose, mouth, and throat. It is imperative that great care be taken to prevent contamination of the lower airway. To insure this, sterile gloves should be worn by the attendant and a sterile catheter should be used each time the airway is suctioned. It is also advisable to change the connecting tubes to the respirator daily.

THE AIRWAY

Endotracheal or tracheostomy tubes placed for many days, particularly with an inflated balloon, can result in serious injury to the trachea. The constant pressure of the bag or impingement of the tube on the trachea ulcerates it and often results in chondritis. The first evidence of this complication occurs after removal of the tube, as healing and scarring result in tracheal stenosis. This complication can be minimized by not inflating the bag too tightly, by deflating the bag periodically, and by using soft tubes made of Silastic or rubber rather than metal. Another important safeguard is to use a flexible corrugated tube to connect the airway to the respirator. This tube acts as a shock absorber to diminish the force driving the airway against the tracheal wall.

Occasionally the constant driving pressure of the respirator can cause very rapid ulceration of the trachea and even injury to the carotid vessels, particularly if the tracheostomy stoma is too low in the neck. It is a good policy to use nasal or oral endotracheal tubes for at least the first 48 hours of ventilatory support and to do tracheostomies under the ideal conditions of the operating room.

A most immediately life-threatening complication during artificial ventilation is obstruction of the airway. The respirator usually can drive air past the obstruction, but the patient is unable to exhale. The offending substance is usually dried secretions, and often the tube must be removed to remove the obstruction. This complication can be suspected if the pressure in the respirator rises or if the patient's chest volume appears to be increasing.

PNEUMOTHORAX

If there is an air leak in the lung or airway due either to trauma or to rupture of a bleb, the positive pressure exerted by the respirator can quickly force air out through the leak, creating a tension pneumothorax. If during artificial ventilation any lung air leak is present, great care must be taken to be sure that closed chest drainage is instituted and functions properly. Should such a leak develop during artificial ventilation, the respirator pressure will rise and the chest will appear hyperinflated, just as when the airway is obstructed.

GASTRIC DILATATION

Sick patients who are being ventilated with a respirator often swallow excessive amounts of air, and they can develop acute gastric dilatation with attendant fall in blood pressure and upper abdominal distension and vomiting. If there is evidence of this, such as large gastric gas bubbles on chest x-ray or abdominal distension, continuous gastric suction is indicated. Often this complication is the result of stimulation of the swallowing reflex by a tube high in the trachea. Using a different shaped tube or repositioning the tube may stop the air swallowing.

OXYGEN TOXICITY

Many patients who require ventilatory support have diffusion blocks, ventilation-perfusion abnormalities, and intrapulmonary shunts. To correct the resultant hypoxemia, the concentration of oxygen in the inspired air mixture is raised. The inspired oxygen concentration should rarely be raised above 50 to 60%, and then only to bring a depressed pO_2 up to 110 mm. Hg. Inspired oxygen concentrations above 50%, a partial pressure of 350 to 400 mm. Hg, lead to the development of oxygen toxicity. This is a progressive syndrome characterized by capillary congestion and proliferation of diffuse fibrosis, edema, and thickening of the alveolar membranes. This progressive process is related to the absolute partial pressure of the inspired oxygen, the duration of the exposure, and perhaps the level of systemic arterial pO_2. If increased concentrations of oxygen are used, the arterial pO_2 should be checked at frequent intervals and only that concentration required to maintain an arterial pO_2 in the 90 to 100 mm. Hg range used. A level greater than this has no therapeutic value, since at this level the hemoglobin is fully saturated with oxygen and the use of higher concentrations risks the complication of oxygen toxicity.

Unfortunately the available respirators do not have foolproof, accurate ways of setting the inspired oxygen content. To protect the patient from excessive inspired oxygen concentrations, the inspired oxygen concentration should be measured with an oxygen meter at periodic intervals.

The great push in the middle 1960's for the development of hyperbaric chambers to treat patients with acute pulmonary problems, coronary occlusion, and peripheral vascular insufficiency has been cut short by the dire consequences of oxygen toxicity. In most types of pulmonary disease with severe hypoxemia and in congenital heart disease and severe hypoxemia the hypoxemia is the result of a left-to-right shunt. Without undue elevation of environmental pressure, the amount of dissolved oxygen that can be added to blood going to perfused and unventilated alveoli is insufficient to overcome the lack of oxygen in the shunted blood and so does not effectively increase the arterial oxygen saturation. It appears at this writing that all but the enthusiasts will limit the therapeutic use of hyperbaric oxygen to the treatment of anaerobic infections such as gas gangrene.

RESPIRATORY ALKALOSIS

One of the troublesome and sometimes dangerous complications of artificial ventilation is acute, severe alkalosis. To suppress the patient's own respiratory drive, some hyperventilation is necessary, lowering pCO_2 to about 35 mm. Hg. If hypoxia is also present, this may not completely suppress the patient's respiratory efforts. Severe respiratory alkalosis or excessive hyperventilation can lead to potassium shifts and ventricular arrhythmias such as tachycardia or fibrillation. These arrythmias are particularly likely to occur if potassium stores are low due to the use of diuretics or following use of a pump oxygenator with a dilute prime. The risk of arrhythmias is compounded further in patients who have been receiving digitalis. It is imperative that these patients receive potassium supplements and that the hyperventilation be corrected.

If patients with chronic hypercapnia and compensatory increase in serum bicarbonate are placed on a ventilator, the acute lowering of serum pCO_2 will cause an acute rise in serum pH. This rise in the pH of the fluids bathing the nervous system can cause twitching convulsions and unconsciousness.

Patients with chronic, borderline respiratory insufficiency and evidence of cor pulmonale are usually treated with digitalis, low-salt diets, and diuretics. When they are seen with respiratory decompensation and hypercapnia, the low-salt diet and diuretic medication have caused an associated metabolic alkalosis. If the patient is placed on a respirator, the increased ventilation lowers the pCO_2 acutely. In these patients the chloride has been depleted by prior excretion by the kidney and by the low-salt diet, and potassium stores have been depleted by the prior diuretic regime. The correction of hypercapnia with the respirator results in an acute rise of cerebrospinal and blood pH due to the high bicarbonate. This alkalosis can cause muscle twitching, hyperactivity, convulsions, and acute cardiac arrhythmias. In such patients the arterial pCO_2 should be lowered slowly and supplementary potassium and chloride should be administered to permit correction of the metabolic alkalosis.

RESPIRATORS AND DERANGED RESPIRATORY MECHANICS

The essential considerations which must be constantly kept in mind in the use of a respirator in patients with deranged respiratory mechanics are as listed below for easy review. Figure 13-6 shows the pressures at various sites in the respiratory system with various types of mechanical derangement.

1. Fall in lung compliance leads to increased stiffness of the lung and progressive collapse of alveoli. This commonly occurs in the posttraumatic lung syndrome, the postpump syndrome, and in postoperative patients. The lungs should be hyperinflated at frequent intervals, and if arterial pO_2 is falling, careful consideration should be given to the use of an expiratory retard to increase the end-expiratory pressure.

2. Increased airway resistance due to airway obstruction by secretions or bronchoconstriction requires greater pressures to inflate and deflate the lungs. The deflation pressure must be provided by the elastic recoil of the lungs and chest wall. If the resistance is high, all air pumped

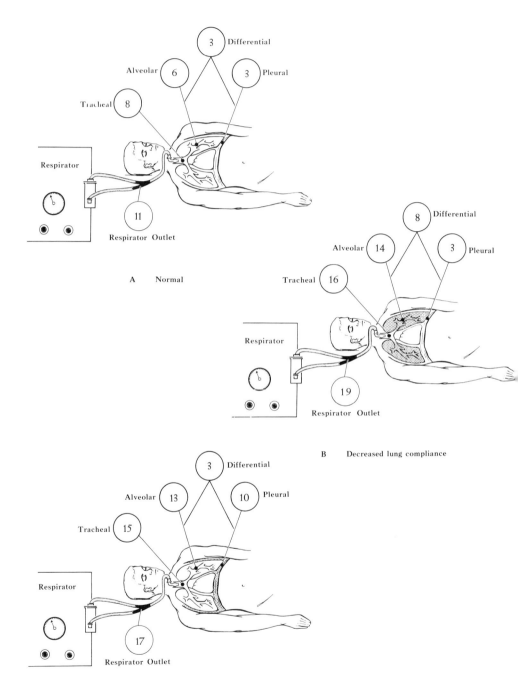

3 Differential

Alveolar 6

3 Pleural

Tracheal 8

Respirator

11

Respirator Outlet

A   Normal

8 Differential

Alveolar 14

3 Pleural

Tracheal 16

Respirator

19

Respirator Outlet

B   Decreased lung compliance

3 Differential

Alveolar 13

10 Pleural

Tracheal 15

Respirator

17

Respirator Outlet

C   Decreased chest wall compliance or obesity

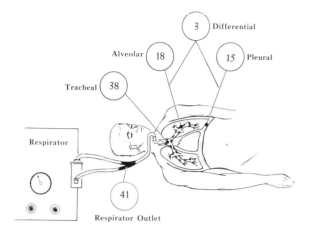

D   Increased resistance

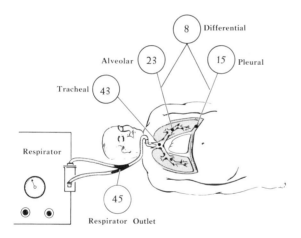

E   Obesity, increased resistance, decreased compliance
         of lungs and chest wall

Fig. 13-6. Pressures at various sites in the airways of patients receiving artificial ventilation illustrating the variations typical of different abnormalities.

in may not be expelled during the expiratory cycle, resulting in an increased end-expiratory lung volume. To minimize this increase in end-expiratory volume, the portion of the respiratory cycle devoted to expiration should be increased. The increase in pressure can result in high intrapleural pressure and lowering of venous return to the heart.

3. If the chest wall compliance is diminished due to limitation of

motion of the rib cage, obesity, or abdominal distension, increased pressures will be required to inflate the lungs. The increase in inflation pressure necessary to move a stiff chest wall will increase the intrapleural pressure and can result in decreased venous return to the heart.

4. During artificial ventilation with a respirator, expired tidal volume, inspired oxygen tension, arterial blood gas, central venous pressure, and systemic arterial pressure must be carefully monitored to assess the adequacy of ventilation and to assure that cardiac output is not being compromised.

14. PULMONARY TRANSPLANTATION

PETER HUTCHIN, M.D.

TRANSPLANTATION of normal organs to replace diseased ones has been an ancient preoccupation of mankind. Since the first experiments performed by surgeon Demikhov in Russia and by Juvenelle in this country, extensive experience with lung transplantation has been accumulated in the past fifteen to twenty years. In 1967 Trummer listed 192 papers dealing with the subject of lung transplantation. Although much insight has been gained into the physiological aspects of pulmonary transplantation, clinical application has been slow. Procurement and preservation of viable lung allografts, selection of patients for transplantation, and prevention of infection in the transplanted lung are major unsolved problems.

TECHNICAL CONSIDERATIONS

In preparation for transplantation of a lung, the recipient's own organ is excised by dividing sequentially the main-stem bronchus, the main pulmonary artery, and the pulmonary veins inside the pericardium. The donor is heparinized prior to removal of his lung to prevent intravascular clotting during performance of the three anastomoses. The donor lung is then removed, leaving a cuff of the left atrium around the opening of the pulmonary veins for subsequent anastomosis to the recipient's left atrium. The bronchus of the donor lung should be divided near its bifurcation, in the case of the left lung, or near the right upper lobe takeoff, in the case of the right lung, to prevent ischemic necrosis of the transplanted main-stem bronchus. In the dog, right lung transplantation is more difficult than left lung transplantation because of the high origin

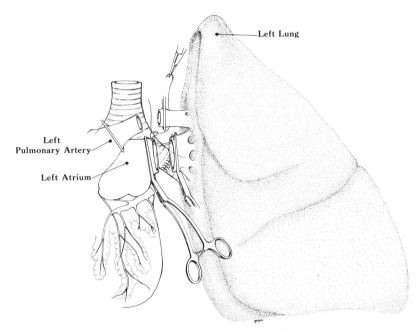

Fig. 14-1. Technique of left lung transplantation. End-to-end anastomosis of distal main-stem bronchus, pulmonary artery, and left atrial cuff is shown. No attempt is made to restore continuity of bronchial arteries and lymphatics. The bronchial anastomosis is performed close to the bifurcation of the left main stem bronchus to prevent ischemic necrosis of the transplanted bronchus. Everting sutures of 4-0 or 3-0 Dacron are used to perform the left atrial anastomosis. This technique results in good intima-to-intima approximation and eliminates raw edges which might predispose to thrombosis of the venous suture line. The pulmonary artery anastomosis may be performed with interrupted or continuous 5-0 or 6-0 sutures. A vein patch across the pulmonary artery anastomosis may be added to ensure a widely patent lumen without constriction.

of the right upper lobe bronchus. During transection of the bronchus, no clamping is done on the lung side of the donor in order to prevent obstruction of the pulmonary lymphatics by ligatures. Prior to implantation of the lung, irrigation of the excised organ may be done through the pulmonary artery using cold Ringer's lactate or some other solution to remove blood and to cool the pulmonary parenchyma.

The transplantation procedure in the left lung is carried out as follows (Fig. 14-1). First the cuff of the left atrium is anastomosed to the recipient's left atrium. Meticulous technique must be used to suture the left atrial cuff to the recipient's left atrium, carefully everting the suture line and preventing obstruction of the pulmonary veins draining the transplant. Elimination of all raw surfaces is of extreme importance to prevent thrombus formation at the suture line in the immediate postoperative period. Venous suture line thrombus formation cannot be readily prevented with heparinization. Should pulmonary venous thrombosis occur, hemorrhagic infarction of the transplanted lung will develop, resulting in death of the recipient. The atrial anastomosis is followed by an end-to-end anastomosis of the pulmonary artery and the bronchus. Continuous or interrupted sutures of 3-0 or 4-0 silk or polyester fiber may be used to reestablish the vascular and bronchial connections. No effort is made to restore continuity of the bronchial arteries and lymphatics.

For reimplantation of the lung, a similar procedure is followed. After the lung has been removed, it is sutured back in its position orthotopically. For lobar transplantation, an anastomosis is made at the level of the lobar bronchus, artery, and vein. In experimental lobar transplantation the remaining lobe or lobes on the side of operation may be removed to facilitate performance of postoperative pulmonary function studies. The venous anastomosis may be conveniently performed between the lobar vein and the left atrium. Antibiotics should be given routinely and continued for several days postoperatively to minimize the occurrence of infection in the transplanted or reimplanted lung.

Operative complications relate to the three suture lines. Bronchial necrosis is not a problem if bronchial arterial blood supply to the main-stem bronchus of the recipient is not interfered with and if the donor's main-stem bronchus is made as short as possible. In the absence of venous suture line complications, pulmonary edema is not a problem if the divided lymphatics are allowed to drain into the pleural space. This drainage is usually minimal and does not require prolonged postoperative chest tube drainage. Circumferential narrowing of the pulmonary artery is a late complication which may result in elevation of pulmonary artery pressure proximal to the anastomosis. It is seen less often when interrupted rather than continuous sutures are used in the construction of this anastomosis. A vein patch sutured across the pulmonary artery anastomosis will minimize the occurrence of this complication.

PULMONARY FUNCTION OF THE REIMPLANTED LUNG

The functional competence of the implanted lung can be best judged from experiments in which the autologous lung is removed and reimplanted. The observed changes in pulmonary function are primarily due to pulmonary denervation, which is a necessary consequence of the operative procedure. Division of lymphatics and bronchial arteries has relatively little effect on pulmonary function. Most of the available information has been obtained from experiments with dogs.

Immediately after operation, ventilation, oxygen uptake, and carbon dioxide elimination are all reduced. Usually ventilation is depressed only slightly, but oxygen and carbon dioxide exchange are depressed, on the average, to one-third of normal. Lung compliance is only slightly decreased. Clinical pulmonary edema may be seen, especially when increased capillary permeability develops as a result of prolonged ischemia. Division of pulmonary lymphatics alone does not result in pulmonary edema unless pulmonary venous obstruction is also present. Moderate systemic arterial desaturation may develop due to right-to-left shunting in scattered areas of atelectasis in the reimplanted lung. This atelectasis probably results from retained secretions secondary to loss of the cough reflex. Systemic arterial oxygenation usually improves as blood flow to the atelectatic areas decreases, but some ventilation-perfusion imbalance may persist until late in the postoperative period. The pulmonary vascular resistance is increased, primarily because of decreased blood flow in the reimplanted lung rather than because of increased pulmonary artery pressure.

The depression of pulmonary function is maximal in the first two to three weeks following reimplantation. Regeneration of the lymphatics and bronchial arteries takes place during this time. The preoperative level of pulmonary function is usually attained by four to six weeks, although the reimplanted lung frequently remains slightly less efficient than normal. Continued ventilation-perfusion imbalance, altered bronchomotor tone, and pulmonary hypertension may be responsible for the incomplete return of function.

The evidence for nerve regeneration following reimplantation procedures is in favor of an inconsistent and always incomplete return of nerve function several months after the operation. The cough reflex,

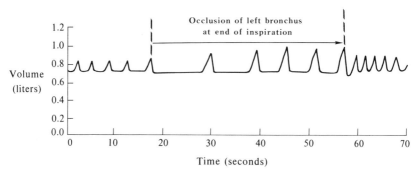

Fig. 14-2. Normal Hering-Breuer reflex in a dog. Spirograph tracing from the right lung. Occlusion of the airway from the left lung at the end of inspiration produces stimulation and continued discharge of pulmonary stretch receptors, resulting in apnea that is followed by resumption of breathing by the right lung at a slower rate and an increased tidal volume.

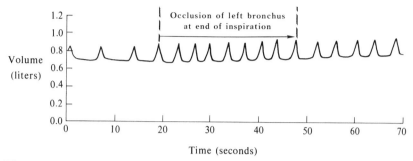

Fig. 14-3. Absent Hering-Breuer reflex after left lung reimplantation. Spirograph tracing from the right lung. Occlusion of the airway from the left lung at the end of inspiration does not stimulate pulmonary stretch receptors, because the afferent vagal fibers have been divided; apnea or slowing of respiration does not occur.

which is mediated by vagal afferent fibers, has not been shown to return in any of the animal preparations studied as late as five years post-operatively. Evacuation of retained secretions depends on ciliary activity of the bronchial epithelium and normal cough reflex from the innervated proximal tracheobronchial tree.

The Hering-Breuer reflex (Figs. 14-2, 14-3) returns only rarely after reimplantation. In the dog, afferent impulses originating in the lungs play an essential role in the regulation of respiration, and contralateral lung reimplantation, pneumonectomy, or pulmonary artery ligation are not readily tolerated because of interference with the normal respiratory pattern. If some time is allowed to elapse after lung reimplantation, survival after contralateral lung ablation may be possible because of the intrinsic periodicity of the respiratory center in the medulla. Dogs with bilateral pulmonary denervation have slow, deep respirations with long interposed pauses, and death from respiratory insufficiency is common. Primates, on the other hand, tolerate complete pulmonary denervation much better. Their respiratory pattern remains normal, because they have a greater periodicity of the respiratory center and are less dependent on the Hering-Breuer stretch reflex. The strength of the Hering-Breuer inflation reflex is especially weak in man, in whom the homeostatic mechanisms concerned with the chemical control of breathing have become more highly developed at the expense of pulmonary reflex control.

Failure of regeneration of nerves in the reimplanted lung may explain some instances of persistence of high pulmonary vascular resistance many months after reimplantation, when anastomotic complications are absent and blood flow in the transplanted lung is apparently normal. Under these conditions, pulmonary hypertension probably represents an interplay of mechanisms which have not been clearly identified. The loss of function of pulmonary vasomotor nerves is difficult to assess, and before changes in pulmonary vasomotor tone can be incriminated, all conceivable passive mechanisms which may affect the vascular caliber must be taken into account. One such mechanism may be related to the sensitivity of denervated bronchi to neural transmitter substances. Bronchograms after pulmonary reimplantation have shown the bronchi to be dilated and to constrict markedly in response to parasympathomimetic drugs. Since bronchomotor tone may affect flow and pressure in the pulmonary artery, abnormalities of pulmonary circulation may be secondary to bronchomotor changes. Reports of pulmonary hypertension in the reimplanted lung have been contradictory. While there is some evidence for an active vasoconstriction of the pulmonary vascular bed after reimplantation, the normal pressures recorded in the pulmonary circulation late in the postoperative period in various animal species and especially in primates are evidence that pulmonary hypertension is not a universal occurrence after lung reimplantation.

In long-term survivors, histological studies of the reimplanted lung have been normal except for lack of complete regeneration of nerve fibers distal to the bronchial transection. Occasionally some distorted, abnormal nerve elements are seen. No evidence of increased distensibility or fibrosis of the pulmonary parenchyma has been seen, and the pulmonary vascular bed has had a normal appearance. The reimplanted immature lung has been shown to continue its growth at an essentially normal rate and to have a relatively normal function.

EXPERIMENTAL LUNG ALLOGRAFTS

While the technical feasibility of lung transplantation has been well established and the reimplanted lung has been proved to be able to sustain life for prolonged periods, lung allografts have not functioned satisfactorily for more than several months after transplantation, even when animal survival has been prolonged with the use of immunosuppressive drugs. Somewhat better success has been obtained in litter mates, which differ less with respect to strong histocompatibility antigens than do unrelated animals. Failure to detect threatened rejection of the lung allograft and infection in the lung transplant in animals receiving high doses of immunosuppressive drugs have been the major obstacles preventing continued long-term function.

In recipients untreated by immunosuppressive drugs, rejection of the allografted lung occurs on the average seven to ten days after transplantation. The earliest pathological change is the appearance of perivenous and, later, periarterial mononuclear infiltrates at about three to five days. As a consequence of the inflammatory changes on the venous side of the pulmonary circulation, alveolar congestion and edema may be present. Progressive involvement of pulmonary arteries at eight to ten days leads to obliteration of the arterial lumen and ischemic necrosis of the allograft. Grossly, the rejected lung is a massively swollen and consolidated organ which may weigh as much as seven times the opposite normal lung.

Immunosuppressive drugs have been variably successful in prolonging lung allograft survival. Azathioprine (Imuran), which has been the mainstay of clinical immunosuppression in kidney transplant recipients, has given somewhat better results that methotrexate. Although some pulmonary function in the transplant has been frequently preserved for three months or rarely longer, neither of these drugs has been successful in preventing rejection of the transplanted lung. On histological examination, the rejected lung from an animal that has received immunosuppressive drugs shows chronic arterial lesions with intimal proliferation and thickening and pulmonary fibrosis. In sacrificed animals there has been a reasonable correlation between the structural integrity of the lung allograft and its function. The lungs that had remained structurally normal had had normal respiratory function, and the lungs which had the most marked changes had been useless in gas exchange.

Detection of threatened rejection in the transplanted lung has been most difficult. In the past, heavy reliance has been placed on differential bronchospirometry to detect abnormalities of oxygen uptake and carbon dioxide elimination in the transplanted lung. The technique is difficult, traumatic, and not always successful. Chest x-rays have not been helpful, since changes due to rejection and common postoperative problems such as atelectasis, congestion, and infection cannot be readily separated. Since a temporary increase in dosage of the immunosuppressive drugs will frequently avert a full-blown rejection, recognition of threatened rejection is of utmost importance. The recently introduced xenon 133 scanning technique permits daily appraisal of ventilation and perfusion of the lung allograft and may be of great usefulness in future studies.

The immune response accompanying lung rejection has not been adequately documented, and the antigenic expression of histocompatibility in lung tissue has not been clearly defined. The lung is known to share antigens with several other organs, including the kidney and the skin. The skin is more antigenic and is rejected before the lung when simultaneous allografts of skin and lung are performed. In some dogs surviving with a lung allograft for one to five years, immunosuppressive therapy could be discontinued with maintenance of pulmonary function as determined by bronchospirometry. The oxygen uptake in such transplants, however, usually has been markedly reduced and probably insufficient to support life. Skin grafts from the animal donating the lung performed after cessation of immunosuppressive therapy have survived longer in animals with viable lung allografts than skin grafts taken from other animals. This suggests that tolerance to the donor antigens might have developed as a result of immunosuppressive treatment.

Prolonged survival of lung allografts in some recipients may be due to chance antigenic similarities. With the development of better tissue typing techniques, selection of the most compatible donor–host combination should be possible and prolonged lung allograft survival become the rule rather than the exception. Use of the heterologous antilymphocyte serum introduced by Levey and Medawar holds promise also. Its mode of action, while not completely understood, appears to permit continued immune response against common bacterial invaders while suppressing cellular immunity against the graft antigens.

CLINICAL LUNG TRANSPLANTATION

In contrast to the extensive animal experience with lung transplantation, human lung transplantation has been carried out in only a few cases. Chronic pulmonary insufficiency, either present at the time of surgery or anticipated as a result of the operative procedure, has been the indication for operation in most patients. Although the transplanted lung functioned temporarily in all recipients, the clinical value of lung transplantation has not been established.

The surgical technique followed was that employed experimentally in animals. The lung donor was heparinized at the time of death, and the lung was perfused with cold dextran solution and intermittently inflated after its removal. There was a remarkable lack of anastomotic complications. All recipients of the lung allografts had difficulty getting rid of pulmonary secretions, and bronchoscopy was frequently necessary to improve the bronchopulmonary toilet. Immunosuppressive drugs were relied on heavily. Infection in the transplanted lung was the predominant terminal event. Immunosuppression appeared to prevent allograft rejection at least in one patient, who died of renal failure eighteen days postoperatively. Lack of tissue histocompatibility and pulmonary infection were the deciding factors in the fatal outcome of the other patients.

Pulmonary function in the transplanted lung was good initially in all patients but deteriorated rapidly in a few days. Evidence of peripheral arterial desaturation with pulmonary arteriovenous shunting was seen. Xenon 133 scanning of the lung was performed in one patient five days postoperatively and demonstrated decreased ventilation in the transplanted lung. Perfusion of the graft was relatively well preserved and preferentially distributed to the upper zone of the lung.

The limited clinical trial with lung transplantation demonstrates many of the unsolved problems present today and points the way to the future. The transplanted lung with an absent cough reflex, exposed, as it continuously is, to contaminated, ambient air, is at maximum risk of developing a pulmonary infection. This risk may be minimized in the future with improved tissue typing and donor selection, the use of heterologous antilymphocyte serum, and less heavy reliance on the currently employed immunosuppressive drugs, which remove all antibacterial defense mechanisms. Careful attention to bronchopulmonary toilet will be required postoperatively to reduce morbidity and mortality from retained secretions. The long-term complications of pulmonary transplantation in the human are presently unknown.

PROCUREMENT AND PRESERVATION

Since the human cadaver lung is most likely to remain the best source of donor pulmonary tissue, development of techniques of cadaver lung procurement and preservation will be necessary. Procurement of viable lung tissue that will assume immediate function after transplantation into the recipient and sterility of the preserved lung are two major technical considerations.

The lung is relatively resistant to anoxia. Two hours or less of ischemia at normal temperature is readily tolerated without detectable impairment of function. If the ischemic lung is ventilated during this time, the period of preservation can be more than doubled, presumably by providing oxygen for continued metabolism of the alveolar cells. Longer survival of the ischemic organ is possible when metabolism is slowed down by the use of hypothermia or metabolic inhibitors.

Surface cooling of the lung is as effective in decreasing the metabolic rate as is perfusion of the pulmonary artery with cold solution. As the temperature of the lung falls, metabolism slows linearly, and at 4°C. it is less than 5% of normal. With hypothermia alone, however, successful preservation for twenty-four hours is achieved in less than 50% of the cases. The addition of continuous ventilation or hyperbaric oxygen (two to three atmospheres) improves the results of hypothermic preservation, but after twenty-four hours function in the preserved lung decreases rapidly. The effects of oxygen under increased pressure are conjectural and probably depend on depression of metabolism by high pressure, since nitrogen or helium can be substituted for oxygen during hypothermic preservation.

Present chemical methods of metabolic inhibition are far less effective than hypothermia in prolonging viability of the ischemic lung. Since critical concentrations of magnesium have an important catalytic effect on many cellular enzyme systems, an excess of magnesium salts has been used to depress the metabolic rate of the pulmonary parenchyma. The reduction of metabolism achieved is comparable to that obtained with mild hypothermia. When the lung is cooled, a synergistic effect may be produced.

Artificial perfusion of the lung during its extracorporeal state holds great potential promise in future attempts at lung preservation. Continuous perfusion prevents thrombosis in the pulmonary vascular tree, provides oxygen and other nutrients for the lung parenchyma, and removes metabolic waste products. In addition, effective cooling of the lung can be achieved. A major obstacle to a successful long-term perfusion has been the maintenance of adequate flow without causing tissue swelling, vasoconstriction, and mechanical blockage of capillaries due to sludging. Asanguinous perfusates such as serum, plasma, or buffered low-molecular-weight dextran are preferable to whole blood when hypothermia is employed, as the increased viscosity of blood at low temperatures interferes with flow in the small vessels and oxygen becomes less readily available to the cells as the hemoglobin dissociation curve shifts to the left. In addition, the buffering effect of oxyhemoglobin is less than that of reduced hemoglobin at low temperatures, and removal of acid waste products of metabolism is less efficient. All the factors producing vasoconstriction and tissue edema during prolonged artificial perfusion have not been fully clarified.

All of the currently available methods of lung preservation incur some degree of functional damage after a relatively short period of time. This damage interferes with the resumption of function by the transplanted lung and may not be completely reversible. Since the manner in which the graft is prepared significantly influences the immediate and long-term results of pulmonary transplantation, further development of methods and techniques of lung preservation will be of the utmost importance.

APPENDIX

THE PHYSICAL BASIS OF RESPIRATION

AN UNDERSTANDING of some of the basic laws of physics and fluid mechanics is essential to an intelligent analysis of respiration. For this reason, this Appendix gives a somewhat simplified review of basic principles, particularly as they are related to physiological processes. This review is, of course, by no means an exhaustive treatment of these subjects. Since the Appendix uses many symbols in various equations, a list of these follows arranged in the order in which they appear in the text.

DEFINITIONS OF SYMBOLS USED

P = Pressure
P_{TM} = Transmural pressure
V = Volume
$\dot{V}$ = First derivative of volume, or flow
$\ddot{V}$ = Second derivative of volume, or rate of change of flow
T = Temperature
R = Resistance
E = Voltage
I = Current
$\dot{I}$ = First derivative of current
l = Length
η = Coefficient of viscosity
α = Resistivity of a substance
r = Radius
A = Area
M = Mass

v = Velocity
F = Force
W = Work
E = Energy
K_E = Kinetic energy
N_R = Reynold's number
d = Density
S = Tension
a = Acceleration
C = Compliance or capacitance
Q = Charge
L = Inductance
Pow = Power
f = Frequency
X_C = Compliant or capacitive reactance
X_L = Inertial or inductive reactance
Z = Impedance
e = Base of natural logarithm 2.73

SUBSCRIPTS:

D.C. = Direct current, steady flow, or pressure
A.C. = Alternating current, pulsatile flow, or pressure
m = Peak or maximum

GAS LAWS AND KINETIC THEORY

The physical properties of gases are basic to an orderly analysis of the process of respiration. The understanding of the transfer and transport of gases by the respiratory mechanism in a biological system is founded upon a sound knowledge of the physics of gases. This section presents a brief review of the gas laws and kinetic theory, with emphasis on the properties of gases in the range of temperature and pressure seen in biological systems.

BOYLE'S AND CHARLES' (GAY LUSSAC'S) LAWS

A characteristic property of a gas is that it fills any space uniformly; therefore, there must be a relationship between the size of the container and the number of gas molecules per unit of volume. Boyle's law states that at a constant temperature the pressure exerted by a given quantity of gas is inversely proportional to the volume of the gas, or, that the product of pressure and volume of a given mass of gas at constant temperature is a constant:

$$P \times V - K$$

Charles' or Gay Lussac's law defines the effect of temperature change: At a constant pressure, the volume of a given mass of gases varies directly as the absolute temperature (degrees centigrade + 273). Stated another way, the volume of a gas at constant pressure will increase by 1/273 for each 1° rise in temperature.

Boyle's law is applicable only if temperature is kept constant, and Charles' law is applicable only if pressure is kept constant, but by combining these two laws, it is possible not only to define the volume of a given mass of gas at any pressure and temperature but also to compute the state that will result from a change in any one of the variables.

To derive the equation of Boyle's and Charles' laws combined, denote initial volume, pressure, and temperature as V_1, P_1, and T_1 and the new values as V_2, P_2, and T_2. Using Boyle's law, a new volume, V_o, can be calculated if the temperature remains constant while the pressure changes from P_1 to P_2.

$$P_1 \times V_1 = P_2 \times V_o \qquad \text{or} \qquad V_o = \frac{P_1 \times V_1}{P_2}$$

Using Charles' law, a further equation can be developed if the new pressure, P_2, is maintained constant.

$$\frac{V_o}{T_1} = \frac{V_2}{T_2} \qquad \text{or} \qquad V_o = \frac{V_2 \times T_1}{T_2}$$

The following equation results when the term V_o is eliminated:

$$\frac{V_2 \times T_1}{T_2} = \frac{P_1 \times V_1}{P_2} \qquad \text{or} \qquad \frac{P_1 \times V_1}{T_1} = \frac{P_2 \times V_2}{T_2}$$

Stated verbally, for a given mass of gas, the pressure times the volume divided by the absolute temperature is a constant. This is called the equation of state of a gas and allows prediction of the third variable when the other two are known.

THE KINETIC THEORY OF GASES

The kinetic theory of gases has been developed to explain the action of gases and to predict variations from the ideal gas laws discussed above. Its basis is the molecular nature of matter.

Solids have a definite shape and volume; liquids have definite volume and no shape. Gases, in contrast, have neither definite shape nor volume; they expand to fill the container. They must be restrained by some force or they will expand indefinitely. In our atmosphere, the restraining force is gravity or an enclosed container.

The kinetic theory postulates that a gas is made up of many molecules which occupy a relatively small part of the total space and which move about randomly, striking one another and the walls of the container. These collisions are perfectly elastic and, therefore, no energy is expended. The pressure of a gas is attributed to the rate of momentum transferred to the container walls by the impact of the molecules. The compressibility of the gas is due to the relatively small size of the molecules compared to the mean free space about them.

Maxwell has shown that the kinetic energy of gas molecules (one-half the mass times the square of the velocity) is the same for all gases at the same temperature. Further, this kinetic energy increases with a rise in temperature. This theory explains both Boyle's and Charles' laws; as the gas decreases in volume, the molecules are closer together and more collisions occur; therefore, the pressure rises (Boyle's law). As the temperature rises, the velocity of the molecules and so the force of their collisions increases and the pressure rises (Charles' law).

THE LAW OF AVOGADRO

The law of Avogadro states that equal volumes of a gas at the same temperature and pressure contain the same number of molecules. This has best been confirmed by the finding that the density or weight per unit of volume of gases is the same as the molecular weight of the gases if the weight of hydrogen is taken as one. Thus, one mol of any gas occupies 22.4 liters at $0°C$. and 760 mm. Hg.

The ideal gas laws do not explain the condensation of gases and vapors into liquids, but gases do not obey the gas laws exactly. The variation from the ideal depends both on the nature and the state of the gas. If the molecules had no mass and did not attract one another, the ideal would be met; but the molecules do have mass and are attracted to one another. It is this interaction between molecules which explains the changes of state. Van der Waal expressed this correction of Boyle's and Charles' ideal gas laws in the equation,

$$P = \frac{KT}{V-b} - \frac{a}{V^2} \quad \text{or} \quad (P + \frac{a}{V^2}) \times (V-b) = KT$$

where b is a function of the volume of the molecules and is subtracted from the total volume of the gas, since the volume occupied by the molecules is not available for the random motion of these bodies. Thus the b term will lead to a greater pressure than Boyle's and Charles' law would predict. The term a/V^2 is Avogadro's number (the number of molecules in a mol of gas) over the square of the volume, and it defines the attractive forces of the molecules. The derivation of this term is beyond the scope of this brief discussion. The term a/V^2 must be subtracted from the pressure, since it acts to slow down the molecules and to diminish the number and force of collisions with the container wall. When the concentration density of the molecules and the speed of travel reach a critical temperature and pressure, the gas becomes a liquid. Only that portion of the molecules with enough energy to escape from these binding forces can get free and exist in the gas or vapor phase.

DALTON'S LAW OF PARTIAL PRESSURES

The discussion up to this point has focused on pure gases. In the biological milieu the atmospheres are mixtures of gases. A plastic bag of one-liter capacity containing one liter of nitrogen at room temperature, 23°C., and at sea level, 760 mm. Hg pressure, has the same number of molecules with the same mean kinetic energy as a similar bag containing one liter of oxygen in the same room at the same temperature. If the oxygen and nitrogen are combined and transferred into one two-liter bag, the number of molecules in the bag will be doubled, the volume will be doubled, and the temperature and total pressure will remain unchanged. The nitrogen molecules will now be distributed in a volume of two liters instead of one. Therefore, the number of collisions by the nitrogen molecules will be cut in half, and so the pressure exerted by the nitrogen alone will be cut in half, to 380 mm. Hg. The same will be true for the oxygen. Boyle's law predicts this change because, since T is constant and V is double, P has to be cut in half.

Instead of holding total pressure constant, the experiment can be changed to keep the volume constant. If two one-liter cylinders are connected together and the contents of one forced into the other, the mixture will have twice the number of molecules of the same mean kinetic energy in one liter of volume. Twice the original pressure will result, because the number of molecular collisions will be twice as frequent. Again, since half of the collisions will be due to nitrogen molecules and half to oxygen molecules, one-half the pressure is attributed to each or each has a partial pressure of 760 mm. Hg, one-half the total pressure of 1,520 mm. Hg.

Dalton's law of partial pressures states: The pressure exerted by a mixture of gases is equal to the sum of the separate pressures which each gas would exert if it alone occupied the whole volume. Expressed algebraically:

$$VP = V (P_1 + P_2 + P_3 + \ldots + P_n)$$

This equation defines the system predicted by Boyle's law and the kinetic theory of gases.

VAPOR PRESSURE

According to the Clausius-Clapeyron equation, the vapor pressure P_V of a vapor in equilibrium with its liquid will increase with increasing temperature. The number of molecules leaving the liquid phase is determined by the energy needed to overcome the binding forces in the liquid; as the temperature rises, the molecules have a higher mean energy, so more escape. All gases that are below their critical temperature, the temperature above which they cannot be liquefied by an increase in pressure, are really vapors. Carbon dioxide, with a critical temperature of 31°C., is thus a vapor at room temperatures.

Although a vapor that is in contact with and in equilibrium with its own liquid phase may appear to disobey the gas laws, vapors do obey all the gas laws. Since the liquid is a source of additional molecules for the vapor phase, as the temperature rises in the liquid, the free energy of the molecules increases, This increase in free energy allows more molecules to escape into the vapor phase, so the vapor pressure of the liquid rises. If a vapor is in equilibrium with its liquid and if both the vapor and its liquid are heated, vapor pressure will be increased because of the added energy of the molecules already in the gas phase (Charles' law) and also because of the additional molecules that have escaped from the liquid phase.

At any given pressure, if an equilibrium has been reached so the number of molecules escaping from the liquid equals those reentering, the gas is called fully or 100% saturated with the vapor. A gas 100% saturated with water vapor at 38°C. will be oversaturated, and droplets of water will form if the temperature is dropped to 31°. If the number of water molecules diminishes, the partial pressure of the gas will diminish. Therefore the partial pressure of water vapor in a gas mixture that is 100% saturated will depend on the temperature of the gas.

If the total barometric pressure is lowered, the partial pressures of the gases not in equilibrium with their liquid phase will fall. However, over the range of barometric pressures compatible with life, the absolute pressure exerted by a vapor in equilibrium with its liquid is little affected, because these relatively small changes in total barometric pressure do not significantly alter the free energy necessary for the escape of molecules from the liquid phase. If the free energy required for escape is unchanged, the number of molecules of vapor in a given volume will be unchanged, so the vapor pressure will remain the same. A corollary to this statement is that the vapor pressure of water in the alveolar air stays the same over the range of atmospheric pressures compatible with life and is unaffected by alterations in intrathoracic pressure. The only thing that alters the vapor pressure in the alveoli is body temperature.

This concept perhaps can be clarified further with an example. At an altitude of 20,000 feet, the barometric pressure is 350 mm. Hg and in the alveolar air 46 mm. Hg pressure, or approximately 14% of the total pressure, is taken up by water vapor. At 64 feet below the surface of the ocean, barometric pressure is twice that at the surface but there is only the same 46 mm. Hg water vapor present in the alveoli, and so water vapor makes up only 3% of the total pressure. On the other hand, the percentage of oxygen remains the same so the partial pressure of oxygen varies from 70 mm. Hg at 20,000 feet to 300 mm. Hg at two atmospheres.

HENRY'S LAW—SOLUTION OF GASES IN LIQUIDS

Henry's law states that the amount of gas dissolved in any liquid is equal to the solubility coefficient of the gas times its partial pressure. Henry's law applies only to free or chemically unbound gas in a dilute solution. The solubility of a gas is defined by the Bunsen absorption coefficient. Some examples of these coefficients for gas in water at 20° C. and one atmosphere pressure are, in cubic centimeters of gas per cubic centimeter of water: oxygen, 0.031; nitrogen, 0.0155; carbon dioxide, 0.872; helium, 0.0088; and nitrous oxide, 0.629. If oxygen is given a value of one, nitrogen is one-half as soluble in water, carbon dioxide twenty-five times more soluble, helium one-fourth as soluble, and nitrous oxide twenty times more soluble. The solubility of the gas in the liquid defines the quantity of gas or the number of cubic centimeters that will be dissolved in a given volume of liquid at any given partial pressure.

From the art of cooking, many of us are aware of the fact that heating a solution increases the solubility of sugar or other compounds in a liquid. The effect of heat on the solubility of a gas is less obvious, since gases are invisible. Heat *reduces* the solubility of a gas in a liquid. Table A-1 shows the effect of heating on the amount of oxygen, nitrogen, and carbon dioxide, dissolved in a 100 cc. volume of water in equilibrium with room air at sea level. One application of Henry's law is to

Table A-1. The Effect of Heat on Solubility of Gases in 100 cc. of Water in Equilibrium with Room Air at Sea Level

Gas	0°C.	20°C.	30°C.	40°C.
O_2	1.03 cc.	0.65 cc.	0.55 cc.	0.49 cc.
N_2	1.85 cc.	1.22 cc.	1.06 cc.	0.95 cc.
CO_2	0.051 cc.	0.026 cc.	0.020 cc.	0.016 cc.

explain the decrease in solubility of gas in a liquid as it is warmed, which leads to the danger of bubble formation in a pump oxygenator of an extracorporeal circulation system if the blood is warmed too fast.

FLUID MECHANICS

Just as the gas laws define equilibrium states of gases and their distribution between gas and liquid media, a set of laws exists which defines the relation of pressure to flow in tubes. Since gases are governed by the same rules of fluid mechanics as are liquids, the same rules fortunately apply to both blood and air flow. The flow of fluid through the vascular system and air through the respiratory system determines in turn the effectiveness of circulation and respiration.

The flow of electric current is analogous to flow of fluids in pipes. An understanding of the electrical analogy is helpful in the analysis of the mechanical phasic flow systems—circulation of blood and exchange of air in the lungs. The theory of flow has been much better worked out for electrical than mechanical flow circuits, and parallel discussion of two analogous systems will reinforce the reader's understanding of each.

FACTORS REGULATING FLOW

The flow of a liquid or gas through a tube requires a force to move it, and this force is called the driving pressure. The driving pressure over any given portion of a pipe—or blood vessel or respiratory passage— is the difference in pressure across that segment. This driving pressure can be determined by subtracting the lower pressure at one end of the segment from the higher pressure at the other end. For example, the pressure driving blood through the lungs is the difference between the pulmonary artery pressure and the left atrial pressure. This is denoted as ΔP and is usually expressed in millimeters of mercury or grams per square centimeter or dynes per square centimeter. The driving pressure is not equal to the pressure on the upstream side of the tube segment under study but is equal to the difference in pressure across the segment. Many inconsistencies in experimental results are due to neglect of this basic concept.

The rate of flow is also dependent on the physical characteristics of the system of pipes. It has proved useful to define this effect by introducing the concept of resistance. It is apparent that the resistance retarding flow through a tube is equal to the driving pressure divided by the flow.

$$R = \frac{P}{\dot{V}}$$

This equation is fundamentally the same as Ohm's law for the flow of current in an electrical circuit, $R = E/I$, or, transposing, $I = E/R$, where I stands for the current (or flow) and E for the voltage (electrical equivalent of pressure). Thus, as pressure or voltage rises, the flow will increase; while increase in resistance will decrease the flow.

The volume of air or blood that can flow through a tube with a given resistance is affected not only by the pressure but also by time and resistance.

$$R = \text{pressure/flow} \qquad \text{Flow} = \text{liters/second}$$

$$R = \frac{P}{\text{liters/second}} \qquad P = \frac{R \times \text{liters}}{\text{seconds}}$$

For any given resistance and pressure, the longer the time available, the larger will be the volume that will flow through the system. For example, the pressure necessary to drive a given volume of blood from the left atrium into the left ventricle through a stenotic mitral valve will be less if the pulse is slow and diastole long.

Electronic or vascular circuits with only one resistance rarely exist. Obviously, the vascular or bronchial trees are not such simple systems, and the manner in which they deviate from the following analogy will be clarified in subsequent sections. In a simple resistance circuit such as a set of rigid pipes, the fluid or current entering the circuit must equal that coming out. If the resistances are connected in series (such as the resistance of the larynx, trachea, bronchi, and alveolar ducts), the flow through each resistance must be the same, and the sum of the pressure drops across the various resistances must equal the pressure drop across the whole circuit.

$$R = \frac{E}{I} = \frac{E_1 + E_2 + E_3}{I} \cdots \qquad R = \frac{P}{\dot{V}} = \frac{P_1 + P_2 + P_3}{\dot{V}} \cdots$$

$$R = \frac{E_1}{I} + \frac{E_2}{I} + \frac{E_3}{I} \cdots \qquad\qquad R = \frac{P_1}{\dot{V}} + \frac{P_2}{\dot{V}} + \frac{P_3}{\dot{V}} \cdots$$

$$R = R_1 + R_2 + R_3 \cdots \qquad\qquad R = R_1 + R_2 + R_3 \cdots$$

Thus the total resistance across a tube circuit with resistances connected in series is the sum of the various individual resistances (Fig. A-1A).

If the resistances are connected in a parallel manner, such as the vascular beds are in the right and left lungs, the pressure across the various resistances will be the same and the total flow passing through the various resistances will be the sum of the various flows. For example,

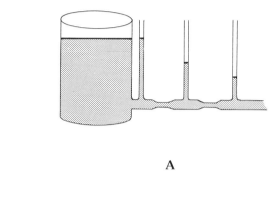

A

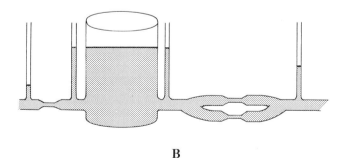

B

Fig. A-1. (A) The difference in height of the liquid level in the vertical tubes represents the drop in pressure due to resistance to flow through the horizontal tube. Since the resistances along the horizontal tube are in series, the pressure drop across the two resistances is the sum of the drop across each.

(B) On the left is depicted the pressure drop across a single resistance, on the right is the pressure drop across two identical resistors connected in parallel. The pressure drop across the two resistors in parallel is one-half that across the single resistance, so the flow is twice as great.

the difference in pressure between the pulmonary artery and the left auricle is the same and the total flow is equal to the sum of flow to each lung (Fig. A-1B). Therefore:

$$I = I_1 + I_2 + I_3 \cdots \qquad\qquad \dot{V} = \dot{V}_1 + \dot{V}_2 + \dot{V}_3 \cdots$$

$$E = E_1 = E_2 = E_3 \cdots \qquad\qquad \Delta P = \Delta P_1 = \Delta P_2 = \Delta P_3 \cdots$$

$$I = \frac{E}{R} = \frac{E}{R_1} + \frac{E}{R_2} + \frac{E}{R_3} \cdots \qquad \dot{V} = \frac{\Delta P}{R} = \frac{\Delta P}{R_1} + \frac{\Delta P}{R_2} + \frac{\Delta P}{R_3} \cdots$$

Divide by E or divide by ΔP and

$$\frac{1}{R} = \frac{1}{R_1} + \frac{1}{R_2} + \frac{1}{R_3} \cdots$$

These equations show that the total resistance of a set of resistances connected in parallel must be smaller than the smallest resistance. In any of the derivations, current can, of course, be interchanged with flow and voltage with ΔP, making the analogy between an electronic circuit and the circulatory or respiratory system complete.

FACTORS DETERMINING RESISTANCE IN A FLUID SYSTEM

In an electronic circuit, the composition, length, cross-sectional area of wire, and temperature determine the resistance. Flow of electricity is termed the *conductance of electricity*, and the ability of a material to conduct electric energy is *conductivity*; the restraining force is the *resistivity*. The same terms are applicable and used in discussion of fluid flow.

The electrical resistivity of a substance is one of its physical characteristics. The resistance is equal to the resistivity times the length over the cross-sectional area. For a round wire where α is the resistivity of the substance,

$$R = \frac{\alpha l}{\pi r^2}$$

In a fluid system, the relation between flow and pressure is defined by Poiseuille's equation:

$$\dot{V} = \Delta P \times \frac{\pi r^4}{8l} \times \frac{1}{\eta}$$

where   r = the radius of the vessel or pipe
             l = the length
             η = coefficient of viscosity (composition)

For laminar or orderly flow, flow is equal to the cross-sectional area of a tube (πr^2) times the mean velocity of fluid flowing. As predicted from the theoretical derivation by Poiseuille's equation, actual measurements have shown that fluid at the wall of the vessel is not moving and that the velocity increases rapidly at first and then more slowly to reach a maximum at the center of the tube. The velocity of the fluid at any point on the radius of the tube is proportional to the square of the distance from the wall. The mean velocity of the fluid is proportional, therefore, to the square of the radius. Since flow equals area times velocity, it can be shown that flow is directly proportional to the fourth power of the radius.

$$\dot{V} = A \times v$$
where $A = \pi r^2$
and $\bar{v} \cong r^2$
Then $\dot{V} \cong \pi r^2 \times r^2 \cong \pi r^4$

In purely laminar flow, fluid is stationary at the edge of a tube, and there is in effect no motion between the fluid and the tube. The only motion is between the stationary fluid at the edge of the tube and the moving fluid. Stagnation does not occur at the edge of the tube in fact because there is always some turbulence in any actual flowing fluid. Poiseuille's equation describes only laminar flow, so no actual system

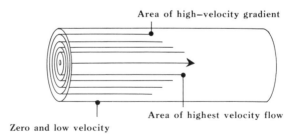

Area of high–velocity gradient

Area of highest velocity flow

Zero and low velocity

Fig. A-2. Pattern of laminar flow in a tube. The flow velocity is zero at the vessel wall and highest at the apex of the cone front. This velocity gradient means the inner layers of fluid are sliding past the outer layers and the force required to make one slide over the other is the function of the viscosity of the fluid. Thus the resistance or ratio of flow to driving pressure is a function of viscosity of the fluid.

meets the assumptions of the equation. However, the equation is still a useful approximation of the interplay of forces. The idea that one layer of fluid slides past another was first expressed by Sir Isaac Newton; using this concept he postulated that the force per unit area tending to impede this sliding (the stress) is directly proportional to the difference in velocity between the two adjacent layers (the shear velocity). This shear velocity is a measure of the viscosity of the fluid (Fig. A-2).

Poiseuille's equation can be restated to define resistance, since resistance is:

$$R = \frac{\Delta P}{\dot{V}}$$

From the equation $\dot{V} = \Delta P \times \dfrac{\pi r^4}{8l} \times \dfrac{1}{\eta}$

$$\frac{1}{\dot{V}} = \frac{1}{\Delta P \dfrac{\pi r^4}{8l\eta}} \qquad \frac{\Delta P}{\dot{V}} = \frac{8l\eta}{\pi r^4}$$

or

$$R = \frac{8l\eta}{\pi r^4}$$

The resistance increases directly as the length of the tube and the viscosity of the fluid, and it decreases as a function of the fourth power of the radius. Thus, with a given pressure head, flow is inversely proportional to the length of tubing and viscosity of fluid and directly proportional to the fourth power of the radius. This latter relationship is very important in small vessels of the size of an arteriole, where a 19% increase in radius leads to a 100% increase in flow.

The viscosity factor is of significance in the vascular tree. In the respiratory tree it is less important, since the viscosity of air is about one-thirtieth that of water at body temperature.

Since the viscosity of a liquid is due to the presence of cohesive forces between molecules, an increase in temperature will decrease the viscosity. The viscosity of a gas does not respond in the same manner to change in temperature. In a gas the molecules are too far apart for significant cohesion to exist between them. Different layers of the gas are flowing at different rates, creating internal friction between the layers due to momentum transfer. This friction determines the viscosity. When the gas is heated, the momentum of particles is higher so the friction increases. As a result, a rise in temperature increases the viscosity of a gas.

Since at the same pressure and temperature a given volume of any gas has the same number of molecules, the force of collisions on the wall of the container must be the same to maintain the same pressure. A gas of less density will have a smaller mass per molecule, and therefore the kinetic energy ($\frac{1}{2}$ Mv^2) will be smaller at any given velocity for this molecule. To maintain the same pressure the velocity will have to be increased. If the velocity is increased, the momentum and, therefore, the friction of layers will go up, and so the viscosity must increase.

A less dense gas such as helium is more viscous than air. Since density does not affect the flow-pressure relationship defined by Poiseuille's law but viscosity does, the substitution of helium for nitrogen in an inspired gas mixture will increase flow resistance. As indicated on page 333, however, there may be a decrease in pressure because of lowering of Reynold's number and elimination of turbulence.

Blood, which consists of red cells of relatively large size suspended in a fluid, does not maintain the same viscosity under different conditions. (It is a non-Newtonian fluid.) It has what is called *anomalous viscosity*. Its apparent viscosity (the ratio of flow of blood to that of water under identical conditions of tubing, size, temperature, and pressure gradient) in small vessels is like that of plasma.

In the aorta, blood viscosity is greater than that of plasma, and as flow rate increases, its viscosity decreases. Axial accumulation of cells in large vessels due to Bernoulli's effect leaves the less viscous plasma as a lubricant along the edges and lowers the viscosity as the rate of flow increases. (The center stream is moving fastest, and so the pressure is lower in the center and the cells have lower pressure on the medial than on the lateral surface.) When the circulation is slowed, as in shock, the axial accumulation is less and the apparent viscosity rises. Actually, the viscosity of blood in the vascular bed varies from two to fifteen times the viscosity of water.

Poiseuille's equation states that in any given tube the pressure should go up as a direct function of the flow through the tube if all of the conditions of the equation are met. These conditions are that the tube be long, straight, smooth, narrow, and round; that the viscosity of the fluid remain unchanged at different rates of flow; and that tube diameter and the geometry of the tube be unaffected by pressure. Unfortunately, none of these conditions can be satisfied in either the vascular system or the bronchial tree. This means that Poiseuille's equation cannot describe accurately but only approximates the relation between flow and pressure in these physiological systems.

CONTINUITY EQUATION

In any closed system of connecting tubes, the total flow at one point must be equal to the flow at every other point upstream or downstream. Flow is equal to cross-sectional area times velocity; therefore, the area times velocity at any one point must be equal to area times velocity at any other point.

$$\dot{V} = A \times v$$
$$\dot{V}_1 = \dot{V}_2$$
$$v_1 A_1 = v_2 A_2$$

This concept is important in the study of biological tube systems, because in additional to functional variations in tube diameter due to changes in pressure and wall tension, there are marked anatomical variations in diameter.

As the cross-sectional area of the vascular bed increases from 2 cm.^{2} in the large vessels, where the speed is 50 cm. per second, to 1,000 cm.^{2} in the myriad of 8 μ diameter capillaries, the speed of blood flow drops to only 0.1 cm. per second. If there is an obstruction in a flow stream such as a stenotic valve or bronchus, the velocity of flow through this area is greatly increased.

WORK AND BERNOULLI'S EQUATION

In a system in which the energy is conserved, the work done is equal to the decrease in potential energy. If fluids are to be moved in a tube system, work must be done. Work is defined as a force moving through a distance.

$$W = F \times l \qquad \text{or} \qquad W = \text{gm.} \times \text{cm.}$$

Pressure is a force per unit area, and the amount of this force is equal to the pressure times the area over which it acts.

$$F = P \times A \qquad \text{or} \qquad F = \frac{\text{gm.}}{\text{cm.}^2} \times \text{cm.}^2$$

Volume is the product of an area times a given length.

$$\Delta V = A \times l \qquad \text{or} \qquad \Delta V = \text{cm.}^2 \times \text{cm.}$$

Therefore, by substituting in the first equation,

$$W = P \times A \times l = \frac{gm.}{cm.^2} \times cm.^3$$

and from the third equation,

$$W = P \times \Delta V = gm. \times cm.$$

If the applied pressure is constant throughout the volume change, work can be measured by the simple multiplication of the applied pressure times the change in volume. In a biological system the driving pressures throughout the period of volume change vary, as does the rate of change of volume, so pressure cannot be simply multiplied by volume change to give work. In this real system both the forcing pressure and the rate at which volume changes (the flow rate) are varying through each cycle. At any instant a certain amount of power is generated by the system. Power is a measure of the ability to do work and in a pressure-volume system is at any instant equal to the product of pressure times the flow rate. The amount of work done in a given period to time (one respiratory cycle) is equal to the sum of all the different amounts of power expended during that period. In terms of calculus, it is the integral of the power available during the cycle.

$$W = \int_{t_1}^{t_2} P \times \dot{V}$$

Energy is the capacity of doing work. Thus an object or system contains energy if it is capable of doing work. Potential energy is energy available to perform work, and in a conservative field of force, work done on a body equals the potential energy expended. The pressure in a fluid system is a measure of the potential energy capable of doing work to move the fluid.

Kinetic energy is the energy of motion. For a body or fluid to gain kinetic energy, that is, to move, work must be done on it to overcome the opposing force, inertia. In a conservative field of force the kinetic energy of a body is equal to the work done on it. The amount of kinetic energy an object possesses is equal to one-half the mass times the velocity squared.

$$KE = \frac{1}{2} Mv^2$$

Kinetic energy or energy of motion can be converted into work by an appropriate mechanical system so that kinetic energy units have the same dimensions as work units, just as do potential energy units. The energy used to overcome friction is not available to do useful work but is dissipated as heat energy.

When a fluid or gas is in motion or flowing, both potential and kinetic energy are present. Bernoulli's equation defines the relationship between the kinetic and potential energy of a flowing fluid based on the principle of conservation of energy. It states that the principle of conservation of energy requires that the energy, E, at any two points in the system be equal. This energy is made up of potential and kinetic energy:

$$E = P\Delta V + \tfrac{1}{2} Mv^2$$

If the fluid flows through a constriction, the cross-sectional area will be smaller, and, therefore, the velocity will have to increase to keep the flow rate the same. As a result, the kinetic energy ($\tfrac{1}{2} Mv^2$) due to velocity must increase and the potential energy or pressure will fall.

The Bernoulli effect is of negligible significance in gas flow because the mass (density) of gas is so low. Both Bernoulli's and Poiseuille's laws have very restrictive conditions. They apply only for streamline or laminar flow, this is, flow in which the particles are moving in parallel paths in an orderly manner. They do not apply under conditions of turbulence or eddies. Under such conditions the potential energy of pressure or the pressure available to drive the fluid down the tube is converted to kinetic energy of motion as the particles of matter swirl about; this kinetic energy is dissipated as heat because the motions are random and disorderly. In other words, turbulence dissipates mechanical energy into heat through random motion. In addition, disorderly flow causes added friction at the wall as well as in the fluid, which converts still more energy to heat. The amount of potential energy converted to heat in a system with turbulence may be very large, and the pressure drop across the system will greatly exceed that predicted by Poiseuille.

REYNOLD'S NUMBER

Since turbulence causes a change in the amount of forward flow that can be achieved by a given driving pressure (amount of potential energy) the conditions which determine whether flow will be laminar (streamline) or turbulent are very important. These factors are the radius of the tube, the velocity, and the ratio of density of fluid to viscosity. They are related in the equation which defines Reynold's number (N_R), a dimensionless quantity which describes the limits of velocity before turbulence occurs.

$$N_R = \frac{2vrd}{\eta}$$

Or, since velocity equals flow divided by cross-sectional area,

$$v = \frac{\dot{V}}{\pi r^2}$$

Substituting the second equation in the first, we have the equation for Reynold's number:

$$N_R = \frac{2\dot{V}d}{\pi r \eta}$$

The Reynold's number expresses the fact that no arbitrarily large part of the work of pressure can be converted into the kinetic energy of directed flow and predicts the conditions under which some of the energy will be dissipated in directionless flow. In most fluids, when the Reynold's number gets in the region of the critical value of 2,000 to 2,300, turbulence can occur; in blood the limit is 1,000. If the flow or geometry is not changed abruptly, however, streamline flow may continue when the Reynold's number is much higher. Likewise, if the flow rate is changing rapidly or if an irregularity of the tube exists, turbulence can intervene at a lower flow rate.

It can be seen from the last equation above that if the flow rate remains the same, since the radius is in the denominator, an increase in radius lowers Reynold's number (decreases the likelihood of turbulence). This is because at a given flow rate, when the radius increases, the velocity of the fluid decreases. Also, it is apparent that for a given velocity of flow, the smaller the radius the less likelihood there is of turbulence occurring. Likewise, for a given radius, the smaller the velocity the less likelihood there is of turbulence.

The radius of the vessels or airways constantly decreases in size as branching occurs, but the total cross-sectional area increases. If the cross-sectional area increases and the mean flow rate in any segment of the system must be the same as that in another, the velocity must slow in the smaller branches. The decrease in radius of the individual tubes and the decrease in velocity of fluid as vascular tree and bronchial tree branch prevent turbulence in small vessels and airways.

A decrease in density of a gas or an increase in the viscosity tends to decrease the Reynold's number (i.e., decrease the likelihood of turbulence). Since the viscosity of blood paradoxically decreases at higher flow rates in the vascular system (see below), the stabilizing effect of viscosity is less effective. In respiratory gas mixtures, the effects of substitution of diluents such as helium for nitrogen will significantly lower the density and raise the viscosity, both of which should make these gases less likely to develop turbulent flow. It is this property of helium, not the change in density of the gas, which creates the apparent decrease in work associated with helium breathing.

LAPLACE EQUATION

In addition to turbulence, another factor which limits the applicability of the principles of Bernoulli and Poiseuille to the biological systems is the elasticity of the vascular and bronchial tubes. The so-called geometric factor, length over radius to the fourth power (l/r^4), is not a constant in an elastic tube system. The radius of these biological tubes is altered by the interaction between the distending force, the intraluminal pressure, and the restraining forces; the pressure surrounding the vessel; and the tensions of the various fibers (muscle, elastic, and collagenous) that make up the vessel wall. The difference between the intraluminal pressure and the surounding pressure is called the transmural pressure (P_{TM}). Transmural pressure is as important a concept to consider in analysis of distending forces on vessels as is the concept of the pressure difference along a pipe system in defining the driving force pushing fluid ahead (Fig. A-3).

If the venous pressure in a system should rise as fast as the arterial pressure, no change in driving pressure, ΔP, would occur. However, there would be a change in transmural pressure. This would distend the vessels, increasing their radii, and increase the flow, due to the

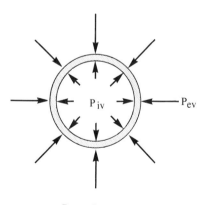

$$P_{tm} = P_{iv} - P_{ev}$$

Fig. A-3. Transmural pressure. The net pressure on the wall of the tube is the difference between the pressure (P_{iv}) within the tube pushing out and the pressure (P_{ev}) outside the tube pushing in. The pressure across (P_{tm}) distending the vessel equals $P_{iv} - P_{ev}$.

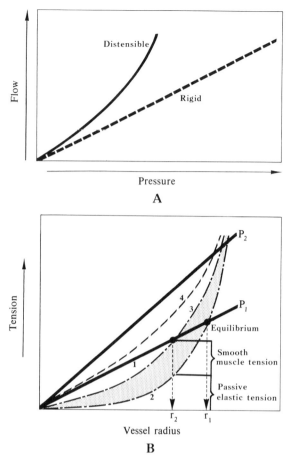

Fig. A-4. (A) Flow-pressure relationships. If flow is laminar in a rigid tube, there is a straight-line relationship; in a distensible tube, as the pressure rises, the tube stretches and the cross-sectional area increases. As a result, flow rises faster than pressure.

(B) This figure depicts the various factors contributing to changes in vessel radius. Curve *1*, the lower solid straight line, is the relationship between radius and tension at a fixed transmural pressure. As defined by the Laplace equation, as the radius increases, the tension in the wall rises for any given pressure.

Curve *2*, the bottom curved line, shows the effects of the elastic tissue contribution to tension in the wall as a function of radius when the transmural pressure is slowly increased. The first part of the curve is horizontal, because the vessel expands easily; as it enlarges, tension rises progressively faster than radius. At pressure P_1 the distending force and tension are in equilibrium when radius is r_1. If the radius were larger or smaller, the two forces would be unbalanced and the vessel would expand or contract to r_1. If the smooth muscle is stimulated to contract, this added tension in the wall would result in a new tension radius curve, curve *3* (middle curved line), and at pressure P_1 the vessel radius would fall to r_2 and flow would decrease. Further contraction of muscle would move the curve up to curve *4*, and at pressure P_1 the vessel would be completely occluded. Before flow could start again, pressure in the vessel would have to rise. If it rose to P_2, flow would restart and a new equilibrium would be established between wall tension, pressure, and radius.

(A & B from Carl F. Rothe, "Fluid Dynamics." In E. E. Selkurt (Ed.), *Physiology.* Boston: Little, Brown, 1963.)

lowered resistance, without any change in the driving force (Fig. A 4A). For this reason it becomes very important to define the distensibility function.

The constricting force in equilibrium with and holding back the distending force is due to the circumferential tension (S), expressed in dynes per unit length of the cylindrical vessel. If the vessel is in a state of equilibrium, the force distending the vessel (P_{TM}) must be restrained by an equal and opposite force in the vessel wall. In an elastic tube, the interrelationship of tension in the wall, transmural pressure, and vessel size will predict the needed wall strength and the effect of change in pressure on radius and thus resistance.

The interrelationship of these opposing forces can be derived by using the principle of so-called virtual work. If the radius is increased by a very small amount, Δr, the work done to stretch the tube must equal the resulting change in potential energy stored as elastic energy in the vessel wall (law of conservation of energy). Since work is the movement of a force through a distance, the work done to increase the radius by Δr is equal to the force P_{TM} acting over the area $2\pi rl$ through a distance Δr. The work will be

$$W = 2\pi rl \times P_{TM}\Delta r$$

Since the vessel will be stretched by this work, the area of the wall will be increasead by an equal amount from $2\pi rl$ to $2\pi rl + 2\pi\Delta rl$. The increase in surface area is $2\pi\Delta rl$. Therefore, the increase in surface energy or the elastic potential energy opposing the pressure equals the change in area times the tension, S.

$$PE = 2\pi Sl\Delta r$$

During equilibrium the work done by the pressure to stretch the vessel must be equal to the added elastic potential energy stored by the vessel wall. Equating the last two equations above,

$$2\pi rl \times P_{TM}\Delta r = 2\pi Sl\Delta r$$

Reducing $\qquad\qquad\qquad P_{TM}r = S$

and, therefore $\qquad\qquad\qquad P_{TM} = \dfrac{S}{r}$

This states that the smaller the tube, the less effect a change in pressure will have on the amount of tension or structural strength required to contain the transmural pressure. Conversely, a dilated vessel will have more tension on its wall at any given pressure than a small one, or a dilated heart will have to produce a greater contractual force to create a given pressure than a small heart. For this same reason, after an aneurysm reaches a critical size, the danger of rupture becomes acute.

The actual size of a given biological tube will be determined by the make-up of its wall. It is interesting that large tubes required to have greater wall tension have greater amounts of elastic tissue which can maintain size without energy expenditure. The elastic fibers serve to contain the general high pressure, while the muscle fibers only actively alter the resistance. As the vessels decrease in size and require less structural strength to contain the pressure, they have relatively less elastic tissue and more muscle.

MECHANICS OF PULSATILE FLOW

The laws of fluid mechanics discussed up to this point can be applied only under very specific conditions, one of which is a steady flow rate. In the biological tube system the flow is phasic (Fig. A-5A). Air flow in and out of the lungs is truly alternating; a given volume flows in and a like volume out. In the vascular system flow is unidirectional in a closed circuit, but it is phasic with surges of pressure and flow in arteries as the ventricle ejects blood. These pulses are mostly damped out by the time blood reaches the capillaries. The flow in the arteries is a pulsed, D.C. flow and its wave pattern is depicted in Figure A-5B.

To make the tracings in Figures A-5A and B, the oscillograph moved the paper from left to right at a given speed while the pen was deflected up or down. The vertical movement of the pen is a function of the flow rate; the greater the excursion from the zero level, the higher the flow at that instant. Thus the horizontal axis records time and the vertical axis flow rate or amplitude.

THE SINE WAVE AND PHASE

A pure sine wave similar to those in Figure A-6A (below) can be traced by attaching a pen to a rotating wheel and drawing a paper under it. The farther the pen is from the axis of the wheel, the greater will be the maximum height or amplitude of the wave. Each time the wheel turns through one complete cycle of 360° (2π radians in algebraic terms), a sine wave is traced. This is a perfectly symmetrical wave equal in its rate and degree of rise and fall. As the disc spins faster, a greater number of such waves will be traced per second, a faster frequency. Such a wave is called a sine wave, because it is defined by the

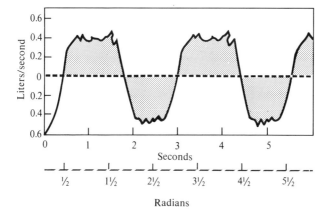

A

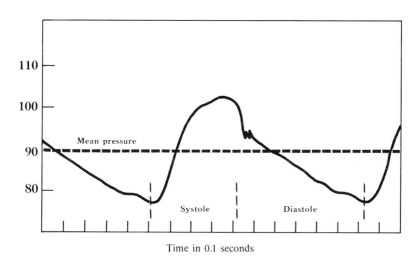

B

Fig. A-5. (A) Typical oscillograph tracing of air flow into and out of the lungs. The horizontal axis can be measured in units of time or as angular velocity radians. The vertical axis is flow rate. At the start of inspiration flow is zero. It rises to a peak flow rate at midinspiration and falls back to zero at end-inspiration; then the direction is reversed during expiration, with a similar pattern of rise and fall. (B) A typical arterial pulse tracing. This pressure wave is really very similar to the respiratory flow wave. Rather than oscillating about zero pressure, it oscillates about the mean arterial pressure of 90 mm. Hg.

trignometric function, sine of an angle. The sine of the angle is equal to the distance the pen has risen above the zero level divided by the distance from the center of the wheel to the pen, OB/CB. The distance from the center of the wheel is equal to maximum amplitude. Therefore, the sine of the angle at any point on the curve is equal to the amplitude at that point over the maximum amplitude. When the pen on the disc is above the zero level, the sine of the angle at any moment will be positive, and when it is below the zero level, it will be negative.

The rate of change of the ratio of the amplitude at any point to the maximum amplitude describes how fast the angle Θ is changing. This is called the *angular velocity* of the sine wave. If the angle increases from zero to Θ in time T, the angular velocity $W = \Theta/T$ radians or Θ degrees in T seconds or W radians or degrees per second. This is another measure of frequency. For example, from Figure 5a one complete cycle of respiration takes three seconds, or the frequency is twenty per minute. If this were a pure sine wave, the angular velocity of the wave would be 2π radians, 360 degrees, in each cycle, or $2\pi/3$ radians per second. The distance along the horizontal axis can therefore also have the dimensions of radians or degrees per second.

In all systems in which fluid is flowing, the pressure and flow waves can be recorded. They both have the same frequency but do not start and finish each cycle at precisely the same moment (Fig. A-6B). Figure A-6C depicts such a system in which a second pen is placed on the disc on another radial line. Thus, the second pen will cross the zero line after the first pen. This is called *phase lag*. The difference between the angle of the curve described by the first pen and that described by the second pen is the *phase shift*. By measuring the number of radians or degrees along the horizontal axis, the number of degrees of difference between the two can be measured. The phase shift is then expressed as a phase angle betwen the two waves. The lag in time between the two curves can be determined by noting the difference in phase, angle, and frequency. For example, if the frequency is $2\pi/3$ radians per second and the phase difference is $\frac{1}{2}\pi$ radians, the time lag between waves is three-quarters of a second.

Physiological wave forms are not pure sine waves (Fig. A-7). They are not precisely symmetrical, and their angular velocity is not constant. However, a complicated wave form such as this can be resolved into a series of sine waves: the fundamental wave at the frequency of respiration plus waves at two, three, four, etc., times this fundamental frequency. Thus with computational techniques these waves can be resolved into their components, permitting use of principles based on sine wave analysis as described below.

FORCING AND IMPEDANCE

In the blood vessels the simple description of flow alternating about zero or flow just in one direction and then in the other does not hold. However, an analogy can be used. If the mean pressure is determined, it is that level at which the excursions above and below the line are equal. The flow and pressure in the bloodstream therefore describe an alternating flow and pressure about a steady, positive flow.

A pressure wave is a measure of the forcing and a flow wave a measure of the movement in a fluid system. For fluid to flow, there must be a force applied to the system to set it in motion and to maintain it in motion. In the vascular and respiratory systems the tubes are elastic and can be stretched, and in the lungs the alveoli must be stretched to accommodate more volume. There is resistance to flow through the tubes, and the liquid has inertia. To set the system in motion, the opposition of each of these elements must be overcome by the driving force. If a given force is applied, the amount of flow resulting will depend on the impediment to flow offered by three elements—the elasticity or compliance, the resistance, and the inertance.*

RESPONSE OF DIFFERENT ORDER SYSTEMS

The way a system will respond when force is applied depends on whether it has only rigidity; or rigidity and friction; or rigidity, friction, and inertia. The formula which covers all circumstances is:

$$F = Sl + R\dot{V} + Ma$$

For a flow system, in which volume is substituted for length, pressure for force, and compliance for stiffness, the equation is:

$$P = \frac{1}{C}\Delta V + R\dot{V} + M\ddot{V}$$

where C = compliance
          ΔV = change in volume
          $\dot{V}$ = flow
          M = mass
          $\ddot{V}$ = rate of change of flow

*In an electrical analog, compliance is equivalent to capacitance and inertance to inductance.

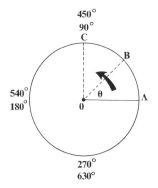

450°
90°
C

B

540°
180°

θ

A

270°
630°

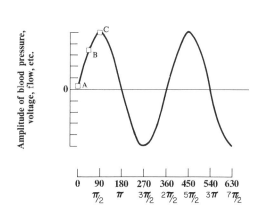

Amplitude of blood pressure, voltage, flow, etc.

0

C

B

A

0   90   180   270   360   450   540   630
     π/2   π   3π/2 2π/2 5π/2 3π   7π/2

Time, degrees or radians

A

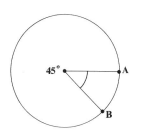

45°   A

B

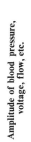

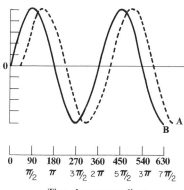

Amplitude of blood pressure, voltage, flow, etc.

0

A

B

0   90   180   270   360   450   540   630
     π/2   π   3π/2 2π   5π/2 3π   7π/2

Time, degrees or radians

B

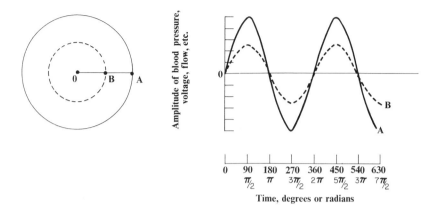

C

Fig. A-6. (A) The principle of tracing a sine wave. If a pen is attached to the disc *A* and paper is drawn from left to right as the disc rotates, a curve as depicted will be transcribed. The amplitude is measured by the distance above or below the zero line. The distance along the horizontal axis can be measured in time, in degrees, or in radians. If the speed at which the disc is spinning (frequency per second) is known, then angles or degrees can be converted to time.

(B) Phase lag or shift. Two curves are inscribed in the same manner as depicted in (A) with one pen 45 degrees away from the other. Pen *A* describes the dotted line which crosses zero at one-sixth of a cycle, 45 degrees, or π radians before the solid line described by pen *B*. The phase lag or shift between curve *A* and *B* is 45 degrees.

(C) Difference in amplitude. In this illustration the two pens are on the same radial line, but *B* is only one-half the distance from the axis as *A*. The curves are exactly in phase, but the amplitude of *A* is twice that of *B*.

$\dot{V}$ is the flow or the rate of change of volume per second $\Delta V/\text{sec.}$, or the first derivative of volume with respect to time. $\ddot{V}$ is the rate of change of flow or the change in volume per second per second $\Delta V/\text{sec.}/\text{sec.}$

A zero-order system is one in which no resistance or inertia is present. Such a system does not exist, but it can be approached in a fluid system if the flow rate is very slow. In a zero-order system all the pressure applied would be used to stretch a vessel (or the lung) to a given size or volume; none would be acting to overcome friction or inertance. In a first-order system resistance and compliance are present, but there is no inertance. Since air is so light and frequency so low in the pulmonary system, the inertance is very small and is usually neglected. For this reason the pulmonary system is often analyzed as a second-order system, a system with only compliance and resistance. In fact, all phasic flow can

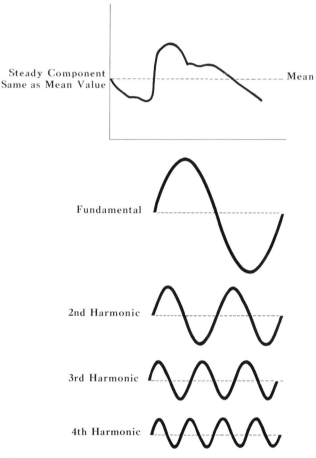

Fig. A-7. Fourier series analysis. Any complex wave form can be separated mathematically into component sine waves of the fundamental frequency and those twice, thrice, etc., the fundamental frequency. Each of these components has a given amplitude and phase and oscillates around the mean pressure. The mean pressure plus the sum of the waves reconstructs the original. In physiological systems, the first five harmonics contain all the useful information. This technique is very useful, since all theoretical flow analysis applies only to sine waves.

only be completely described as a third-order system, one with resistance, compliance, and inertance.

The same principles apply to electrical systems.

$$E = \frac{1}{C} \times Q + RI + L\dot{I}$$

where E = voltage
     C = capacitance
     Q = charge
     R = resistance
     I = current
     $\dot{I}$ = rate of change in current

and where $\dot{I}$ is the first derivative of current flow with respect to time.

To understand the effect of the pulsatile flow on the forcing required, it is best to analyze the effect of each of the retarding factors separately. The usual method of measuring the impediment to flow in the vascular tree is to calculate the mean pressure and mean flow. Then, mean pressure divided by flow equals the resistance. If one attempts to turn this around and use the resistance and cardiac output (mean flow) to back-calculate for the forcing or pressure that will be required, the predicted pressure is different from the measured pressure required.

RESISTANCE IN A PULSATILE SYSTEM

The reason for the discrepancy described above can best be understood by considering the amount of power or energy that will be dissipated in moving the fluid. The simplest theoretical case is a system with only resistance and no compliance or inertance. In such a system the power dissipated will be turned to heat. For the steady flow state, i.e., for mean pressure and flow, the level of power dissipated as heat will be equal to the product of flow rate times pressure:

$$\text{Pow}_{\text{D.C.}} = \text{P}_{\text{D.C.}} \times \text{V}_{\text{D.C.}}$$

The power dissipated in a pure A.C. circuit is equal to maximum amplitude of the pressure wave (Pm) times maximum amplitude of flow wave ($\dot{\text{V}}$m) over two, multiplied by the cosine of the phase angle between the two.

$$\text{Pow}_{\text{A.C.}} = \frac{\text{P}_{\text{m}} \times \dot{\text{V}}_{\text{m}}}{2} \text{Cos } \Theta$$

If there is only resistance in the system, the phase of the two waves, flow and pressure, will be exactly the same and Θ will be zero. The cosine of zero is one; thus, the power dissipation for the pulsatile wave equals (Pm $\times$ $\dot{\text{V}}$m)/2. In pulsed D.C. flow the potential energy converted to heat is the sum of that due to A.C. flow and that due to D.C. flow.

Thus in pulsed D.C. flow more energy is required to overcome friction for a given volume of fluid to be moved than if the flow and pressure were not pulsatile. The amount of potential energy converted to heat by a given resistance in a pulsatile system is not affected by frequency but only by the amplitude of pulse and pressure waves. The portion of total power dissipated as heat due to pulsation in a phasic D.C. system depends on the relationship of the mean pressure to the pulse pressure.

During pulsatile flow, when an elastic element is added to the system, it absorbs some of the potential energy represented by pressure on the pulse upstroke, when the elastic element is stretched; thus, the system can accommodate more volume. On the downstroke the vessel or alveolus contracts, using the potential energy stored to express the stored volume. Thus there is no net gain or loss of volume, just a damping of the surges of flow and pressure.

The inertance has a similar effect during upstroke. Some potential energy or pressure is expended and converted to kinetic energy as the system is accelerated. During downstroke, as the system slows, the kinetic energy is converted back to potential energy. A resistance converts potential energy to heat and it is lost to the system; this is not true in compliance or inertance, where the energy is stored or transformed and the flow wave altered. The alteration induced by compliance and inertance is called reactance. If the type of compliant unit and inertance are known, their effect on the system can be determined. The total effect of the resistance and compliant and inertant reactance is called the *impedance*.

The effect of the resistance, elasticity, and inertance in the phase and amplitude of flow pressure waves requires understanding of the interplay of these three factors when the system is phasic. Resistance has been defined earlier as having the effects of interconnecting resistances in series or parallel. The way resistance, compliance, and inertance are arranged in the circuit is as important in a phasic flow system as whether resistance is in parallel or series in a D.C. system.

ELASTICITY AND COMPLIANCE

The elastic nature of the biological system acts to smooth surges of pressure by expanding the walls of the vessels, bronchi, and alveoli as the pressure rises and then contracting the walls again as the pressure falls. This elastic quality is analogous to a capacitor in an electrical system. The elastic element never allows any flow through it, but the flow of air just surges in during a rise in pressure and out during a fall. Thus, during rises in pressure, the vessels or alveoli store volume and potential energy. A capacitor in an electrical circuit does exactly the same thing during periods of rise in voltage; it stores charge and, when the voltage decreases, it releases the charge. For a given unit rise in pressure, the amount of volume that can be absorbed is a function of the physical characteristics of the elastic element.

The distensibility, or, in physiological terms, the compliance of a tube or an alveolus is defined as the added volume which can be accommodated for any given increment in pressure.

$$V = C \times P$$

$$C = \frac{V}{P}$$

$$P = \frac{1}{C} V$$

The compliance is a function of the size of the elastic elements and the distensibility of these elements. More precisely stated, $C = KV$ in which K is a constant that depends on the type, arrangement, and volume of the elastic elements. It is important to reemphasize that a fluid cannot flow through these compliant elements; it can only surge in during one phase of pressure change and out during the other. Only if there is physical rupture or destruction of the system can blood or gas flow through these elements.

Any biological system is made up of many different compliant elements. The effects of these combinations are the reverse of the effects of combinations of resistances. When a group of compliances or capacitors is connected in series, the total compliance or capacitance is less than that of the smallest element (similar to resistance in parallel).

Series compliance: $\dfrac{1}{C} = \dfrac{1}{C_1} + \dfrac{1}{C_2} + \dfrac{1}{C_3}$

When compliances are connected in parallel, the total compliance is equal to the sum of the various compliances (two lungs can accommodate more air at any given distending pressure than one can).

INERTANCE

When a mass of any kind is accelerated or started to move, a certain force is required to overcome the inertia to get it started. The mass impedes the motion, and the greater the mass, the larger the impedance to acceleration.

$$X_L = \frac{1}{2} Mv^2$$

The effects of inertia will be manifest only when the fluid flow is changing with respect to time. That is, the rate of flow must be phasic or alternating. When inductances are added, they are similar to resistors.

Series: $$L = L_1 + L_2 + L_3 \cdots$$

Parallel: $$\frac{1}{L} = \frac{1}{L_1} + \frac{1}{L_2} + \frac{1}{L_3} \cdots$$

REACTANCE AND IMPEDANCE

The nature of reactance can be defined much as Ohm's law defines resistance. The amount of volume stored in a compliant element will depend on the pressure and the time during which this pressure is applied. Since flow is the rate of change of volume, at a fast frequency more fluid will flow because the volume flows in and out of the compliant element more often per unit of time. Thus reactance is affected by frequency as well as by the compliance. The relation between flow, pressure, and compliance is:

$$\dot{V} = P(2\pi f C)$$

$$2\pi f C = \frac{\dot{V}}{P}$$

$$\frac{\dot{V}}{P} = \frac{1}{2\pi f C}$$

$$X_C = \frac{1}{2\pi f C}$$

The reactance term X_C is used rather than resistance, since the reactance does not dissipate energy as heat but only transforms it during the phasic changes in flow and pressure. The above relationship predicts that the compliant reactance falls as the frequency and compliance increase, since each of these is in the denominator.

Inertial reactance has a different relationship. It is derived as follows:

$$\dot{V} = \frac{P}{2\pi f L}$$

$$\frac{P}{\dot{V}} = 2\pi f L$$

$$X_L = 2\pi f L$$

The inertial reactance increases as the frequency and mass increase.

If all three elements are present, they all affect the relationship between flow and pressure. In a series circuit the relationship is:

$$P = \dot{V}\sqrt{R^2 + X^2}$$

$$\frac{P_m}{\dot{V}_m} = \sqrt{R^2 + X^2}$$

where P_M and $\dot{V}_M$ equal the maximum amplitudes of the pressure and flow waves. If the expressions for inertia and compliance are substituted for X, the phase relationship between X_C and X_L will be known.

In a purely compliant system (Fig. A-8), as the fluid starts to flow into the compliant element, the pressure across the element will be at a minimum and pressure will rise to a maximum as flow stops at maximum volume. Since flow maximum occurs when pressure is at a minimum in a system with only compliant reactance, flow leads pressure by 90°.

The effect of pure inductance on the relationship between the flow and pressure waves is the opposite. To start the flow and overcome the inertia, the forcing pressure will have to be at its maximum and the flow rate will steadily increase as the accelerating pressure falls to zero; so, in this instance, pressure leads flow by 90 degrees. Thus if the reactances due to pure compliance and pure inertance are 180 degrees out of phase, they will have opposing effects on the systems, and, if present together, the net effect will be the difference between the two. If the values for compliant and inertial reactance are substituted, the impedance Z equals:

$$Z = \sqrt{R^2 + \left(2\pi f L - \frac{1}{2\pi f C}\right)^2}$$

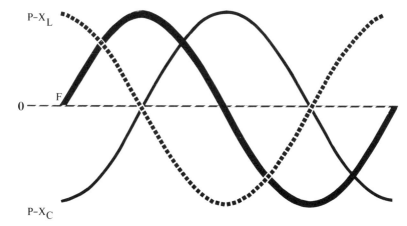

Fig. A-8. Phase relationship between flow wave (*heavy line*) and pressure (*thin line*) in a system with only reactance. With a pure capacitative reactance, the pressure (*thin line*) lags 90 degrees behind flow; that is, its peak pressure is reached one-quarter of a cycle after peak flow is reached. With a pure inductive reactance, the peak pressure (*dotted line*) is reached 90 degrees or one-quarter cycle before the peak pressure. If both inductance and capacitance are present, the resultant phase difference between flow and pressure and amplitude of the pressure wave will depend on the relative values of X_L and X_C and R.

The relationship of impedance, resistance, and reactance in a series circuit thus has the relationship of the sides of a right triangle.

$$Z^2 = R^2 + X^2$$

If any two of the three values are known, the third can be calculated from the above geometric relationship. (Fig. A-9). Using trigonometry, similar calculations can be made. If Z and R are known, then cos Θ equals R/Z, so the phase angle between the flow and pressure waves can be calculated. If R and X are known, the phase angle can be calculated using the tangent function, and if X and Z are known, the sine function will give the phase angle. Likewise, if the phase angle between flow and pressure and the impedance are known, the reactance and resistance can be determined.

This concept can be used further to predict the amplitude of the flow wave at any given frequency if the amplitude of the pressure or forcing wave is held constant while the impedance is increased.

$$Z = \frac{P}{\dot{V}} \qquad \text{if } P = K \qquad \text{and } \dot{V} = \frac{K}{Z}$$

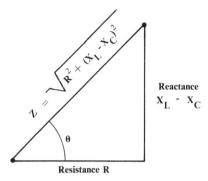

Fig. A-9. Geometric representation of the relationship between compliance, resistance, and reactance in a series circuit. If the phase angle and any one of the three quantities—reactance, resistance, or compliance—is known, the others can be calculated using the appropriate trigonometric function to define the relationship between the known and unknown. For example, sin Θ equals X/Z.

The amplitude of the flow wave will be proportional to $1/Z$ times the pressure. To hold flow constant at a given frequency as the impedance rises, pressure amplitude will have to rise in proportion to the rise in impedance. In other words, a greater driving force will be required to maintain a constant flow if the impeding force increases.

Since the reactance associated with compliance and inertance is affected by frequency, the impedance must be frequency-dependent. Thus any such system will have a time constant—the amount of time it takes the system to respond to any given forcing.

An example of a first-order system containing compliance and resistance would be an alveolus with its connecting bronchial tube. If the pressure pushing air into the alveolus is zero and is instantaneously raised to P_I, how fast will the pressure in the alveolus rise with respect to time, or, how long will it take the pressure to equal the forcing pressure? This relationship can be determined by using calculus to solve with respect to time the equation:

$$P = R\dot{V} + \frac{1}{C}\Delta V$$

which can be written:

$$P = R\frac{dV}{dt} + \frac{1}{C}\Delta V$$

Integrating this equation,

$$P_o = P_I(1 - e^{-t/RC})$$

where P_I equals the forcing pressure; P_O the pressure in the alveolus at any time, t; and e the base of natural logarithms, or 2.73.

Expressed in words, this equation states that the pressure in the alveolus at any given time after the application of the pressure will be equal to the initial pressure times a factor which is affected by the elapsed time, the resistance, and the compliance. The term $-t/RC$ will equal one when the time is equal to the product of the resistance times the compliance. If the exponent factor $-t/RC$ equals one, then the expression $1 - e^{-t/RC}$ equals $(1 - 2.73^{-1})$ or $\left(1 - \dfrac{1}{2.73}\right)$ or 0.63. Then, at a time when t equals RC, the pressure in the alveolus will have risen to 63% of the forcing pressure; and in three times RC, P_o will be 95% of P_I. The product of RC is therefore called the time constant, since it predicts how fast the system will respond to a forcing. The more elastic a vessel is or the higher the resistance, the longer it will take to completely respond to a given forcing.

A system with inertance also is affected by time. The formula in this case is:

$$P_I = P_o(1 - e^{-tR/L})$$

It is from these formulas that the frequency response of systems is determined. This time dependence is described in terms of the phase of the responding wave as compared to the input, a clinical example of which would be the blood pressure in the brachial artery compared to the blood pressure in the aortic root.

The time constant concept is of very real importance in predicting how biological systems will react. For example, if various regions of the lung have different time constants, the distribution of air to these various regions will be different. Those with short time constants will fill more completely and will empty completely before those with a long time constant.

An illustration of the practical use of the concept of impedance and phase angle is its use to analyze the resistance and compliance in the respiratory system. If the flow maximum and pressure maximum are known as well as the phase angle between the waves, then:

$$Z = \frac{P_m}{F_m}$$

and
$$\cos \Theta = \frac{R}{P_m/F_m}$$

or
$$R = \frac{\cos 2\Theta \times P_m}{F_m}$$

or
$$\sin \Theta = \frac{1/2\pi f C}{P_m/F_m}$$

$$\sin \Theta = \frac{F_m}{P_m \times 2\pi f C}$$

$$C = \frac{F_m}{P_m \times 2\pi f \sin \Theta}$$

In this manner, from an analysis of flow and transpulmonary pressure curves compliance and resistance of the lung can be determined.

Similar studies are possible in the vascular circuit, though they are much more complicated since the inertance cannot be ignored and the compliance is in parallel rather than in series with the resistance. The important fact is that by using electronic circuit theory and taking advantage of rather than ignoring the dynamic nature of fluid and airflow, much better descriptions and consequently improved understanding of biological flow systems are possible.

REFERENCES

REFERENCES

CHAPTER 1: FUNCTIONAL ANATOMY

FENN, W. O., and RAHN, H. (Eds.). *Handbook of Physiology*, Section 3: *Respiration*. Washington, D.C.: American Physiological Society, 1964.

    IRVING, L. Comparative Anatomy and Physiology of Gas Transport Mechanisms. Vol. I, Chap. 5, p. 177.

    KRAHL, V. E. Anatomy of the Mammalian Lung. Vol. I, Chap. 6, p. 213.

    WEIBEL, E. R. Morphometrics of the Lung. Vol. I, Chap. 7, p. 285.

    AGOSTONI, E. Action of Respiratory Muscles. Vol. I, Chap. 12, p. 377.

ENGEL, S. *Lung Structure*. Springfield, Ill.: Thomas, 1962.

KROGH, A. The rate of diffusion of gases through animal tissues with some remarks on the coefficient of invasion. *J. Physiol.* 52:391, 1919.

MILLER, W. S. *The Lung*. Springfield, Ill.: Thomas, 1937.

WEIBEL, E. R., and GOMEZ, D. M. Architecture of the human lung. *Science* 137:577, 1962.

CHAPTER 2: BLOOD GASES AND ACID-BASE BALANCE

FENN, W. O., and RAHN, H. (Eds.). *Handbook of Physiology*, Section 3: *Respiration*. Washington, D. C.: American Physiological Society, 1964.

    ROUGHTON, F. J. W. Transport of Oxygen and Carbon Dioxide. Vol. I, Chap. 31, p. 767.

    FORSTER, R. E. Rate of Gas Uptake by Red Cells. Vol. I, Chap. 32, p. 827.

ASTRUP, P. A new approach to acid-base metabolism. *Clin. Chem.* Vol. 7, No. 1, Feb., 1961.

BARCROFT, J. *The Respiratory Function of the Blood*. Cambridge: The University Press, 1914.

BARCROFT, J. *The Respiratory Function of the Blood. Part II. Haemoglobin*. Cambridge: The University Press, 1928.

BRACKETT, N. C., JR., COHEN, J., and SCHWARTZ, W. B. Carbon dioxide titration curve of normal man: Effect of increasing degrees of acute hypercapnia on acid-base equilibrium. *New Eng. J. Med.* 272:6, 1965.

Current concepts of acid-base measurement: Report of the New York Academy of Sciences Conference, Nov. 23–24, 1964. *Ann. N.Y. Acad. Sci.* 133:1, 1966.

DAVENPORT, H. W.   *The ABC of Acid-Base Chemistry* (4th ed.). Chicago: University of Chicago Press, 1958.

HILL, R. L., and FELLOWS, R. E.   Recent developments in hemoglobin structure and function. *Physiol. Physicians* Vol. 2, No. 9, Sept., 1964.

HUCKABEE, W. E.   Henderson vs. Hasslebach. *Clin. Res.* 9:116, 1961.

PERUTZ, M. F.   The hemoglobin molecule. *Sci. Amer.* 211:64 (Nov.), 1964.

PETERS, J. P., and VAN SLYKE, D. D.   Hemoglobin and Oxygen. In *Quantitative Clinical Chemistry*. Baltimore: Williams & Wilkins, 1931. P. 518. (Also published as *Hemoglobin and Oxygen: Carbonic Acid and Acid-Base Balance*. Baltimore: Williams & Wilkins, 1931.)

PITTS, R. F.   *Physiology of the Kidney and Body Fluids*. Chicago: Year Book, 1963.

ROUGHTON, F. J. W.   The Chemistry of Respiration. In D. J. C. CUNNINGHAM and B. B. LLOYD (Eds.), *The Regulation of Human Respiration*. Philadelphia: Davis, 1963. P. 33.

SCHWARTZ, W. B., BRACKETT, N. C., JR., and COHEN, J. J.   The response of extracellular hydrogen ion concentration to graded degrees of chronic hypercapnia: The physiologic limits of the defense of pH. *J. Clin. Invest.* 44:291, 1965.

WINTERS, R. W.   Terminology of acid-base disorders. *Ann. Intern. Med.* 63:873, 1965.

WINTERS, R. W., ENGEL, K., and DELL, R. B.   *Acid Base Physiology in Medicine: A Self-Instruction Program*. Cleveland, Ohio: The London Company, 1967.

CHAPTER 3:   VENTILATION

FENN, W. O., and RAHN, H. (Eds.)   *Handbook of Physiology,* Section 3: *Respiration*. Washington, D.C.: American Physiological Society, 1965.

TENNEY, S. M. and LAMB, T. W.   Physiological Consequences of Hypoventilation and Hyperventilation. Vol. II, Chap. 37, p. 979.

BRISCOE, W. A.   Lung Volumes. Vol. II, Chap. 53, p. 1345.

AUCHINCLOSS, J. H., JR.   Ventilatory Disturbances in Disease. Vol. II, Chap. 68, p. 1553.

COMROE J. H., JR., FORSTER, R. E., II, DuBOIS, A. B., BRISCOE, W. A., and CARLSEN, E.   *The Lung: Clinical Physiology and Pulmonary Function Tests* (2d ed.). Chicago: Year Book, 1962. Chap. 2, p. 7; Chap. 3, p. 27.

CHAPTER 4:   MECHANICAL PROPERTIES OF THE RESPIRATORY SYSTEM

FENN, W. O., and RAHN, H. (Eds.).   *Handbook of Physiology*, Section 3: *Respiration*. Washington, D.C.: American Physiological Society, 1964, 1965.

FENN, W. O.   Introduction to the Mechanics of Breathing. Vol. I, Chap. 10, p. 357.

MEAD, J., and MILIC-EMILI, J.   Theory and Methodology in Respiratory Mechanics with Glossary of Symbols. Vol. I, Chap. 11, p. 363.

AGOSTONI, E. Action of Respiratory Muscles. Vol. I, Chap. 12, p. 377.

AGOSTONI, E., and MEAD, J. Statics of the Respiratory System. Vol. I, Chap. 13, p. 387.

MEAD, J., and AGOSTONI, E. Dynamics of Breathing. Vol. I, Chap. 14, p. 411.

RADFORD, E. P., JR. Static Mechanical Properties of Mammalian Lungs. Vol. I, Chap. 15, p. 429.

DUBOIS, A. B. Resistance to Breathing. Vol. I, Chap. 16, p. 451.

OTIS, A. B. The Work of Breathing. Vol. I, Chap. 17, p. 463.

MARSHALL, R. Objective Tests of Respiratory Mechanics. Vol. II, Chap. 55, p. 1399.

CARO, C. G., BUTLER, J., and DUBOIS, A. B. Some effects of restriction of chest cage expansion on pulmonary function in man: An experimental study. *J. Clin. Invest.* 39:573, 1960.

CLEMENTS, J. A. Surface tension in the lungs. *Sci. Amer.* 207:120, 1962.

MEAD, J. Mechanical properties of lungs. *Physiol. Rev.* 41:281, 1961.

OTIS, A. B., MCKERROW, C. B., BARTLETT, R. A., MEAD, J., MCILROY, M. B., SELVERSTONE, N. J., and RADFORD, E. P. Mechanical factors in distribution of pulmonary ventilation. *J. Appl. Physiol.* 8:427, 1956.

PATTLE, R. E. Surface lining of lung alveoli. *Physiol. Rev.* 45:48, 1965.

SHARP, J. T., HENRY, J. P., SWEANY, S. K., MEADOWS, W. R., and PIETRAS, R. J. Effects of mass loading the respiratory system in man. *J. Appl. Physiol.* 19:959, 1964.

WIDDICOMBE, J. G. Regulation of tracheobronchial smooth muscle. *Physiol. Rev.* 43:1, 1963.

CHAPTER 5: PULMONARY CIRCULATION

HAMILTON, W. F., and DOW, P. (Eds.). *Handbook of Physiology,* Section 2: *Circulation.* Washington, D.C.: American Physiological Society, 1963.

SPENCER, M. P., and DENNISON, A. B., JR. Pulsatile Blood Flow in the Vascular System. Vol. II, Chap. 25, p. 839.

FISHMAN, A. P. Dynamics of the Pulmonary Circulation. Vol. II, Chap. 48, p. 1667.

FENN, W. O., and RAHN, H. (Eds.). *Handbook of Physiology,* Section 3: *Respiration.* Washington, D.C.: American Physiological Society, 1964, 1965.

MEAD, J., and WHITTENBERGER, J. L. Lung Inflation and Hemodynamics. Vol. I, Chap. 18, p. 477.

GREENE, D. G. Pulmonary Edema. Vol. II, Chap. 70, p. 1585.

ADAMS, W. R., and VEITH, I. (Eds.). *Pulmonary Circulation.* New York: Grune & Stratton, 1959.

AVIADO, D. M. *The Lung Circulation*: I. *Physiology and Pharmacology*; II. *Pathologic Physiology and Therapy of Diseases.* Oxford: Pergamon, 1965.

BLOUNT, S. G., JR., and VOGEL, J. H. K. Pulmonary hypertension. *Mod. Conc. Cardiovasc. Dis.* 36:61, 1967.

BRODY, J. S., STEMMLER, E. J., and DuBois, A. B. Longitudinal distribution of vascular resistance in the pulmonary arteries, capillaries, and veins. *J. Clin. Invest.* 47:783, 1968.

DALY, W. J., KRUMHOLZ, R. A., and ROSS, J. C. The venous pump in the legs as a determinant of pulmonary capillary filling. *J. Clin. Invest.* 44:271, 1965.

DRINKER, C. K. *Pulmonary Edema and Inflammation: An Analysis of Processes Involved in the Formation and Removal of Pulmonary Transudates and Exudates.* Cambridge, Mass.: Harvard University Press, 1945.

FISHMAN, A. P. Respiratory gases in the regulation of the pulmonary circulation. *Physiol. Rev.* 41:214, 1961.

HARVEY, R. M., ENSON, Y., BETTI, R., LEWIS, M. L., ROCHESTER, D. F., and FERRER, M. I. Further observations on the effect of hydrogen ion on the pulmonary circulation. *Circulation* 35:1019, 1967.

LEVINE, O. R., MELLINS, R. B., SENIOR, R. M., and FISHMAN, A. P. The application of Starling's law of capillary exchange to the lungs. *J. Clin. Invest.* 46:934, 1967.

MENON, N. D. High-altitude pulmonary edema: A clinical study. *New Eng. J. Med.* 273:66, 1965.

MILNOR, W. R., BERGEL, D. H., and BARGAINER, J. D. Hydraulic power associated with pulmonary blood flow and its relation to heart rate. *Circ. Res.* 19:467, 1966.

ROOS, A. Poiseuille's Law and Its Limitations in Vascular Systems. In R. F. GROVER (Ed.), *Progress in Research in Emphysema and Chronic Bronchitis: Normal and Abnormal Pulmonary Circulation.* Basel: Karger, 1963. P. 32.

STAUB, N. C., NAGANO, H., and PEARCE, M. L. Pulmonary edema in dogs, especially the sequence of fluid accumulation in the lungs. *J. Appl. Physiol.* 22:227, 1967.

CHAPTER 6: DIFFUSION

FENN, W. O., and RAHN, H. (Eds.). *Handbook of Physiology*, Section 3: *Respiration.* Washington, D.C.: American Physiological Society, 1964, 1965.

    FORSTER, R. E. Diffusion of Gases. Vol. I, Chap. 33, p. 839.

    FORSTER, R. E. Interpretation of Measurements of Pulmonary Diffusing Capacity. Vol. II, Chap. 59, p. 1453.

FORSTER, R. E. Exchange of gases between alveolar air and pulmonary capillary blood: Pulmonary diffusing capacity. *Physiol. Rev.* 37:391, 1957.

CHAPTER 7: COORDINATION OF VENTILATION AND PERFUSION

FENN, W. O., and RAHN, H. (Eds.). *Handbook of Physiology*, Section 3: *Respiration.* Washington, D.C.: American Physiological Society, 1964, 1965.

    BOUHUYS, A. Distribution of Inspired Gas in the Lungs. Vol. I, Chap. 29, p. 715.

RAHN, H., and FARHI, L. E.   Ventilation, Perfusion, and Gas Exchange—The V_A/Q Concept. Vol. I, Chap. 30, p. 735.

RILEY, R. L., and PERMUTT, S.   The Four-Quadrant Diagram for Analyzing the Distribution of Gas and Blood in the Lung. Vol. II, Chap. 56, p. 1413.

BATES, D. V.   Measurement of Regional Ventilation and Blood Flow Distribution. Vol. II, Chap. 57, p. 1425.

WEST, J. B.   The Effect of Uneven Blood Flow in the Lung on Regional Gas Exchange. Vol. II, Chap. 58, p. 1437.

COMROE, J. H., JR.   Pulmonary Gas Exchange. In D. J. C. CUNNINGHAM and B. B. LLOYD (Eds.), *The Regulation of Human Respiration*. Philadelphia: Davis, 1963. P. 45.

MEAD, J.   Mechanical properties of lungs. *Physiol. Rev.* 41:281, 1961.

WEST, J. B.   The Effect of Uneven Blood Flow in the Lung on Regional Gas Exchange. In R. F. GROVER (Ed.), *Progress in Research in Emphysema and Chronic Bronchitis: Normal and Abnormal Pulmonary Circulation*. Basel: Karger, 1963. P. 200.

WEST, J. B.   *Ventilation/Blood Flow and Gas Exchange*. Philadelphia: Davis, 1965.

CHAPTER 8:   CHEMICAL AND REFLEX REGULATION OF RESPIRATION

FENN, W. O., and RAHN, H. (Eds.).   *Handbook of Physiology*, Section 3: *Respiration*. Washington, D.C.: American Physiological Society, 1964, 1965.

WANG, S. C., and NGAI, S. H.   General Organization of Central Respiratory Mechanisms. Vol. I, Chap. 19, p. 487.

KELLOGG, R. H.   Central Chemical Regulation of Respiration. Vol. I, Chap. 20, p. 507.

CAMPBELL, E. J. M.   Motor Pathways. Vol. I, Chap. 21, p. 535.

LAMBERTSEN, C. J.   Effects of Drugs and Hormones on the Respiratory Response to Carbon Dioxide. Vol. I, Chap. 22, p. 545.

COMROE, J. H., JR.   The Peripheral Chemoreceptors. Vol. I, Chap. 23, p. 557.

WIDDICOMBE, J. G.   Respiratory Reflexes. Vol. I, Chap. 24, p. 585.

DEJOURS, P.   Control of Respiration in Muscular Exercise. Vol. I, Chap. 25, p. 631.

DEFARES, J. G.   Principles of Feedback Control and Their Application to the Respiratory Control System. Vol. I, Chap. 26, p. 649.

OTIS, A. B.   Quantitative Relationships in Steady-State Gas Exchange. Vol. I, Chap. 27, p. 681.

CHERNIACK, R. M.   Work of Breathing and the Ventilatory Response to CO_2. Vol. II, Chap. 60, p. 1469.

BULGER, R. J., SCHRIER, R. W., AREND, W. P., and SWANSON, A. G.   Spinal-fluid acidosis and the diagnosis of pulmonary encephalopathy. *New Eng. J. Med.* 274:433, 1966.

CUNNINGHAM, D. J. C., and LLOYD, B. B. (Eds.).   *The Regulation of Human Respiration*. Philadelphia: Davis, 1963.

DEJOURS, P.   *Respiration* (L. Farhi, Trans.). London; New York: Oxford University Press, 1966. "Neurogenesis—The Ventilatory System," p. 127, and "Regulation of Ventilation," p. 148.

GRAY, J. S. *Pulmonary Ventilation and Its Physiological Regulation.* Springfield, Ill.: Thomas, 1950.

MITCHELL, R. A., and SEVERINGHAUS, J. W. Cerebrospinal fluid and the regulation of respiration. *Physiol. Physicians* Vol. 3, No. 3, March, 1965.

POSNER, J. B., and PLUM, F. Spinal-fluid pH and neurologic symptoms in systemic acidosis. *New Eng. J. Med.* 277:605, 1967.

ROBIN, E. D. Abnormalities of acid-base regulation in chronic pulmonary disease, with special reference to hypercapnia and extracellular alkalosis. *New Eng. J. Med.* 268:917, 1963.

CHAPTER 9: THE ENERGY COST (WORK) OF BREATHING

FENN, W. O., and RAHN, H. (Eds.). *Handbook of Physiology*, Section 3: *Respiration.* Washington, D.C.: American Physiological Society, 1964, 1965.

    OTIS, A. B. The Work of Breathing. Vol. I, Chap. 17, p. 463.

    CHERNIACK, R. M. Work of Breathing and the Ventilatory Response to CO_2. Vol. II, Chap. 60, p. 1469.

COURNAND, A., RICHARDS, D. W., JR., BADER, R. A., BADER, M. E., and FISHMAN, A. P. The oxygen cost of breathing. *Trans. Ass. Amer. Physicians* 67:162, 1954.

KRIEGER, I., and WHITTEN, C. F. Work of respiration in bronchiolitis. *Amer. J. Dis. Child.* 107:386, 1964.

MILIC-EMILI, J., and PETIT, J. M. Mechanical efficiency of breathing. *J. Appl. Physiol.* 15:359, 1960.

OTIS, A. B. The work of breathing. *Physiol. Rev.* 34:449, 1954.

PETERS, R. M. Work of breathing following trauma. *J. Trauma* 8:915, 1968.

PETERS, R. M., and HEDGPETH, E. M., JR. Acid-base balance and respiratory work. *J. Thorac. Cardiovasc. Surg.* 52:649, 1966.

PETERS, R. M., HEDGPETH, E. M., JR., and GREENBERG, B. G. The effect of alterations in acid base balance on pulmonary mechanics. *J. Thorac. Cardiovasc. Surg.* 57:303, 1969.

SHARP, J. T., HENRY, J. P., SWEANY, S. K., MEADOWS, W. R., and PIETRAS, R. J. The total work of breathing in normal and obese men. *J. Clin. Invest.* 43:728, 1964.

WIDDICOMBE, J. G., and NADEL, J. A. Airway volume, airway resistance, and work and force of breathing: Theory. *J. Appl. Physiol.* 18:863, 1963.

CHAPTER 10: THE EFFECTS OF ENVIRONMENT AND THE LEVEL OF ACTIVITY

THE ATMOSPHERE—AIR POLLUTION—SMOKING

FENN, W. O., and RAHN, H. (Eds.). *Handbook of Physiology*, Section 3: *Respiration.* Washington, D.C.: American Physiological Society, 1965.

    STOKINGER, H. E. Pollutant Gases. Vol. II, Chap. 42, p. 1067.

    ROOT, W. S. Carbon Monoxide. Vol. II, Chap. 43, p. 1087.

COOPER, K. H., GEY, G. O., and BOTTENBERG, R. A. Effects of cigarette smoking on endurance performance. *J.A.M.A.* 203:189, 1968.

GOLDSMITH, J. R., and LANDAW, S. A. Carbon monoxide and human health. *Science* 162:1352, 1968.

PETERS, J. M., and FERRIS, B. G., JR. Smoking and morbidity in a college-age group. *Amer. Rev. Resp. Dis.* 95:783, 1967.

PETERS, J. M., and FERRIS, B. G., JR. Smoking, pulmonary function, and respiratory symptoms in a college-age group. *Amer. Rev. Resp. Dis.* 95:774, 1967.

HIGH ALTITUDE

FENN, W. O., and RAHN, H. (Eds.). *Handbook of Physiology*, Section 3: *Respiration.* Washington, D.C.: American Physiological Society, 1965.
    LUFT, U. C. Aviation Physiology—The Effects of Altitude. Vol. II, Chap. 44, p. 1099.
    CLAMANN, H. G. Space Physiology. Vol. II, Chap. 45, p. 1147.

ARIAS-STELLA, J., and SALDAÑA, M. The terminal portion of the pulmonary arterial tree in people native to high altitudes. *Circulation* 28: 915, 1963.

BARCROFT, J., BINGER, C. A., BOCK, A. V., DOGGART, J. H., FORBES, H. S., HARROP, G., MEAKINS, J. C., and REDFIELD, A. C. Observations upon the effect of high altitude on the physiological processes of the human body, carried out in the Peruvian Andes, chiefly at Cerro de Pasco. *Philosoph. Trans. Roy. Soc. London*, Series B, 211:351, 1922.

ROTH, E. M. Gas physiology in space operations. *New Eng. J. Med.* 275: 144, 1966.

HYPERBARIC ENVIRONMENTS

FENN, W. O., and RAHN, H. (Eds.). *Handbook of Physiology*, Section 3: *Respiration.* Washington, D.C.: American Physiological Society, 1965.
    BEHNKE, A. R., JR. Inert Gas Narcosis. Vol. II, Chap. 41, p. 1059.
    BEHNKE, A. R., JR., and LANPHIER, E. H. Underwater Physiology. Vol. II, Chap. 46, p. 1159.

Committee on Hyperbaric Oxygenation. *Fundamentals of Hyperbaric Medicine.* Washington, D.C.: National Academy of Sciences–National Research Council, 1966 (Pub. No. 1298).

WHIPPLE, H. E. (Ed.). Hyperbaric oxygenation. *Ann. N.Y. Acad. Sci.* 117:647, 1965.

DROWNING

FENN, W. O., and RAHN, H. (Eds.). *Handbook of Physiology*, Section 3: *Respiration.* Washington, D.C.: American Physiological Society, 1965.
    GREENE, D. G. Drowning. Vol. II, Chap. 47, p. 1195.

CRAIG, A. B., JR. Causes of loss of consciousness during underwater swimming. *J. Appl. Physiol.* 16:583, 1961.

DAVIS, J. H. Fatal underwater breath holding in trained swimmers. *J. Forensic Sci.* 6:301, 1961.

ELAM, J. O., RUBEN, A. M., and GREENE, D. G. Resuscitation of drowning victims. *J.A.M.A.* 174:13, 1960.

HADDY, T. B., and DISENHOUSE, R. B. Acute pulmonary edema due to near-drowning in fresh water. *J. Pediat.* 44:565, 1954.

SWANN, H. G. Mechanism of circulatory failure in fresh and sea water drowning (Editorial). *Circ. Res.* 4:241, 1956.

EXERCISE

FENN, W. O., and RAHN, H. (Eds.). *Handbook of Physiology*, Section 3: *Respiration*. Washington, D.C.: American Physiological Society, 1965. ASMUSSEN, E. Muscular Exercise. Vol. II, Chap. 36, p. 939.

SALTIN, B., BLOMQVIST, G., MITCHELL, J. H., JOHNSON, R. L., JR., WILDENTHAL, K., and CHAPMAN, C. B. Response to exercise after bed rest and after training. *Circulation* 37 (Suppl. 7):1, 1968.

SLEEP AND ANESTHESIA

FENN, W. O., and RAHN, H. (Eds.). *Handbook of Physiology*, Section 3: *Respiration*. Washington, D.C.: American Physiological Society, 1965. SEVERINGHAUS, J. W., and LARSON, C. P., JR. Respiration in Anesthesia. Vol. II, Chap. 49, p. 1219.

BELVILLE, J. W., HOWLAND, W. S., SEED, J. C., and HOUDE, R. W. The effect of sleep on the respiratory response to carbon dioxide. *Anesthesiology* 20:628, 1959.

FINK, B. R. Influence of cerebral activity in wakefulness on regulation of breathing. *J. Appl. Physiol.* 16:15, 1961.

FINK, B. R., HANKS, E. C., NGAI, S. H., and PAPPER, E. M. Central regulation of respiration during anesthesia and wakefulness. *Ann. N.Y. Acad Sci.* 109:892, 1963.

REED, D. J., and KELLOGG, R. H. Changes in respiratory response to CO_2 during natural sleep at sea level and at altitude. *J. Appl. Physiol.* 13:325, 1958.

REED, D. J., and KELLOGG, R. H. Effect of sleep on hypoxic stimulation of breathing at sea level and altitude. *J. Appl. Physiol.* 15:1130, 1960.

CHAPTER 11: AGE, HABITUS, AND DEGENERATIVE DISEASE

AGING

FENN, W. O., and RAHN, H. (Eds.). *Handbook of Physiology*, Section 3: *Respiration*. Washington, D.C.: American Physiological Society, 1965. BRISCOE, W. A. Lung Volumes. "Effect of Age on Lung Volumes." Vol. II, Chap. 53, p. 1360. RICHARDS, D. W. Pulmonary Changes Due to Aging. Vol. II. Chap. 66, p. 1525.

DILL, D. B., HORVATH, S. M., and CRAIG, F. N. Responses to exercise as related to age. *J. Appl. Physiol.* 12:195, 1958.

FRANK, N. R., MEAD, J., and FERRIS, B. G., JR. The mechanical behavior of the lungs in healthy elderly persons. *J. Clin. Invest.* 36:1680, 1957.

OBESITY

AMAD, K. H., BRENNAN, J. C., and ALEXANDER, J. K.   The cardiac pathology of chronic exogenous obesity. *Circulation* 32:740, 1965.

DEMPSEY, J. A., REDDAN, W., BALKE, B., and RANKIN, J.   Work capacity determinants and physiologic cost of weight-supported work in obesity. *J. Appl. Physiol.* 21:1815, 1966.

DEMPSEY, J. A., REDDAN, W., RANKIN, J., and BALKE, B.   Alveolar-arterial gas exchange during muscular work in obesity. *J. Appl. Physiol.* 21:1807, 1966.

HOLLEY, H. S., MILIC-EMILI, J., BECKLAKE, M. R., and BATES, D. V.   Regional distribution of pulmonary ventilation and perfusion in obesity. *J. Clin. Invest.* 46:475, 1967.

KAUFMAN, B. J., FERGUSON, M. H., and CHERNIACK, R. M.   Hypoventilation in obesity. *J. Clin. Invest.* 38:500, 1959.

NAIMARK, A., and CHERNIACK, R. M.   Compliance of the respiratory system and its components in health and obesity. *J. Appl. Physiol.* 15: 377, 1960.

ABDOMINAL DISTENSION

FENN, W. O., and RAHN, H. (Eds.).   *Handbook of Physiology*, Section 3: *Respiration*. Washington, D.C.: American Physiological Society, 1965.
GAENSLER, E. A.   Lung Displacement: Abdominal Enlargement, Pleural Space Disorders, Deformities of the Thoracic Cage. "Abdominal Enlargement." Vol. II, Chap. 73, p. 1624.

ABELMANN, W. H., FRANK, N. R., GAENSLER, E. A., and CUGELL, D. W.   Effects of abdominal distension by ascites on lung volumes and ventilation. *Arch. Intern. Med.* 93:528, 1954.

GEE, J. B. L., PACKER, B. S., MILLEN, J. E., and ROBIN, E. D.   Pulmonary mechanics during pregnancy. *J. Clin. Invest.* 46:945, 1967.

CHEST DEFORMITIES

FENN, W. O., and RAHN, H. (Eds.).   *Handbook of Physiology*, Section 3: *Respiration*. Washington, D.C.: American Physiological Society, 1965.
GAENSLER, E. A.   Lung Displacement: Abdominal Enlargement, Pleural Space Disorders, Deformities of the Thoracic Cage. Vol. II, Chap. 73, p. 1623.

BERGOFSKY, E. H., TURINO, G. M., and FISHMAN, A. P.   Cardiorespiratory failure in kyphoscoliosis. *Medicine* 38:263, 1959.

BEVEGARD, S.   Postural circulatory changes at rest and during exercise in patients with funnel chest, with special reference to factors affecting the stroke volume. *Acta Med. Scand.* 171:695, 1962.

CARO, C. G., and DUBOIS, A. B.   Pulmonary function in kyphoscoliosis. *Thorax* 16:282, 1961.

FABRICIUS, J., DAVIDSEN, H. G., and HANSEN, A. T.   Cardiac function in funnel chest. *Danish Med. Bull.* 4:251, 1957.

FINK, A., RIVIN, A., and MURRAY, J. F.   Pectus excavatum. An analysis of twenty-seven cases. *Arch. Intern. Med.* 108:427, 1961.

FISHMAN, A. P., TURINO, G. M., and BERGOFSKY, E. H.   Disorders of the respiration and circulation in subjects with deformities of the thorax. *Mod. Conc. Cardiovasc. Dis.* 27:449, 1958.

HANSEN, J., and JACOBY, O.   The respiratory function before and following surgery in cases of funnel chest. *Acta Chir. Scand.* 111:226, 1956.

RAVITCH, M. M.   Pectus excavatum and heart failure. *Surgery* 30:178, 1951.

DEGENERATIVE LUNG DISEASE

FENN, W. O., and RAHN, H. (Eds.).   *Handbook of Physiology*, Section 3: *Respiration*. Washington, D.C.: American Physiological Society, 1965.
  DuBOIS, A. B.   Obstructions of the Airway and Restrictions of Lung Expansion. Vol. II, Chap. 63, p. 1505.
  AUCHINCLOSS, J. H., JR.   Ventilatory Disturbances in Disease. Vol. II, Chap. 68, p. 1553.
  BECKLAKE, M. R.   Pneumoconioses. Vol. II, Chap. 71, p. 1601.

LENFANT, C., and PACE, W. R., JR.   Alterations of ventilation to perfusion ratios distribution associated with successive clinical stages of pulmonary emphysema. *J. Clin. Invest.* 44:1566, 1965.

LOPEZ-MAJANO, V., TOW, D. E., and WAGNER, H. N., JR.   Regional distribution of pulmonary arterial blood flow in emphysema. *J.A.M.A.* 197:81, 1966.

ROGERS, R. M., DuBOIS, A. B., and BLAKEMORE, W. S.   Effect of removal of bullae on airway conductance and conductance volume ratios. *J. Clin. Invest.* 47:2569, 1968.

PULMONARY EMBOLUS

FRED, H. L., AXELRAD, M. A., LEWIS, J. M., and ALEXANDER, J. K.   Rapid resolution of pulmonary thromboemboli in man: An angiographic study. *J.A.M.A.* 196:1137, 1966.

LEVY, S. E., STEIN, M., TOTTEN, R. S., BRUDERMAN, I., WESSLER, S., and ROBIN, E. D.   Ventilation-perfusion abnormalities in experimental pulmonary embolism. *J. Clin. Invest.* 44:1699, 1965.

SABISTON, D. C., JR., and WAGNER, H. N., JR.   The diagnosis of pulmonary embolism by radioisotope scanning. *Ann. Surg.* 160:575, 1964.

SASAHARA, A. A.   Pulmonary vascular responses to thromboembolism. *Mod. Conc. Cardiovasc. Dis.* 36:55, 1967.

WAGNER, H. N., JR., and JONES, R. H.   Massive pulmonary embolism. *Physiol. Physicians* Vol. 3, Feb., 1965.

CHAPTER 12:   THE EFFECT OF INJURY ON PULMONARY FUNCTION

POSTOPERATIVE RESPIRATORY FUNCTION

BRYANT, L. R., SPENCER, F. C., GREENLAW, R. H., PRATHNADI, P., and BOWLIN, J. W.   Postoperative changes in regional pulmonary blood flow. *J. Thorac. Cardiovasc. Surg.* 53:64, 1967.

CLOWES, G. H. A., JR., ALICHNIEWICZ, A., DEL GUERCIO, L. R. M., and GILLESPIE, D. The relationship of postoperative acidosis to pulmonary and cardiovascular function. *J. Thorac. Cardiovasc. Surg.* 39:1, 1960.

COLES, J. C., BUTTIGLIERO, J. R., and GERGELY, N. F. Pulmonary vascular resistance following thoracotomy. *Arch. Surg.* (Chicago) 91:55, 1965.

ELLISON, L. T., DUKE, J. F., III, and ELLISON, R. G. Pulmonary compliance following open-heart surgery and its relationship to ventilation and gas exchange. *Circulation* 35 (Suppl. 1):217, 1967.

ELLISON, R. G., HALL, D. P., TALLEY, R. E., and ELLISON, L. T. Analysis of ventilatory and respiratory function after 82 thoracic and nonthoracic operations. *Amer. Surg.* 26:485, 1960.

GEHA, A. S., SESSLER, A. D., and KIRKLIN, J. W. Alveolar–arterial oxygen gradients after open intracardiac surgery. *J. Thorac. Cardiovasc. Surg.* 51:609, 1966.

HEDLEY-WHYTE, J., CORNING, H., LAVER, M. B., AUSTEN, W. G., and BENDIXEN, H. H. Pulmonary ventilation-perfusion relations after heart valve replacement or repair in man. *J. Clin. Invest.* 44:406, 1965.

KINNEY, J. M., and ROE, C. F. Caloric equivalent of fever: I. Patterns of postoperative response. *Ann. Surg.* 156:610, 1962.

OKINAKA, A. J. Postoperative pattern of breathing and compliance. *Arch. Surg.* (Chicago) 92:887, 1966.

PALMER, K. N. V., GARDINER, A. J. S., and MCGREGOR, M. H. Hypoxaemia after partial gastrectomy. *Thorax* 20:73, 1965.

PETERS, R. M., WELLONS, H. A., JR., and HTWE, T. M. Total compliance and work of breathing after thoracotomy. *J. Thorac. Cardiovasc. Surg.* 57:348, 1969.

THUNG, N., HERZOG, P., CHRISTLIEB, I. I., THOMPSON, W. M., JR., and DAMMANN, J. F., JR. The cost of respiratory effort in postoperative cardiac patients. *Circulation* 28:552, 1963.

CHEST CAGE INJURIES

MALONEY, J. V., JR., SCHMUTZER, K. J., and RASCHKE, E. Paradoxical respiration and "Pendelluft." *J. Thorac. Cardiovasc. Surg.* 41:291, 1961.

PETERS, R. M. Work of breathing following trauma. *J. Trauma* 8:915, 1968.

ATELECTASIS AND RUPTURED BRONCHUS

PETERS, R. M., BENSON, W. R., and SCHULTZ, E. H. The effect of prolonged atelectasis or ischemia upon the lungs of growing dogs. *J. Thorac. Cardiovasc. Surg.* 49:179, 1965.

PETERS, R. M., LORING, W. E., and SPRUNT, W. H. Traumatic rupture of the bronchus: A clinical and experimental study. *Ann. Surg.* 148:871, 1958.

PETERS, R. M., LORING, W. E., and SPRUNT, W. H. An experimental study of the effect of chronic atelectasis on pulmonary and bronchial blood flow. *Circ. Res.* 7:31, 1959.

PETERS, R. M., and ROOS, A. The effects of atelectasis on pulmonary blood flow in the dog. *J. Thorac. Surg.* 24:389, 1952.

PLEURAL COMPLICATIONS

GOBBEL, W. G., JR., RHEA, W. G., JR., NELSON, I. A., and DANIEL, R. A., JR. Spontaneous pneumothorax. *J. Thorac. Cardiovasc. Surg.* 46:331, 1963.

GRAHAM, E. A. *Some Fundamental Considerations in the Treatment of Empyema Thoracis.* St. Louis: Mosby, 1925.

RAVITCH, M. M., and FEIN, R. The changing picture of pneumonia and empyema in infants and children. *J.A.M.A.* 175:1039, 1961.

PULMONARY INFECTION

ALEXANDER, J. K., TAKEZAWA, H., ABU-NASSAR, H. J., and YOW, E. M. Studies on pulmonary blood flow in pneumococcal pneumonia. *Cardiovasc. Res. Cent. Bull.* 1:86, 1963.

COLP, C. R., PARK, S. S., and WILLIAMS, M. H., JR. Pulmonary function in pneumonia. *Amer. Rev. Resp. Dis.* 85:808, 1962.

LINDSKOG, G. E., LIEBOW, A. A., and GLENN, W. W. L. *Thoracic and Cardiovascular Surgery with Related Pathology.* New York: Appleton-Century-Crofts, 1962. Chap. 8, p. 176.

MARSHALL, R., and CHRISTIE, R. V. The visco-elastic properties of the lungs in acute pneumonia. *Clin. Sci.* 13:403, 1954.

PULMONARY RESECTION

FENN, W. O., and RAHN, H. (Eds.). *Handbook of Physiology*, Section 3: *Respiration.* Washington, D.C.: American Physiological Society, 1965.
    SCHILLING, J. A. Pulmonary Resection and Sequelae of Thoracic Surgery. Vol. II, Chap. 67, p. 1531.

COURNAND, A., RILEY, R. L., HIMMELSTEIN, A., and AUSTRIAN, R. Pulmonary circulation and alveolar ventilation-perfusion relationships after pneumonectomy. *J. Thorac. Surg.* 19:80, 1950.

PETERS, R. M., ROOS, A., BLACK, H., BURFORD, T. H., and GRAHAM, E. A. Respiratory and circulatory studies after pneumonectomy in childhood. *J. Thorac. Surg.* 20:484, 1950.

PETERS, R. M., WILCOX, B. R., and SCHULTZ, E. H. Pulmonary resection in children: Long-term effect on function and lung growth. *Ann. Surg.* 159:652, 1964.

WELLONS, H. A., JR., and PETERS, R. M. Effect of pneumonectomy on the mechanics of breathing. *Surg. Forum* 18:205, 1967.

SHOCK LUNG

GERST, P. H., RATTENBORG, C., and HOLADAY, D. A. The effects of hemorrhage on pulmonary circulation and respiratory gas exchange. *J. Clin. Invest.* 38:524, 1959.

HENRY, J. N., McARDLE, A. H., SCOTT, H. J., and GURD, F. N. A study of the acute and chronic respiratory pathophysiology of hemorrahagic shock. *J. Thorac. Cardiovasc. Surg.* 54:666, 1967.

PETERS, R. M. Respiratory aspects of the dynamics of septic shock in man. In *Transactions of the Conference on the Dynamics of Septic Shock in Man.* Boston: Little, Brown. In press.

SEALY, W. C., OGINO, S., LESAGE, A. M., and YOUNG, W. G., JR. Functional and structural changes in the lung in hemorrhagic shock. *Surg. Gynec. Obstet.* 122:754, 1966.

TERZI, R. G., and PETERS, R. M. The effect of large fluid loads on lung mechanics and work. *Ann. Thorac. Surg.* 6:16, 1968.

WIGGERS, H. C., and INGRAHAM, R. C. Hemorrhagic shock: Definition and criteria for its diagnosis. *J. Clin. Invest.* 25:30, 1946.

WILCOX, B. R., and CROOM, R. D., III. Effects of maintaining normal pulmonary perfusion on the lung in hemorrhagic shock in dogs. *J. Surg. Res.* (Suppl. I: Current Topics in Surgical Research.) In press.

WILLWERTH, B. M., CRAWFORD, F. A., YOUNG, W. G., JR., and SEALY, W. C. The role of functional demand on the development of pulmonary lesions during hemorrhagic shock. *J. Thorac. Cardiovasc. Surg.* 54:658, 1967.

FAT EMBOLISM

COLLINS, J. A., GORDON, W. C., JR., HUDSON, T. L., IRVIN, R. W., JR., KELLY, T., and HARDAWAY, R. M., III. Inapparent hypoxemia in casualties with wounded limbs: Pulmonary fat embolism? *Ann. Surg.* 167:511, 1968.

COLLINS, J. A., HUDSON, T. L., HAMACHER, W. R., ROKOUS, J., WILLIAMS, G., and HARDAWAY, R. M., III. Systemic fat embolism in four combat casualties. *Ann. Surg.* 167:493, 1968.

CHAPTER 13: RESPIRATORS

ARTIFICIAL RESPIRATION

BRYANT, L. R. Mechanical respirators: Their use and application in lung trauma. *J.A.M.A.* 199:149, 1967.

CLOWES, G. H. A., JR., COOK, W. A., VUJOVIC, V., and ALBRECHT, M. Patterns of circulatory response to the use of respirators. *Circulation* 31 (Suppl. 1):157, 1965.

HUTCHIN, P., and PETERS, R. M. The influence of altered pulmonary mechanics on the adequacy of controlled ventilation. *Ann. Thorac. Surg.* 7:302, 1969.

PETERS, R. M., and HUTCHIN, P. Adequacy of available respirators to their tasks. *Ann. Thorac. Surg.* 3:414, 1967.

SMITH, A. C., SPALDING, J. M. K., and WATSON, W. E. Stimuli to Spontaneous Ventilation after Prolonged Artificial Ventilation. In D. J. C. CUNNINGHAM and B. B. LLOYD (Eds.), *The Regulation of Human Respiration.* Philadelphia: Davis, 1963. P. 409.

WHITTENBERGER, J. L. (Ed.). *Artificial Respiration: Theory and Applications.* New York: Hoeber, 1962.

OXYGEN TOXICITY

FENN, W. O., and RAHN, H. (Eds.). *Handbook of Physiology*, Section 3: *Respiration*. Washington, D.C.: American Physiological Society, 1965. LAMBERTSEN, C. J. Effects of Oxygen at High Partial Pressure. Vol. II, Chap. 39, p. 1027.

DAVIES, H. C., and DAVIES, R. E. Biochemical Aspects of Oxygen Poisoning. Vol. II, Chap. 40, p. 1047.

CLAMANN, H. G. Space Physiology. "Increased Oxygen Percentage." Vol. II, Chap. 45, p. 1149.

BEHNKE, A. R., JR., and LANPHIER, E. H. Underwater Physiology. Vol. II, Chap. 46, p. 1159.

DAVIES, R. E. Oxygen Toxicity at Near-Normal Partial Pressures. In *Physiology in the Space Environment*, Vol. II: *Respiration*. Washington, D.C.: National Academy of Sciences–National Research Council (Publ. No. 1485 B), 1967. p. 93.

PONTOPPIDAN, H., and BERRY, P. R. Regulation of the inspired oxygen concentration during artificial ventilation. *J.A.M.A.* 201:11, 1967.

WHIPPLE, H. E. (Ed.). Hyperbaric oxygenation: Section II. Oxygen. *Ann. N. Y. Acad. Sci.* 117:727, 1965.

CHAPTER 14: PULMONARY TRANSPLANTATION

BLUMENSTOCK, D. A. Transplantation of the Lung: Current Status. In J. DAUSSET, J. HAMBURGER, and G. MATHE (Eds.), *Advance in Transplantation*. Baltimore: Williams & Wilkins, 1968. P. 681.

FLAX, M. H., and BARNES, B. A. The role of vascular injury in pulmonary allograft rejection. *Transplantation* 4:66, 1966.

HOMATAS, J., BRYANT, L., and EISEMAN, B. Time limits of cadaver lung viability. *J. Thorac. Cardiovasc. Surg.* 56:132, 1968.

MARSHALL, R., and GUNNING, A. J. The long-term physiological effects of lung reimplantation in the dog. *J. Surg. Res.* 6:185, 1966.

NAKAE, S., WEBB, W. R., THEODORIDES, T., and SUGG, W. L. Respiratory function following cardiopulmonary denervation in dog, cat, and monkey. *Surg. Gynec., Obstet.* 125:1285, 1967.

STRIEDER, D. J., BARNES, B. A., ARONOW, S., RUSSELL, P. S., and KAZEMI, H. Xenon 133 study of ventilation and perfusion in normal and transplanted dog lungs. *J. Appl. Physiol.* 23:359, 1967.

TRUMMER, M. J. Bibliography of lung transplantation. *Transplantation* 5:747, 1967.

APPENDIX: THE PHYSICAL BASIS OF RESPIRATION

FENN, W. O., and RAHN, H. (Eds.). *Handbook of Physiology*, Section 3: *Respiration*. Washington, D.C.: American Physiological Society, 1964. RADFORD, E. P., JR. The Physics of Gases. Vol. I, Chap. 3, p. 125. GILBERT, D. L. Cosmic and Geophysical Aspects of the Respiratory Gases. Vol. I, Chap. 4, p. 153.

HIRSCHFELDER, J. O., CURTISS, C. F., and BIRD, R. B. *The Molecular Theory of Gases and Liquids*. New York: Wiley, 1954.

INDEX

Abdomen
 abnormalities and respiration, 232
 distention
  effects, 234–235
  respirator use and, 299
 muscles in respiration, 61
Accessory muscles in breathing, 3
Acetylcholine
 bronchomotor effects, 96
 vasomotor effects, 113
Acid(s)
 defined, 17
 measure of strength, 17
Acid-base balance, 26–40
 changes, chemoreceptors and, 180–
  181, 181–183
 disturbances, 26–30
  compensatory changes, 28, 29
  differential diagnosis, 29–40
  etiology in classification, 27, 28–
   29
  terminology of, 27–30
 hemoglobulin in, 22–24
 laboratory assessment, 30–33
Acidemia, pulmonary vessels and, 130–
  131
Acidosis, 26
 defined, 27
 metabolic, 27, 28
  cardiac insufficiency and, 284,
   285–287
  in drowning, 220–222
  in shock, 271, 277, 278
  therapy, 185, 278
  ventilation and, 185
 mixed, 29
  effects of, 286–287
 respiratory, 28–30

bronchoconstriction, 96
 diagnosis, 35
 emphysema, 237–239
 respiratory insufficiency and, 186,
  285–286
 and work of breathing, 191–193,
  210–211
Activity. *See* Exercise
Age and respiration, 95, 231–232
 airways and, 99–100, 231
 breathing work and, 188
 compliance and, 75, 81–83, 231
 lung volume and, 100, 232
 minute ventilation and, 232
 narcotic effects on respiration and,
  227
 pulmonary vascular bed size and,
  132
 residual capacity and, 83, 231, 232
 resistance and, 231
 tidal volume and, 232
 ventilation-perfusion ratio and, 177–
  178
 vital capacity and, 232
Air. *See also* Gas(es); *and specific gas*
 alveolar
  composition, 42, 43, 44, 45
  residual volume and, 48–51
  respiratory cycle and, 48–51
  unequal impedance and, 98
 atmospheric, described, 213–214
 expired, 42, 43, 44, 48
 inspired
  altitude and oxygen in, 218–219
  breathing mechanics and, 95, 96
  gas composition of 42–43, 44, 48
  temperature, 42

Air—*Continued*
    mixing of inspired and alveolar, 157–158
    movement in hyperventilation, 5
    nasal passages and, 41–42
    phasic flow, 338, 339
    in pleural cavity, 84, 85, 86, 87. *See also* Pneumothorax
    pollution, effects of, 95, 96, 214–217, 238
    upper airways and, 42
    water vapor in, 42, 43, 44, 45
Airway(s), 5–6. *See also* Airway resistance; *and specific structure*
    age and, 99–100, 231
    air in, 42, 45, 46, 48
    complications with artificial ventilation, 298–299
    functional anatomy, 5–6
    lung size and, 99-100
    obstruction and breathing work, 188
    pressure, 66–67
        barometric pressure and, 67
        pleural pressure and, 64, 65, 67
    role in ventilation, 41–42
    size
        age and, 99–100
        intrapleural pressure and, 93
    volume of conducting, 46
Airway resistance, 89, 90–97
    age and, 100, 232
    anesthesia and, 224
    arterial pCO_2 and, 96
    breathing and, 91–92
    bronchial size and, 91, 92–95, 225
    bronchomotor tone and, 91, 95–97, 225
    coughing and, 102, 252
    dead space and, 96
    distribution, 92
    distribution of ventilation and, 161–164
    drugs and, 96
    in emphysema, 238
    exercise and, 101
    inflammation and, 91, 100
    lung compliance and, 94–95
    position and, 94
    postoperative, 250–252
    smog and, 95, 96
    smoking and, 95, 96
    sulfur dioxide and, 215
    tidal volume and, 291–292
Alkalosis
    defined, 27
    metabolic, 27–28

    respiratory, 28
        artificial ventilation and, 300–301
        blood gas in, 40
Allografts, experimental lung, 310–312
Alloxan, vasomotor tone and, 113
Altitude. *See also* Barometric pressure
    carbon monoxide poisoning and, 217
    composition of inspired air and, 42–43
    effects of below sea level, 219–220
    lung cysts and pneumothorax and, 241
    minute ventilation and, 184
    oxygen saturation and, 43
    partial pressure of oxygen and, 40
    pulmonary hypertension and, 129–130
    resistance and blood viscosity and, 109
    ventilation and, 53, 218–219
Alveolar air. *See* Alveolar ventilation; Alveoli, gases
Alveolar ventilation, 46
    adequacy of, 52–53
    anesthesia and, 226–227
    blood gases and, 53, 113, 210, 211
    coordination of ventilation and perfusion, 157
    dead space and, 46–48, 169–170
    estimation of, 52
    hyperventilation, 45
    hypoventilation, 53, 131
    minute ventilation and, 48
    needs, 52–53
    residual volume and, 48–51
Alveoli. *See also* Alveolar ventilation
    age and, 231
    air mixing in, 146, 147, 157–158
    anatomy of, 7, 149
    capillary-alveolar interface, 117–120, 149
        diffusing capacity, 150–155
        distortions, 155
        gas diffusion across, 148–150
        surface area, 149
    diffusion in, 148–149, 150–155
    in emphysema, 158, 238
    formation, 60
    gas(es), 8, 149
        carbon dioxide, 43, 44, 45
            arterial carbon dioxide vs., 171–174, 243–244
        nitrogen, 43
            arterial nitrogen vs., 173–174
        oxygen, 43, 44, 45

arterial oxygen vs., 170–174, 272
pulmonary vasomotor tone and, 113
residual volume and, 48–51
respiratory cycle and, 48–51
inflation of deflated, 74, 75, 265, 279
loss of surfactant effect and, 73
membrane distortions, 155
number and lung compliance, 75
pressure. *See* Intraalveolar pressure
surface area, 8, 149
surface tension, 70–71, 72, 73
Anemia
blood flow and, 152
diffusing capacity and, 152, 154
Anesthesia, 190–191
airway resistance and, 224
alveolar ventilation and, 226–227
anesthetic gases, effects of, 228
arterial gas concentrations and, 227
compliance and, 225–226
hyperinflation in, 73
metabolic rate and, 224
residual volume and, 49, 51
respiration control in, 179
synergistic effects of drugs and anesthetics, 228–229
vasomotor effects on bronchi, 224
Angiography, pulmonary, 174
Angular velocity of sine wave, 340
Anion, defined, 16
Ankylosing spondylitis, 235
Anomalous viscosity, 330
Anoxia, lung resistance to, 313
Anticholinesterases, bronchomotor response to, 96
Aorta, pressure pulse wave of, 106
Aortic bodies, 180, 183
Apnea, 191, 224
Arteries. *See* Blood vessels; *and specific artery*
Arterioles, 104
Artificial ventilation. *See also* Respirator(s)
breathing work in, 203–204
in cardiac dysfunction, 242
chest wall resistance in, 90
complications, 298–301
in drowning, 221, 222
open chest and, 294–296
pressure-volume relations in, 203–204
in pulmonary edema, 127
sedation with, 191
surfactant effect and, 73

ventilatory response restoration with, 193
Ascites, 79–80, 234
Asphyxia, in drowning, 221–222
Astrup method of blood analysis, 31
Atelectasis, 264–265. *See also* Microatelectasis
anesthesia and, 226
defined, 264
in drowning, 221, 222
lung compliance and, 75
pneumothorax and, 84
pulmonary circulation and, 105
ventilation and, 105
ventilation-perfusion ratio and, 165, 166, 177
Atherosclerosis, pulmonary hypertension and, 129
Atmosphere. *See* Air
Atmospheric pressure. *See* Barometric pressure
Atrium
left, pressure in, 107, 108
right
control of filling, 107
gas distribution in vessels entering, 157
pressure in, 107
Atropine, bronchomotor response to, 96, 224, 225
Avogadro, law of, 320–321

Barometric pressure. *See also* Altitude
airway pressure and, 67
alterations, 218–220
alveolar pressure and, 63–64
below sea level, 219–220
inspired oxygen pressure with altitude change and, 218–219
pleural pressure and, 64, 65
respiration pressure and, 55
vapor pressure and, 322–323
Baroreceptors, 180
Base, defined, 17
"Bends," 220
Bernoulli's effect, 108, 330
conditions for, 333, 335
work and, 331–333
Bicarbonate
artificial ventilation and serum, 301
as buffer, 18–22
chemoreceptors and changes in, 180–181
hydrogen ion concentration and carbonic acid ratio to, 19–22

Bicarbonate—*Continued*
in respiratory acidosis, 28
standard blood, 31–32
Blood
acid-base balance parameters of arterial, 35, 37–40
chemical analysis methods, 30 33
gases. *See* Carbon dioxide, blood;
Oxygen, blood
pH of, 18, 24
principal functions, 9
standard bicarbonate, 31–32
viscosity
flow rate and, 109–110, 330
hematocrit and, 109–110
whole-blood buffer base, 31
Blood flow. *See also* Flow; Pulmonary
circulation
in anemia and polycythemia, 152
blood pressure and, 110, 111, 112
blood vessel size and, 110, 111
in shock, 154
ventilation-perfusion ratio and, 165–
170
viscosity and, 109–110, 330
Blood pressure. *See also* Pulmonary
hypertension
arterial systemic, 96, 108
cardiac function and, 106-107
chemoreceptor stimulation and,
180
monitoring, in respirator patients,
293–294, 295
pulmonary
arterial, 108, 110, 111, 112
blood flow and, 110, 111, 112
blood vessel size and, 110, 111
capillary size and, 116, 117
position and, 114
shock and, 272
venous, 108
Blood vessels
arterial-alveolar gas differences
carbon dioxide, 171–174
nitrogen, 173–174
oxygen, 170–174
cardiac output and, 105
distensibility and flow-pressure relations, 141–142
impedance and flow-pressure relations, 144
pressure pulse wave, 106
pulsatile flow in, 338, 339
regeneration following pulmonary
transplantation, 308

size
intravascular pressure, 110, 111
resistance and, 110
vasomotor control, 110, 112–113
Blood volume
lung compliance and, 74–75
in pulmonary circulation, factors in,
113–114
replacement, cautions in shock, 274–
275, 277–278, 278–279
Body fluids, pH of, 21
Bohr effect, 14
Boyle's law, 318, 319
Breathing. *See also* Breathing work;
Dyspnea; Expiration; Inspiration; Ventilation; *and specific*
topic
airway resistance and, 41, 91–92
alveolar air composition and cycle,
48–51
apnea, 191, 224
chemical control, 179–187
cigarette smoking and, 217–218
diaphragmatic paralysis and, 256–
257
exercise and dynamics of, 100–102
fetal mechanics, 81–83
hyperventilation and, 191
lung laceration and, 258
nasal passages in, 5, 41–42
in natural vs. induced sleep, 224
ozone and, 216
in pneumothorax, 258, 259
pressure-volume relations in, 58, 198,
201–202, 205
pure oxygen, 51
rate. *See* Respiratory rate
respiratory tract pressure in, 92–94
shallow, results of, 249, 250–251
sulfur dioxide and, 214
ventilatory reserve calculation, 54
Breathing work, 195–211
in artificial respiration, 203–204
cardiac insufficiency and, 242
compliance and, 199–200, 201
cough and, 252
disease and, 196
elastic component of, 199–202, 203–
204, 205, 206
emphysema and, 238
helium and, 335
Hering-Breuer reflex and, 187–188
mechanical work, 197–209
calculation of, 206, 208–209
metabolic rate and, 209–211
obesity and, 233, 234

oxygen cost of, 196-197
postoperative, 252–253
prediction, at given ventilation level, 209
pulmonary resection and, 268–269
resistance and, 202–203
respiratory rate and, 202–203
in shock, 277
spontaneous breathing, 199–203
ventilatory response and, 191–193
work on lung, 198–206, 207
Bronchi
anatomy of, 6–7, 95–96
area of, 6
branching, 60
bronchomotor tone
airway resistance and, 91, 95–97, 225
drugs and, 96, 224, 225
inspiration and, 7–8
obstruction
atelectasis and, 265
lung compliance and, 75
rupture, 260
size, 91, 92–95
resistance and, 100
transmural pressure and, 94
transection, in pulmonary transplantation, 305, 306
Bronchial arteries, 104–105
in bronchiectasis, 263
collaterals, 105
Bronchiectasis, 266–267
Bronchioles
anatomy of, 7, 96
constriction and anatomical dead space, 96-97
proprioceptors of, 187
Bronchospirometry, differential, 174
Bunsen absorption coefficient, 323–324

Capillaries. *See also* Pulmonary capillaries
systemic vs. pulmonary, 116
Carbon dioxide. *See also* Carbon dioxide, blood
alveolar, 43, 44, 45
pulmonary vasomotor tone and, 113
residual volume and, 48–51
anesthesia and response to, 224
arterial-alveolar differences, 171–174, 243–244
in atmosphere, 214
carbonic acid and partial pressure of, 21

dissociation curve, 38, 171
excretion, 43
Haldane effect and, 24
hydration of, 16, 22, 23, 24
inspired vs. expired air, 48
production and ventilatory requirements, 209–210
Carbon dioxide, blood
absorption curve, 24–26
alveolar-arterial differences, 171–174, 243–244
alveolar ventilation and increased, 210, 211
anesthesia and, 227
bronchomotor response to, 96
dissociation curves, 38
distribution in whole blood, 22
hydration of, 16, 22, 23, 24
partial pressure
arterial blood, 22
venous blood, 10, 22
postoperative, 248
sleep and, 224
solubility coefficient, 6, 9
transport at rest, 9
ventilation control and, 183–187, 190, 191–193
Carbon monoxide
diffusing capacity measurement, 151
dissociation curve of hemoglobin and, 15–16
poisoning, 216–217
Carbonic acid
as buffer, 18–22
dissociation, 18, 19, 22
excretion, 16
formation, 22, 23, 24
hydrogen ion concentration and ratio to bicarbonate, 19–22
partial pressure of carbon dioxide and, 21
Carbonic anhydrase, 22, 24
Cardiac disease. *See* Heart disease; *and specific condition*
Cardiac output
exercise and, 222, 223
increasing, 105–106, 143, 144
shock and, 272, 274
vascular bed and, 105
Carotid bodies, 180, 183
Cation, defined, 16
Central nervous system
disease
respiration and, 223
respirators in, 282–283

Central nervous system—*Continued*
  respiration control and, 179, 181–183
Cerebrospinal fluid
  composition determination, 182
  hydrogen ion concentration, 182–183
  respiration and, 183–187
Charles' (Gay Lussac's) law, 319, 322
Chemical regulation of respiration, 183–187, 189–190
Chemoreceptors, 179–187
  central nervous system, 181–183
  peripheral, 180–181
  proprioceptive reflexes and, 187
  response of, 179
Chest. *See also* Pneumothorax
  air entrance into, 84
  artificial respiration and open, 294–296
  in breathing, 1–5
  force-pressure factors in, 198–204
  chest cage injuries, 253–264
    bleeding in, 260–261
    complications, 287–288
    crushing injuries, 253–255
    diaphragmatic paralysis and, 256–257
    intrathoracic complications, 258–267
    lung laceration and, 258–260
    lung mechanics and, 257
    penetrating, 255–256
    respirators in, 287–288
    ventilation-perfusion ratio and, 177, 178
  compliance, 76–81
    age and, 81–83, 231, 232
    anesthesia and, 225
    chest wall mass and, 76
    deformities and, 80–81
    gravity and, 76–80
    obesity and, 233–234
    position and, 225–226
    postoperative, 249
  deformities
    compliance and, 80–81
    respirator use in, 284
    results of, 232, 235–237
  drainage, 261–263, 264, 287
  inertance of wall, 88–89
  mechanical dysfunction, 283–287
  muscles, 3–5
    compliance and, 76
    in expiration, 5
    in inspiration, 3–5
    motion and, 60–61

resistance of tissue of wall, 89, 90
shape, changes in, 2, 3
size
  age and, 81, 82
  changes in, 2, 61
  pleural pressure and, 84
  stretching, pressure for, 65–68
Circulation. *See* Pulmonary circulation; Systemic circulation
Clausius-Clapeyron equation, 322
Cold. *See* Temperature
Collagen fibers, lung, 68–69
Compliance, 58, 59. *See also* Chest, compliance; Lung(s), compliance
  age and, 231
  anesthesia and, 225–226
  breathing work and, 188, 199–200, 201
  coordination of ventilation and perfusion and, 159–164
  defined, 64
  distribution of air and, 159–164
  elasticity and, 346–347
  phasic flow systems and, 346
  pleural space and, 83–88
  postoperative, 249, 250
  reactance and, 348
  resistance and, 97
  sum of units of, 65, 66, 347
Conductance, defined, 99–100. *See also* Resistance(s)
Continuity equation, 331
Cor pulmonale
  production, 131
  pulmonary embolism and, 133
  therapy, 239, 301
Cough
  abdominal muscles in, 61
  failure, results of, 252
  mechanics of, 102
  opening collapsed alveoli and, 265
  reflex, lung reimplantation and, 308–309
  respiratory muscles and, 102
  transmural pressure and, 102
Crushing chest cage injuries, 253–255
Cyclopropane, respiratory effects, 228

Dalton's law of partial pressure, 321–322
Dead space
  alveolar, 169, 170
  anatomical, 169, 170
    age and, 232
    anesthesia and, 224

bronchiole constriction and, 96–97
defined, 46
physiological, measurement of, 169–170
role of, 47, 48
Decompression, 219, 220
Deflation reflex, 187–188
Density, turbulence and, 335
Diabetic acidosis, 26
Diaphragm
curvature of, 81, 82
motion, 3, 61
effects of inhibition, 86–87, 256–257
volume of chest cavity and, 4
muscle relaxation and position, 3–4
Diffusion of gases, 1, 145–155
distance and effectiveness of, 146
Fick's law, 145–146
gas mixing in alveoli and, 146, 147
of gas to blood, 148–150
Graham's law, 145, 146–147
Henry's law, 9, 11, 146, 147, 323–324
pulmonary diffusing capacity, 150–155
rate, into or out of liquids, 146–148
Digitalis, use of, 239
Disease. See also Heart disease; and specific condition
degenerative lung, 105, 132
respiratory response to, 223–224
Drainage, chest, 261–263, 264, 287
Drinker respirator, 67, 281
Drowning, 220–222
Drugs. See also specific drug
bronchomotor mechanisms and, 96, 224, 225
effects of barbiturates, 228
immunosuppressive, allograft survival and, 311, 312
narcotic, 228–229
postoperative use, 253
respiration and, 190–191, 227–228
synergisms of, 228–229
Dyspnea
development of, 196
exercise and, 210, 223
metabolic rate and, 210
obesity and, 233
paroxysmal nocturnal, 125–126

Elasticity, 88
compliance and, 346–347

geometric factor in elastic tube system, 335
lung, 68–79
elastic fibers and, 68–69
expiration force and, 93–94
surface tension and, 71
residual capacity and, 292
Electrolyte solution, defined, 17
Emboli. See also Pulmonary emboli
pulmonary hypertension and, 129, 132–133
ventilation-perfusion ratio and, 167–170
Emphysema
air mixing in, 158
breathing in, 95
diffusion in, 149, 154
increasing ventilation in, 191
lung compliance and, 74
obstructive, 217–218, 237–239
bullae with, 240–241
development of, 237–238
effects of, 238–239
therapy, 239
pulmonary hypertension and, 129, 132
respiratory insufficiency in, 259
smoking and, 217–218
subcutaneous, 260
ventilation-perfusion ratio in, 177–178
Empyema
management, 264
postresection, 270
Endotoxins, vasomotor tone and, 113
Endotracheal tube
effects of insertion, 224
use with respirators, 290, 298
Energy. See also Breathing work
defined, 332
kinetic, 332–333
potential, 333
sources in respiration, 57, 59–62
Epinephrine
bronchomotor effects, 96, 224
vasomotor effects, 113
Esophagus, rupture of, 260
Ether, respiratory effects, 228
Exercise, 43
airway resistance and, 101
breathing dynamics and, 101–102
diffusion surface area and, 149
dyspnea and, 210, 223
expiration and, 101

Exercise—*Continued*
  hemoglobin concentration and, 15
  hyperventilation and, 189
  increased levels, response, 222–223
  inspiratory reserve and, 101
  lung volume and, 101
  normal adaptations to, 222
  postoperative, 253, 270
  pulmonary blood volume and, 113, 114
  pulmonary vessels and, 112
  residual capacity and, 101
  respiratory muscles, 101–102
  respiratory rate and, 101
  tidal volume and, 101
  ventilation and, 101
  ventilation-perfusion ratio and, 164, 175
  work capacity and, 233
Expiration
  cough and, 102
  exercise and, 101
  lung elastic recoil and, 93–94
  lung stretching at, 205, 206, 207
  muscles in, 93–94
    abdominal, 61
    chest, 4–5
    intercostals, 60
  normal breathing cycle, 100–101
  obstruction to, 53–54
  pressure-volume change in, 201–202, 203
  quiet, described, 61
  respiratory tract pressure in, 68, 93–94
  ventilation related to, 45–48
Expiratory reserve volume, 45, 46
Expired air, 43, 44, 48
  in shock lung syndrome, 279
  open thoracotomy and, 294

Feedback, in respiration control, 190
Fetus
  breathing mechanics, 81–83
  lung compliance, 82–83
Fibrosis
  alveolar membrane in, 155
  breathing work in, 188
  lung compliance and, 74
Fibrothorax, 263–264
Fick's law of diffusion, 145–146
Fixed acid, defined, 26, 27
Fixed base, defined, 27
Flow. *See also* Blood flow; Flow-pressure relations
  continuity equation, 331

  factors regulating, 324–327
  force and response of system, 341, 343–345
  phasic, 338, 339
  prediction of flow wave amplitudes, 350–351
  pulsatile
    compliance and, 346
    inertance and, 346, 347–348
    mechanics of, 338–353
    resistance in system, 345–346
    transmural pressure and, 335, 336, 337
    turbulence and, 333, 334
    viscosity and, 330
Flow-pressure relations, 325, 327–329, 330, 335–338
  impedance and, 144, 349–350
  kinetic energy changes and, 141
  power dissipation, 142–144
  in pulmonary circulation. *See* Pulmonary circulation, flow-pressure relations
  in systemic circulation, 106–107
  turbulent flow, 141
  vessel distensibility and, 141–142
Fluid(s)
  basic principles of mechanics, 324–353
  drainage from chest, 261–263, 264
  effusion from pulmonary capillaries, 120–121, 122–124
  exchange in pulmonary capillaries, 117–122
  in pleural space
    control of, 85, 86–87
    effects of, 84
    rate of gas diffusion into or out of, 146–148
  resistance determination in system, 327–330
  solution of gases in, 323–324
  transudation to lungs in shock, 274, 275
Force
  impedance and, 341
  to overcome inertia, 347–348
  in respiration, 57–59, 61–62
  system response to, 341, 343–345
Foreign body aspiration, 266
Fourier series analysis, 97–98, 344
Functional residual volume, defined, 45, 46

Gas(es). *See also* Air; Carbon dioxide; Gas(es), blood; Gas ex-

change; Oxygen; *and specific topic*
diffusion, 1, 145–155. *See also* Diffusion of gases
gas laws, 318–319, 320–324. *See also specific law*
kinetic theory of, 319–320
mixing with blood, 157–158
parallel ventilation theory of distribution, 159–164
pressure in pneumothorax, 84, 86
solution in liquids, 323–324
transfer, concepts of, 145
vapor pressure, 322–323
Gas(es), blood. *See also* Carbon dioxide, blood; Oxygen, blood
alveolar ventilation and, 53, 113
analysis of abnormalities in, 33, 35, 37–40
composition of, 43, 44, 45
arterial, 44
entering right atrium, 157
as indications for respirator use, 282, 283, 284, 290–291
pulmonary vasomotor tone and, 113
venous, 43, 44, 45
in ventilatory insufficiency, 35, 37
mixing with blood, 157–158
pressure, 84, 86
transport at rest, 9
Gas exchange
alveoli in, 8
diffusion in, 1, 145–155. *See also* Diffusion of gases
disease and, 223–224
energy cost. *See* Breathing work
required by exercise, 222–223
Gastric dilatation, 235, 299
Gay Lussac's (Charles') law, 319, 322
Graham's law, 145, 146–147
Gravity, compliance and, 76–80

Haldane effect, 24
Halothane, 228
Head injuries, therapy for, 283
Heart. *See also* Heart disease; Heart failure; *and specific topic*
arrythmias, hyperventilation and, 300–301
atrium
filling, 107
pressure in, 107, 108
blood pressure and function of, 106–107
energy output, 195

massage, for pulmonary embolus, 244
myocardium, 107, 124
output. *See* Cardiac output
oxygen consumption, 196
as pulmonary circulation pump, 1–2, 9, 105–107
rate
cardiac output and, 105–106
chemoreceptor stimulation and, 180
stroke volume and cardiac output, 105–106, 143, 144
ventricle
filling pressure, 133–134, 140
output control, 107
pulse, 106–107
Heart disease
congenital
diffusing capacity in, 152
pulmonary hypertension in, 134–140
cyanotic
bronchial circulation and, 105
hematocrit and pulmonary circulation in, 109–110
diffusing capacity and, 152, 154
lung function and, 241–242
mitral insufficiency, 134
mitral stenosis, 75, 113–114, 125, 134, 154, 155, 176, 241
myocardial infarction, 284
precautions in surgery, 241–242
pulmonary hypertension and, 128, 134–140
Heart failure
deterioration in, 284–285
diffusing capacity, 155
pulmonary blood pressure and, 113–114, 241
pulmonary blood volume and, 113–114
respirators in, 284, 285
ventilation-perfusion ratio and, 176
Helium, work of breathing, 335
Hematocrit, blood viscosity and, 109–110
Hemoglobin
acid-base balance and, 23–24
acid-titration curve, 23–24
carbon monoxide saturation, in poisoning, 216–217
chemical composition, 10–11
dissociation curve
carbon monoxide and, 15–16

Hemoglobin, dissociation curve—Continued
 oxygen-hemoglobin, 11–15
 pH and, 14
 gas diffusion from alveolus to, 148–149
 molecular arrangement and oxygen release, 24
 oxygen combination with, 11
 oxyhemoglobin, 11–15, 23, 24, 180, 184
 variations in concentration, 15
Hemothorax, 260–261, 263–264, 270
Henderson equation, 18–22
Henderson-Hasselbach equation, 20–22, 31
Henry's law, 9, 11, 146, 147, 323–324
Hering-Breuer reflex, 187–188
 lung reimplantation and, 309
 normal, 308
Histamine, vasomotor response to, 96, 113
Hood's paradoxical reflex, 188
Hooke's law for elastic bodies, 68
Hydrogen ion concentration (H+).
  See also pH
 cerebrospinal fluid, 182–183
 respiration and, 183–187
 chemoreceptors and changes in, 180–181, 182–183
 defined, 17
 pH and, 17–19
 ratio of carbonic acid to salts of bicarbonate and, 19–22
Hydrogen ions, metabolic sources of, 26
Hydrostatic pressure
 fluid effusion from capillaries and, 120–121
 pulmonary capillaries, 119–120
Hydrothorax, 260–261
Hyperbaric environments
 in cadaver lung maintenance, 313
 compensation for, 219–220
 effects and dangers of, 300, 313–314
Hypercapnia, 34, 35
 anesthesia and, 227
 artificial ventilation in, 301
 bronchomotor response to, 96
 hypoxia without, 24–25, 39
 ventilatory response to, 187
Hyperinflation
 aging, 232
 during anesthesia, 73, 226, 227
 in opening collapsed alveoli, 265
 for respirator patients, 73

Hyperkinetic pulmonary hypertension, 128
Hyperventilation, 45
 ability, physical conditioning and, 232–233
 acid-base disturbance correction and, 186
 air movement in, 5
 airway resistance and, 92
 apnea and, 191
 arterial-alveolar carbon dioxide differences and, 171
 blood gas composition in, 38, 39
 bronchomotor response to, 96
 diffusion and, 149, 152
 effects of excessive, 300–301
 exercise and, 189, 223
 nitrogen washout tests and, 159
 oxygen saturation and, 165–167
 for reduced oxygen pressure, 219
 in shock, 271, 272, 277, 279
 stimulus to, 186–187
 water loss in, 42
Hypocapnia, correction of, 187
Hypothermia
 in cadaver lung maintenance, 313–314
 oxygen dissociation curve and, 14–15
 respiratory effects, 224, 229
 stress of, 15
Hypoventilation
 alveolar, 53, 131
 arterial-alveolar carbon dioxide differences and, 171, 172, 173
 diagnosis, 35, 36
Hypoxemia
 acidosis and, 286
 altitude and, 39, 130, 218
 atelectasis and, 177
 bronchomotor response to, 96
 carbon monoxide and, 216
 cardiac disease and, 241
 coordination of ventilation and perfusion and, 165–167, 170
 diffusion and, 37, 40, 152
 drowning and, 221
 emphysema and, 177, 238
 exercise and, 152, 223
 hypoventilation and, 35
 obesity and, 177–178, 234
 pneumonia and, 177
 postoperative, 176, 248, 252
 pulmonary emboli and, 243
 pulmonary edema and, 124
 pulmonary hypertension and, 130

shunt and, 37–38, 165–167
without hypercapnia, 24–25, 39
Hysteresis, lung, 73

Immune response, lung allograft rejection and, 310–312
Impedance, 97–99
force and, 341
mass and, 348
pressure-flow relationships and, 144, 349–350
reactance and, 348–353
theoretical background of concept, 97
unequal, effects of, 98
Inertance
phasic flow systems and, 346, 347–348
in respiratory mechanics, 58, 59, 60
respiratory system, 88–89
Inertia, defined, 332
Infection(s). *See also specific infection*
bronchiectasis and, 266, 267
as complication of artificial ventilation, 298
in esophageal rupture, 260
intrathoracic complications, 258–267
metabolic rate and, 284–285
pulmonary, 105, 131–132, 284–285
Inflation reflex, 187–188
Injury, 55, 223, 247–279. *See also specific injury, site, topic*
Inspiration
alveolar pressure at, 68
bronchi and, 7–8
bronchomotor response to, 96
chest muscles in, 3–5
in cough, 102
intercostal muscles in, 59–60
lung stretching at, 205, 206, 207
normal breathing cycle, 100
open pneumothorax and, 255
pressure-volume changes in, 198, 201–202, 203–204
quiet, described, 61
respiratory tract pressure in, 92–94
Inspiratory reserve volume
defined and normal values, 45, 46, 101
postoperative, 248
Inspired air, 48
altitude and composition of, 218–219
mixing with alveolar air, 158
ventilation related to, 45–48
Intercostal muscles in breathing, 3

expiration, 60
inspiration, 59–60
Intraalveolar pressure, 62
alterations in, 62
alveolar size in, 70–71
atmospheric pressure and, 63–64
inspiration vs. expiration, 68
pulmonary capillary pressure and, 117–120
pulmonary capillary size and, 116, 117
surface tension and, 70–71, 72, 73
Intraesophageal pressure, 62
Intrapleural pressure, 62
airway pressure and, 64, 65, 67
airway size and, 93
atmospheric pressure and, 64, 65
body surface pressure and, 67
changes in child vs. adult, 81–83
end-inspiratory vs. end-expiratory, 68
in expiration, 93–94
lung volume and, 83–84
measurement of, 61–62
negative, effects of, 84, 85, 86
normal, at relaxation, 83
Iron porphyrin of hemoglobin, 10–11
Isoproterenol
bronchomotor effects, 96, 224
vasomotor effects, 113

Kidneys, acid-base balance and, 16, 26
Kinetic energy
conversion to work, 332–333
defined, 332
flow-pressure relations and changes, 141
potential energy and, 333
Kinetic theory of gases, 319–320
Kyphoscoliosis, 235
Kyphosis, 237

Lacerations, lung, 258–260
Lactic acid formation, 26
Laplace's law, 70, 72, 82, 335–338
Larynx, 5–6
Lung(s). *See also* Alveoli; *and specific topic, e.g.,* Lung compliance; Ventilation
acid-base balance and, 16
acid excretion, 26
aging process of, 81–83, 95, 100, 231, 232
air in
impedance and, 98
mixing, 157–158
bronchial arteries and, 104–105

Lung(s)—*Continued*
  cadaver, handling for transplant, 313–314
  circulation. *See* Pulmonary circulation
  collapse, 259
    compliance and, 294, 295
    in shock lung, 296
    toleration of, 264–265
  compliance. *See* Lung compliance
  cysts
    barometric pressure changes and, 219, 220, 241
    bullae with obstructive emphysema, 240–241
    respiratory effects, 239–241
    type and development of, 239–240
  damage, high oxygen concentration and, 275
  degenerative disease, 105, 132. *See also specific disease*
  dynamic properties of, 88–102
  elasticity, 68–76, 93–94
  experimental allografts, 310–312
  forces in holding, 86–88
  function, 56–59
    disease and. *See specific disease*
    control of, 6
    of reimplanted lung, 307–310, 312–313
  hemorrhage, in shock, 273
  hysteresis of, 73
  immune response, 311–312
  impedance and air distribution in, 98
  inertance, 88–89
  infections
    bronchial circulation in, 105
    respirator use in, 284–285
    vascular bed and, 131–132
  inflammation, diffusion and, 154, 155
  inflation, 68, 69, 120, 281
  laceration in chest injury, 258–260
  lymphatics, 122
  mechanics, 88–102
    age and, 232
    chest wall injuries and, 257
    exercise and, 100–102
    postoperative, 249–252
    respirators and, 301–304
    respirators in dysfunctions, 283–287
    in shock lung syndrome, 275–277
    size and, 99–100
    tidal volume and, 297

  nerve regeneration in reimplantation, 308–310
  perfusion and position, 158
  pleural space
    compliance and, 83–88
    function as interface, 87–88
  pressure. *See* Intrapleural pressure
  pulmonary function tests, 53–54
  recoil
    expiration force and, 93–94
    surface tension and, 71
  resection. *See* Pulmonary resection
  resistance, 89, 90, 91
    determination, 98
    parallel ventilation theory, 159–164
    in shock, 276
  shock and, 272–277, 279, 296. *See also* Shock lung syndrome
  stretching, 65–68
  structure
    altitude and, 130
    compliance and, 74–76
    emphysema and, 238
    smoking and, 217–218
  surfactant and, 69–74
  surface tension and, 71
  tissue loss, pressure and, 131
  transplantation, 305–314. *See also* Pulmonary transplantation
  volume, 6. *See also specific volume, e.g.,* Residual volume; Tidal volume
    age and, 100
    closed pneumothorax and, 258
    compliance and, 279
    defined, 45, 46
    determination at rest, 75–76
    exercise and, 101
    pleural pressure and, 83–84
    unequal impedance and, 98
  work on, in breathing, 198–206, 207
Lung compliance, 65, 68–76, 295–296
  age and, 81–83, 231
  airway resistance and, 94–95
  anesthesia and, 226
  collapse and, 294, 295
  cough effectiveness and, 102
  coordination of ventilation and perfusion and, 159–164
  determination, 67, 68, 98
  distribution of airway and, 159–164
  elastic work of breathing and, 199–200, 201
  in fetus, 82–83
  gravity and, 76

parallel ventilation theory, 159–164
pleural space and, 83–88
postoperative, 249–250
shallow breathing and, 249
shock and, 275, 276, 277, 279
static and dynamic, 68
structure and, 74–76
surfactant and, 69–74
ventilation and differences in, 163–164
Lymphatic system of lung, 122

Marie-Strümpell arthritis, 80
Mass, impedance and, 348
Maximum breathing capacity (MBC), 54
Mechanical work, calculation of, 206, 208–209
Mechanics, 55–102
of cough, 102
early theories, 55
elastic components and, 60, 63–68
glossary of terms, 56
lung. *See* Lung, mechanics
postoperative musculoskeletal, 248–249
of pulsatile flow, 338–352
respirators and deranged, 301–304
Mediastinum, 5, 255–256, 259
Metabolic acid-base balance disturbances, 27–28, 29
Metabolic acidosis, 27, 28
cardiac insufficiency and, 284, 285–287
in drowning, 221, 222
in shock, 277, 278
therapy, 185–186, 278
ventilation and, 185
Metabolic alkalosis, 27–28
Metabolic rate
anesthesia and, 224
carbon monoxide poisoning and, 216–217
energy cost of breathing and, 209–211
infections and, 284–285
injury and, 209, 247
postoperative, 247
respiration and, 223
Methoxyflurane, respiratory effects, 228
Microatelectasis, 265
anesthesia and, 226
intrapulmonary shunts and, 273
shallow breathing and, 249
ventilation-perfusion ratio and, 176–177

ventilatory support in, 288
Minute ventilation, 45–46
age and, 232
altitude and, 184
alveolar ventilation related to, 48
anesthesia and, 224
calculation of, 52
defined, 45
in dyspnea, 196
gas exchange and, 48
requirement and metabolic rate, 209–210
respiratory rate and, 51–52
sleep and, 224
Mitral insufficiency, 134
Mitral stenosis
diffusing capacity and, 154, 155
lung compliance and, 75
pulmonary blood pressure and, 113–114, 241
pulmonary blood volume and, 113–114
pulmonary edema in, 125
pulmonary vascular resistance in, 134
ventilation-perfusion ratio and, 176
Mixed acidosis, 286–287
Morphine, respiratory effects, 227
Mountain sickness, 120, 126
Musculoskeletal system. *See also* specific topic
chest muscles, 3–5
deformities, 235–237
postoperative mechanics, 248–249
respiration and abnormalities, 284
Myocardium
malfunction and pulmonary circulation, 107
in pulmonary edema, 124
respirator use in infarction, 284
Myoglobin, 12, 13, 14

Narcotics. *See* Drugs, narcotic
Neomycin, anesthetic agents and, 228
Nerve regeneration after pulmonary transplantation, 308–310
Neurogenic pulmonary edema, 124
Newtonian fluid, defined, 108
Newton's first law of motion, 56, 329
Nitrogen
alveolar, 43
arterial-alveolar differences, 173–174
atmospheric, 214
narcosis, 220
toxicity, 220
Nitrogen dioxide, as air pollutant, 215

Nitrogen washout tests, 158–159
Nitrous oxide, diffusing capacity, 150–151
Non-Newtonian fluids, 330
Norepinephrine
 bronchomotor effects, 96
 vasomotor effects, 113

Obesity
 postraumatic cardiopulmonary complications and, 248, 249
 respiratory mechanics in, 80, 131, 177, 178, 233–234
 surgery and, 253
Obliterative pulmonary hypertension, 129, 132
Obstruction
 airway
  in artificial ventilation, 299
  breathing work and, 188
  in atelectasis, 264, 265
  to expiration, 53–54
  pulmonary artery, 243, 244
Obstructive emphysema, 237–239, 240–241
Obstructive pulmonary hypertension, 129, 132–133
Occlusion
 arterial
  bronchomotor response to, 96
  capillary surface area and, 149
  lung mechanics and, 161
  ventilation-perfusion ratio and, 167–170
 bronchial, lung compliance and, 75
Ohm's law, 325
Oncotic pressure of plasma proteins, 118
Oxygen
 alveolar, 43, 44, 45, 51, 113
 alveolar-arterial differences in, 170–174, 272
 alveolar residual volume and, 48–51
 anoxia, resistance to, 313
 in artificial respiration, 299–300
 atmospheric, 214
 blood. *See also* Hypoxemia
  alveolar-arterial differences in, 170–174, 272
  anesthesia and, 227
  chemoreceptors and, 180
  different concentrations of, 157
  dissociation curve, 11–15
  partial pressure of, 9–10, 11, 12
   altitude and, 40, 218–219

dissociation curve and, 12–14
  myoglobin and, 14
 postoperative, 176, 248, 252
 saturation and oxygen tension, 13
 solubility coefficient, 6, 9, 11
 states carried in, 11
 transport at rest, 9
 ventilation control and, 190, 191–193
 breathing pure, 51
 combination with hemoglobin, 11
 consumption, 43
  ventilation and, 196–197
  ventilatory requirements and, 209–210
 dissociation curve
  oxygen-hemoglobin, 11–15
  partial pressure and, 12–14
  temperature and, 14–15
 hemoglobin concentration and pressure of, 15
 hemoglobin release of, 24
 hyperbaric
  in cadaver lung maintenance, 313
  compensation for, 219–220
  effects and dangers, 300, 313–314
 hypoxemia, 96, 124, 130
 hypoxia, 24–25, 39, 130, 286
 inspired vs. expired air, 48, 300
 oxygen cost of breathing, 196–197
 partial pressure, 40
  altitude and, 218–219
  dissociation curve and, 12–14
  myoglobin and, 14
 saturation
  altitude and, 43
  hyperventilation and, 165–167
 toxicity, 275
  in artificial respiration, 299–300
  at high concentrations, 220
Oxygen capacity, defined, 11, 152
Oxygen content, defined, 11–12
Oxygen debt, 196–197, 223
Oxygen saturation
 defined, 12
 oxygen tension and, 11, 13
Oxygen tension
 defined, 11
 oxygen saturation and, 11, 13
Oxygen therapy
 in emphysema, 239
 postoperative, 249, 252
 for pulmonary edema and emboli, 245
 residual volume and, 49

in shock, 272, 279
Oxyhemoglobin
  acid-titration curve, 23
  dissociation, 11–15, 24, 180, 184
Ozone, as air pollutant, 216

Pain, respiratory effects, 79, 80, 189, 228
Paradoxical reflex of Hood, 188
Paradoxical respiration, 254, 255, 258
Parallel ventilation theory, 159–164
Parietal pleura, 5, 259–260
Paroxysmal nocturnal dyspnea, 125–126
Partial pressure. *See also under specific gas*
  Dalton's law of, 321–322
  diffusion and, 149
Patent ductus arteriosus, 128, 134–137
Pectus carinatum, 80, 236
Pectus excavatum, 80, 236
Penetrating chest cage injuries, 255–256, 258–260. *See also* Pneumothorax
Perfusion. *See also* Ventilation-perfusion ratio
  in cadaver lung maintenance, 314
  position and lung, 158
Peripheral chemoreceptors, 180–181
pH. *See also* Hydrogen ion concentration (H+)
  of blood, 18, 24
  of body fluids, 21
  changes, peripheral chemoreceptors and, 180–181
  defined, 17–18
  hemoglobin dissociation and, 14
  hydrogen ion concentration and, 17–19
Phase
  lag, 340, 343
  shift, 340, 343
  sine waves and, 338, 340
Phasic flow, 338, 339
Pickwickian syndrome, 131
Pilocarpine, 96
Pleura, 5, 258, 259–260
Pleural pressure. *See* Intrapleural pressure
Pneumonectomy. *See* Pulmonary resection
Pneumonia
  age and tolerance to, 231
  breathing work in, 188
  lobar, 265–266
  respiratory function in, 265, 285

sequellae, 266
  therapy, 265–266, 285
  ventilation-perfusion ratio and, 177
Pneumothorax, 84
  altitude and, 219, 241
  in artificial ventilation, 299
  atelectasis and, 84
  barometric pressure changes and, 219, 220
  chest organ rupture and, 260
  closed, 258–260
  complications, 260–264
  diagnosis, 259
  diffusing capacity and, 154
  gas pressure in, 84, 86
  lung bullae and, 240, 241
  lung volume and, 258
  open, 255–256, 257–258
  tension, 259, 260, 287
  toleration of
    age and, 231
    open, 255–256
  size of opening and, 259
  treatment, 257–258, 287
Poiseuille's law, 91, 108, 140, 141, 327–329, 330
  conditions for, 333, 335
Poliomyelitis, respirators in, 282–283, 289
Pollution, atmospheric, 214–217
  breathing mechanics and, 95, 96
  emphysema and, 238
Polycythemia, 152, 154
Position
  airway resistance and, 94
  changing, in shock, 279
  chest compliance and expiratory reserve volume and, 76–77, 78, 79–80
  diffusing capacity and, 152
  lung perfusion and, 158
  pulmonary blood volume and, 113–114
  pulmonary capillary hydrostatic pressure and, 121, 122
  pulmonary edema and, 125–126
  pulmonary flow-pressure relations and, 114–115
  Trendelenburg, effects of, 225–226
  ventilation-perfusion ratio and, 174–175
Postoperative period, 247–253
  breathing work in, 252–253
  cardiac surgery, respirators in, 284, 285
  care in, 253, 268–269

Postoperative period—*Continued*
  incidence of pulmonary complica-
    tions, 248
  lung mechanics in, 248, 249–252
  metabolic rate in, 247
  musculoskeletal mechanics in, 248–
    249
  pulmonary circulation in, 252
  ventilation and blood gases in, 248
Posture. *See* Position
Potential energy, 333
Power
  defined, 332
  flow-pressure relations and dissipa-
    tion of, 142–144
Precapillary pulmonary vessels, 104
  surfactant and, 120
  systemic vessels vs., 2
  vasomotor control, 110, 112
Pressure. *See also* Pressure-flow rela-
    tions; *and specific type of*
    pressure
  defined, 331
  in respiratory mechanics, 55, 58, 59,
    324
    air entrance into system, 63–64,
      281
    atmospheric pressure and, 55
    for lung and chest expansion, 65–
      68, 198–204
    pressure-volume relations in, 58,
      198, 201–204, 205
Pressure-controlled respirators, 289,
    297–298
Pressure-flow relations, 325, 327–329,
    330
  kinetic energy and, 141
  power dissipation and, 142–144
  pulmonary circulation. *See* Pul-
    monary circulation, pressure-
    flow relations
  systemic circulation, 106–107
  turbulent flow and, 141, 333, 334
  vascular impedance and, 144
  vessel distensibility and, 141–142
Proprioceptors, 179, 187
Pulmonary arteries
  anatomy, 103–104
  ligation, effects of, 104–105
  obstruction, 243, 244
    bronchomotor response to, 96
    capillary surface area and, 149
    lung resistance differences in, 161
    ventilation-perfusion ratio and,
      167–170

  pressure in, 108
    exercise and, 112
    flow and, 112
    radius and, 110, 111
  pressure pulse wave, 106
  vasomotor nerves, 105
Pulmonary capillaries, 5, 104
  alveolar-capillary interface, 117–120.
    See also Alveoli, capillary-
    alveolar interface
  blood flow in, 116, 117
  fluid effusion from, 120–121, 122
  fluid exchange and, 117–122
  lung inflation and, 120
  permeability in pulmonary edema,
    124
  position and, 121, 222
  pressure
    alveolar pressure and, 117–120
    pulmonary edema and, 122–124
  size, control of, 116, 117
  surface area and diffusion, 149
Pulmonary capillary wedge pressure,
    108
Pulmonary circulation, 103–144. *See*
    also Pulmonary arteries; Pul-
    monary capillaries; Pulmo-
    nary hypertension; Pulmonary
    veins
  abnormal dynamics, 107, 122–140
  blood volume, 113–114
  bronchial circulation and, 104–105,
    267
  bronchiectasis and, 266–267
  capillary, 116–122
  exercise and, 222, 223
  flow-pressure relations, 103, 106–
    115, 127, 140–144
    geometric factors, 110–114
    kinetic energy changes, 141
    position and, 114–115
    power dissipation and, 142–144
    turbulent flow, 141
    vascular impedance and, 144
    vessel distensibility and, 141–142
    viscosity and, 108–110
  functional anatomy, 2, 103–107
  kyphoscoliosis and, 236
  lung collapse and, 264–265
  postoperative, 252
  precapillary vessels, 2, 104, 110, 112,
    120
  pulmonary hypertension and, 128
  reserve, 127
  resistance in, 108, 144
  vascular bed, 104

vasomotor control, 105, 110, 112–113
  blood and alveolar oxygen and, 113
  drugs and, 113
  vessels, 103–104, 104–105
Pulmonary edema, 122–127
  acute mountain sickness and, 126
  breathing work in, 188
  cor pulmonale and, 132–133
  diffusing capacity in, 154–155
  in drowning, 221, 222
  etiology, 122–124, 126–127
  fluid effusion in, 122–124
  hypoxemia and, 124
  mitral stenosis and, 125
  neurogenic, 124
  position and, 125–126
  pulmonary emboli and, 244–245
  pulmonary hypertension and, 132–133
  pulmonary transplantation and, 307, 308
  therapy, 124, 127
Pulmonary emboli, 242–245
  bronchial circulation and, 105
  bronchomotor response to, 96
  characteristics, 242–243
  clinical and laboratory signs, 243–244
  diffusing capacity and, 154
  hypoxemia and, 243
  pathophysiology, 243
  pulmonary edema and, 244–245
  pulmonary hypertension and, 129, 132–133
  therapy, 244
Pulmonary function tests, 53–54
Pulmonary hypertension, 127–140
  classification, 127
  clinical syndromes associated with, 129
  emphysema and, 132
  in heart disease, 128, 134–140, 241–242
  hyperkinetic, 128
  left ventricular filling pressure and, 133–134
  lung reimplantation and, 307, 309–312
  lung tissue loss and, 131–132
  mountain sickness and, 130
  obliterative, 129, 132
  obstructive, 129, 132–133
  passive, 127–128
  pulmonary embolus and, 244, 245

vasomotor factors and, 128, 129–131, 132, 133–134
  ventilation-perfusion ratio and, 170
Pulmonary infections, 105, 131–132, 284–285. *See also specific condition*
Pulmonary resection, 267–271
  adjustments following lobectomy, 270
  amounts tolerated, 269
  in children, 270–271
  complications, 270
  diffusing capacity and, 154
  lung compliance and, 75
  postoperative period, 268–269
  pulmonary function and, 267–268, 269
  pulmonary pressure and, 131
  shifts following, 269–270
Pulmonary transplantation, 305–314
  cadaver lung handling for, 313–314
  clinical, 312–313
  complications, 312–313
  experimental allografts, 310–312
  history, 305
  operative complications, 307
  reimplantation, 307
    lung function after, 307–310, 312–313
  technique, 305–307, 312
Pulmonary veins
  anatomy, 104
  vasomotor nerves, 105
Pulsatile flow, 338, 339
  compliance and, 346
  inertance and, 346, 347–348
  mechanics, 338–353
  resistance in system, 345–346
Pulse
  cardiac output and rate, 143, 144
  pulmonary vascular bed, 142–144
  systemic vs. pulmonary circulation, 106–107
  tracing arterial, 338, 339
Pyothorax, 260, 261, 264

Reactance
  compliance and, 348
  defined, 348
  impedance and, 348–353
  initial, 349
Reflexes
  chemoreceptor control of proprioceptive, 187
  following lung reimplantation, 308–309
  in respiration regulation, 187–189

Reserve volume
age and, 231, 232
inspiratory vs. expiratory, 45
lungs, 45, 75, 231, 232
position and expiratory, 78
Residual capacity
age and, 83
bronchial size and, 94
elastic recoil and, 291
exercise and, 101
Residual volume
age and, 232
alveolar air and blood gases and, 48–51
defined, 45
normal values, 45, 46
obesity and, 233
position and, 76–77, 78, 79–80
resistance and, 291
Resistance(s)
addition of parallel, 91
airway. *See* Airway resistance
circulatory system
blood vessel radius and, 110
blood viscosity and, 109
pulmonary circulation, 108, 144
compliance and, 97
determining, in fluid system, 327–330
flow and, 325–327
Poiseuille's equation in defining, 329
in pulsatile system, 345–346
in respiratory mechanics, 41, 58, 59, 60, 89–97
age and, 231
breathing work and, 41, 90, 91, 188, 202–203, 204, 206, 207
bronchial size and, 100
chest wall, 89, 90
lung, 89, 90, 91
determination, 98
parallel ventilation theory, 159–164
in shock, 276
residual volume and, 291
sources of, 89–97
Respirator(s), 281–304. *See also* Artificial ventilation
choice of, factors in, 290
complications in use, 282, 298–301
deranged respiratory mechanics and, 301–304
development of, 281
hyperinflation for respirator patients, 73
indications for use, 282–288
inflation pressure in shock, 276–277
in injury, 284, 287–288
limitations of, 297–298, 300
in open pneumothorax, 257–258
operation principles, 288–289, 290–296
in pneumonia, 265–266
postoperative use, 253, 268–269
requirements for proper use, 291–296
special considerations in infants and children, 296–297
types, 288–290
Respiratory acidosis, 28. *See also* Acidosis, respiratory
diagnosis, 35
respiratory insufficiency and, 285–286
Respiratory alkalosis, 28
artificial ventilation and, 300–301
blood gas in, 40
Respiratory insufficiency. *See also* Acidosis, respiratory
diaphragmatic paralysis and, 257
emphysema and, 239
in pneumothorax, 259
respiratory acidosis and, 285–286
therapy, 301
Respiratory muscles
conditioning and, 101–102, 222, 223
control of contraction, 189
cough and, 102
energy output, 195, 233, 234. *See also* Breathing work
force, 61–62
function of, 59–62
intrapleural pressure and expiratory, 93–94
oxygen consumption, 196
ventilation and, 59–62
Respiratory rate
breathing work and, 188, 202–203, 209
chemoreceptor stimulation and, 180
exercise and, 101, 222
pressure to overcome resistance and, 90, 91
respirator use and, 291
ventilation adequacy and, 51–52
Reynold's number, 333–335
Ribs
anatomy, 2
congenital deformities of, 236–237
fractures
lung lacerations and, 258–260
respiration and, 253, 255
respirators in, 288

movement, chest cavity and, 2–3, 4
    removal, results of, 257
Scoliosis, 80–81
Septal defects, pulmonary hyperten-
    sion in, 128, 134–135, 137,
    138, 139
Seroche, 130
Serotonin, vasomotor effects, 113
Severinghaus glass electrode in blood
    analysis, 31
Shock
    acidosis and, 26
    blood flow and, 109, 110, 154
    blood viscosity and, 109, 110
    breathing work in, 277
    capillary surface area and, 149
    diffusing capacity and, 154
    fluid therapy, cautions with, 274–
        275, 277–278, 278–279
    lung collapse and, 296
    respiratory complications, 271–272
    ventilation and, 276–277
    ventilation-perfusion ratio and, 175–
        176
Shock lung syndrome, 241, 271–279
    clinical picture, 271–272, 273–274
    experimental studies, 272–273
    in humans, 273–275
    progression, 279
    pulmonary mechanics in, 275–277
    therapy, 274–275, 277–279
Shunts
    cardiac
        diffusing capacity and, 152
        pulmonary hypertension and, 129,
            134, 137
    intrapulmonary
        microatelectasis and, 273
        pulmonary resection and, 269
        trunk injury and, 273
    vascular
        anesthesia and, 227
        in bronchiectasis, 267
        measurement, 170
        ventilation-perfusion   ratio   and,
            165–167
    ventilatory
        measurement, 170
        ventilation-perfusion   ratio   and,
            167–170
Siegaard-Andersen nomogram, 33, 36
Sine waves, 338, 340, 342–343, 344
Sleep, respiration in natural, 189–190,
    191, 224
Smog, airways and, 95, 96

Smoking
    airways and, 95, 96
    emphysema and, 238, 239
    nitrogen dioxide in cigarette smoke,
        215
    pollutants in cigarette smoke, 217
    ventilation-perfusion ratio and, 177
Spine
    muscle groups and respiration, 60
    respiratory effects of deformities,
        235–236
Spondylitis, ankylosing, 235
Starling law of the heart, 107
Starling resistor, 116, 117, 176
Sternum
    anatomy, 2
    deformities and respiration, 235–237
Stroke volume, cardiac output and,
        105–106, 143, 144
Subcutaneous emphysema, 260
Sulfur dioxide, 215
Sulfur trioxide, 215
Surfactant
    artificial ventilation and, 73
    compliance and, 69–74
    equilibrium in lung, 71–72
    fluid effusion and, 121
    functions of, 74
    loss of effects, 73, 74
        pulmonary edema and, 127
        shock lung syndrome and, 273
    pericapillary pressure and, 120
    regeneration, shallow breathing and,
        249
Surgery
    cardiac, precautions in, 241–242
    conditioning and elective, 233
    obesity and risk, 233, 234, 253
    postoperative period. See Postopera-
        tive period
    respiratory complications, 55
    smoking and risk, 253
    thoracic
        cosmetic, for chest deformities, 237
        diffusing capacity and, 154
        for emphysema, 239
        hemothorax and, 263, 264
        for pulmonary embolus, 244
        pulmonary function and, 268
        pulmonary pressure after, 131
        pulmonary transplantation, 305–
            314. See also Pulmonary
            transplantation
        respiratory effects, 226
        rib resection results, 257
    as trauma, 247

Surgery—*Continued*
ventilation-perfusion ratio and, 176–177, 178
ventilatory ability and, 54
Symbols, definitions of, 317–318
Systemic circulation, 105–107
arterioles, 104
blood volume and position, 113–114
flow-pressure relations in, 106–107

Tachypnea, narcotics and, 228
Tank respirators, 281, 289
Temperature. *See also* Hypothermia
cadaver lung maintenance, 313–314
carbon dioxide absorption curve and, 25–26
of inspired air, 42
oxygen dissociation and, 14–15
respiratory effects of hypothermia, 224, 229
solubility of gas in liquid and, 323–324
ventilation and, 189
viscosity and, 329–330
Tension pneumothorax, 259, 260, 287
Thorax. *See* Chest
Thrombosis, pulmonary hypertension and, 129, 133
Tidal volume
age and, 81, 232, 297
breathing work and, 188, 209
chemoreceptor stimulation and, 180
defined, 45
elastic work and, 199–203
exercise and, 101, 122
lung mechanics and, 297
normal values, 45, 46
pulmonary resection and, 267–268
respirator use and, 290, 291–292, 293
in shock, 275
Total lung volume, defined and normal values, 45, 46. *See also* *disease entity*
Trachea
air in, 42, 43, 44
anatomy, 6, 95–96
Tracheostomy tube, use with ventilators, 290, 298–299
Transmural pressure
bronchial diameter and, 94
cough and, 102
described, 335
flow and, 335, 336, 337
intravascular pressure and, 110, 111

pulmonary capillary size and, 116, 117
Trendelenburg position, effects of, 225–226
Tube size, flow-pressure relations and, 335–338
Tuberculosis, effects of pulmonary, 266
Turbulence
air mixing and, 158
flow-pressure relations and, 141, 333, 334
velocity and, 334
viscosity and, 334–335

Underventilation. *See* Hypoventilation

Vagotomy, effects of, 224
Van Slyke-Neil apparatus for blood analysis, 31
Vapor pressure, 322–323
Vasomotor factors
blood vessel size and, 110, 112–113
chemoreceptor stimulation and, 180
lung reimplantation and, 310
in pulmonary edema, 124, 125
in pulmonary hypertension, 128, 129–131, 132, 133–134
Vasomotor nerves, pulmonary, 105
Velocity
angular, of sine wave, 340
flow, viscosity and, 108–109
Ventilation, 41–54. *See also* Alveolar ventilation; Hyperventilation; Hypoventilation; Minute ventilation; Ventilation-perfusion ratio
ability, surgery and, 54
absent, with normal blood flow, 165–167
altitude and, 184, 218–219
assessment of adequacy, 51–54
breathing reserve calculation, 54
breathing work and, 191–193, 209
bronchoconstriction and, 225
in cadaver lung maintenance, 313–314
chemical regulation, 179–187
compliance and, 163–164
diagnosis of insufficiency, 35, 37
disease and, 237–241
exercise and, 101, 189, 222–223
gas-blood mixing and, 157–158
hypercapnia and, 187
metabolic alkalosis and, 28, 185–186
metabolic rate and, 209–210
muscular activity and, 59–62, 233

musculoskeletal deformities and, 235–237
narcotics and, 227–228
natural sleep and, 224
normal, with no blood flow, 167–170
obesity and, 233–234
oxygen consumption and, 196–197
pain and, 189
postoperative, 248
pulmonary emboli and, 243–244
of reimplanted lung, 307–308
rib fractures and, 253, 255
shock and, 276–277
stimulation of, 181, 189
temperature and, 189
uneven
  nitrogen washout tests in, 158–159
  parallel ventilation theory, 159–164
Ventilation-perfusion ratio, 155, 157–178
alveolar-arterial oxygen differences, 170–174
anesthesia and, 227
control of, 157
defined, 164
disease and, 175–178
emphysema and, 238
exercise and, 164, 175, 222, 223
incoordination of, 157, 158–164, 252
measurement of, 174–175
position and, 174–175
postoperative, 252
in pulmonary edema, 124
pulmonary resection and, 268
regional differences in, 174–175
right-to-left shunts and, 165–167
ventilatory shunt and, 167–170
Ventilators. See Respirator(s)

Ventricle
filling pressure, 133–134, 140
output control, 107
pulse, left vs. right, 106–107
Venules, pulmonary, 104
Vertebrae, 2
Virtual work, principle of, 337–338
Visceral pleura, 5, 259–260
Viscosity
anomalous, 330
flow and, 108–109, 330
flow-pressure relations and, 108–110
hematocrit and blood, 109–110
temperature and, 329–330
turbulence and, 334–335
Vital capacity
abnormalities, 53–54
age and, 232
defined, 45
measurement, 53
normal values, 45, 46, 53
Volume. See also specific volume
defined, 331
Volume-controlled respirators, 289–290, 297–298

Water vapor, air
altitude and, 43, 44, 45
inspired vs. expired, 42
Work
Bernoulli's equation and, 331–333
defined, 197, 331
kinetic energy conversion to, 332–333
measurement, 332
mechanical
  in breathing, 197–209. See also Breathing work
  calculation of, 206, 208–209
virtual, principle of, 337–338